T0323391

Advance praise for *Philosophy of Psychedelics*

This excellent, well-argued, book is required reading for anyone with interests in philosophy of mind, philosophy of psychology, and philosophy of psychiatry. It presents the first book-length argument for the effectiveness of psychedelic therapy and provides an account of how this effectiveness may be understood from within cognitive neuroscience. Everyone should read this book!

Richard Brown, Humanities Department,
LaGuardia Community College,
CUNY & M.S. program in Cognitive Neuroscience
at the Graduate Center, CUNY

Philosophy of Psychedelics is really two books in one. It provides an easily understood, scholarly and detailed review of psychedelic science, spanning phenomenology, psychology, neuroscience, and medical therapeutics. But setting this book apart from other recent books in this rapidly emerging field of inquiry, Chris Letheby takes his philosopher's scalpel to addressing intriguing philosophical implications of psychedelic research including the unsettling question of whether the claimed benefits from psychedelic experiences require the induction of delusional beliefs. This very readable volume should be of interest to scientists, philosophers, as well as those simply curious about recent the renaissance in psychedelic science and therapeutics.

Roland R. Griffiths, Ph.D. Director,
Center for Psychedelic and Consciousness Research,
Professor, Departments of Psychiatry and Neuroscience,
Johns Hopkins University School of Medicine

Philosophy of Psychedelics is a terrific, intellectually meticulous study of the nature, meaning, and effects of psychedelic experiences. The discussion ranges over the mind-brain relation, transformative experiences, the ethics of psychedelic therapy, and whether psychedelics help us to see the nature of things as they really are or just produce uplifting and therapeutically positive hallucinations. Chris Letheby is a wise and careful guide to the current state of psychedelic therapy and sets very high standards for philosophers who want to follow him in thinking responsibly about this intriguing area of research.

Owen Flanagan is James B. Duke, Professor of Philosophy
at Duke University, and the author of
How to Do Things with Emotions Princeton 2021.
Philosophy of Psychedelics

INTERNATIONAL PERSPECTIVES IN PHILOSOPHY AND PSYCHIATRY

Series editors
Bill (K.W.M.) Fulford, Lisa Bortolotti, Matthew Broome, Katherine Morris, John Z. Sadler, and Giovanni Stanghellini

Philosophy of Psychedelics

Chris Letheby

Lecturer in Philosophy
The University of Western Australia

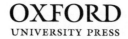

OXFORD
UNIVERSITY PRESS

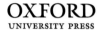

OXFORD
UNIVERSITY PRESS

Great Clarendon Street, Oxford, OX2 6DP,
United Kingdom

Oxford University Press is a department of the University of Oxford.
It furthers the University's objective of excellence in research, scholarship,
and education by publishing worldwide. Oxford is a registered trade mark of
Oxford University Press in the UK and in certain other countries

© Oxford University Press 2021

The moral rights of the author have been asserted

First Edition Published in 2021

Impression: 5

Published in the United States of America by Oxford University Press
198 Madison Avenue, New York, NY 10016, United States of America

British Library Cataloguing in Publication Data

Data available

Library of Congress Control Number: 2020949256

ISBN 978–0–19–884312–2

DOI: 10.1093/med/9780198843122.001.0001

Printed and bound by
CPI Group (UK) Ltd, Croydon, CR0 4YY

Acknowledgements

My deepest thanks are due to Philip Gerrans, Gerard O'Brien, and Jon Opie, without whom this book would not have been written. I am also indebted to Lisa Bortolotti and Thomas Metzinger for timely advice, encouragement, and assistance.

I am extremely grateful to Miri Albahari and Roland Griffiths for their generosity in reading the entire manuscript and providing detailed comments. For reading and commenting on sections of the manuscript, I would like to thank Sam Baron, Sascha Fink, Owen Flanagan, Remco Heesen, Nin Kirkham, Aidan Lyon, Michael Rubin, and Clas Weber. Needless to say, any errors that remain are my responsibility.

Finally, and with apologies to anyone I have forgotten, I would like to thank my stellar editorial team at Oxford University Press: Martin Baum, Janine Fisher, and Charlotte Holloway.

This research was partially supported by the Australian Government through the Australian Research Council's *Discovery Projects* funding scheme (project DP190101451). The views expressed herein are those of the author and are not necessarily those of the Australian Government or Australian Research Council.

The epigraph at the start of Chapter 3 is reproduced from Jane Dunlap, *Exploring Inner Space: Personal Experiences under LSD-25*, p. 166. Copyright © 2003, Harcourt, Brace & World.

The epigraph at the start of Chapter 4 is reproduced from William A. Richards, 'Mystical and archetypal experiences of terminal patients in DPT-assisted psychotherapy', *Journal of Religion and Health, 17*(2), p. 120, DOI: https://doi.org/10.1007/BF01532413 Copyright © 1978, Springer Nature.

The epigraph at the start of Chapter 5 is reproduced from Huston Smith, *Cleansing the Doors of Perception: The Religious Significance of Entheogenic Plants and Chemicals*, p. 15. Copyright © 2003, Sentient Publications.

The epigraph at the start of Chapter 6 is reproduced from *The Poems of Emily Dickinson: Variorum Edition*, edited by Ralph W. Franklin, Cambridge, Mass.: The Belknap Press of Harvard University Press, Copyright © 1998 by the President and Fellows of Harvard College. Copyright © 1951, 1955 by the President and Fellows of Harvard College. Copyright © renewed 1979, 1983 by the President and Fellows of Harvard College. Copyright © 1914, 1918, 1919, 1924, 1929, 1930, 1932, 1935, 1937, 1942 by Martha Dickinson Bianchi. Copyright © 1952, 1957, 1958, 1963, 1965 by Mary L. Hampson.

Contents

Abbreviations

11D-ASC	11 Dimensions of Altered States of Consciousness
5-HT	serotonin (5-hydroxytryptamine)
5-HT2A	serotonin-2a
5-MeO-DMT	5-methoxy-N,N-dimethyltryptamine
AAQ-II	Acceptance and Action Questionnaire II
ACC	anterior cingulate cortex
ACT	Acceptance and Commitment Therapy
AIC	anterior insular cortex
ASC	altered state of consciousness
BDNF	brain-derived neurotrophic factor
CEQ	Challenging Experiences Questionnaire
CTM	computational theory of mind
DBT	Dialectical Behavioural Therapy
DMN	Default Mode network
DMT	N,N-dimethyltryptamine
DPD	depersonalisation disorder
DPT	dipropyltryptamine
EBI	Emotional Breakthrough Inventory
EBO	experience of body ownership
EEG	electroencephalography
EQ	Experiences Questionnaire
FDA	(U.S.) Food and Drug Administration
FFMQ	Five Facet Mindfulness Questionnaire
fMRI	functional magnetic resonance imaging
HPPD	hallucinogen persisting perception disorder
LSD	lysergic acid diethylamide
MAAS	Mindful Attention Awareness Scale
MAT	Metaphysical Alief Theory
MBQ	Metaphysical Belief Questionnaire
MBSR	Mindfulness Based Stress Reduction
MBT	Metaphysical Belief Theory
MDMA (or "Ecstasy")	3,4-methylenedioxymethamphetamine
MEG	magnetoencephalography
MEQ	Mystical Experience Questionnaire
mPFC	medial prefrontal cortex
NMDA	N-methyl-D-aspartate
NYU	New York University
OCD	obsessive-compulsive disorder
PCC	posterior cingulate cortex

PCP	phencyclidine
PET	positron emission tomography
PHC	parahippocampal cortex
PIC	posterior insular cortex
PIQ	Psychological Insight Questionnaire
PMIR	Phenomenal model of the intentionality relation
PP	predictive processing
PSM	phenomenal self-model
RCT	randomised controlled trial
REBUS	RElaxed Beliefs Under pSychedelics
RSC	retrosplenial cortex
SN	Salience Network
SSRI	selective serotonin reuptake inhibitor
TPJ	temporoparietal junction
TPN	task-positive network
TRD	treatment-resistant depression
vmPFC	ventromedial prefrontal cortex

1
Introduction

The unacceptability of psychedelic therapy … stems in part at least from this fundamental empirical fact: Through the psychedelic experience persons tend to accept beliefs which are at variance with the usual conception of the 'scientific world view'.

Willis Harman, 'The issue of the consciousness expanding drugs'.

Something very strange is happening in psychiatry. Clinicians and researchers are becoming increasingly interested in a 'new' experimental treatment, with some suggesting it might herald a 'new paradigm' in the treatment of disorders such as anxiety, depression, and addiction (Nichols et al. 2017, Schenberg 2018). If promising initial results are borne out, this new treatment may significantly outperform existing pharmacological and psychological therapies in terms of rapidity and efficacy. And yet this treatment has a number of properties that, from the standpoint of mainstream philosophy and science, can only be described as extremely weird.

First, although it is a drug treatment, there is no daily dosing regimen of the kind familiar from existing antidepressant and antipsychotic medications. Patients receive one dose (or very few doses) of the drug—albeit with considerable interpersonal support and preparation—and then, in successful cases, their symptoms dramatically decrease for many months; no re-dosing required. Second, although it is *in some sense* a drug treatment, it's far from clear that the drug itself is the direct cause of clinical improvement. Rather, it seems that the drug is merely a catalyst for a brief but intense conscious experience, and it is this experience that causes therapeutic effects. Third, and most weirdly, the kind of experience that seems to lead to the best outcomes is one that patients describe as 'mystical' or 'spiritual'. Many patients given this treatment report transcendent experiences of 'oneness', 'cosmic' consciousness, or 'ego dissolution', and evidence suggests that these patients show the greatest clinical improvement.

I am referring, of course, to *psychedelic therapy*: the treatment of psychiatric disorder by the supervised administration of 'hallucinogenic' serotonin-2a agonist substances such as lysergic acid diethylamide (LSD), psilocybin (the active ingredient in 'magic' mushrooms), and N,N-dimethyltryptamine (DMT; a key psychoactive constituent of the Amazonian beverage ayahuasca). Given their widespread reputation as psychotomimetic (psychosis-mimicking) or psychotogenic (psychosis-generating) chemicals, the very idea of using psychedelics to *treat* mental illness may seem absurd

(Osmond 1957, Carhart-Harris et al. 2016a). However, these drugs were studied and prescribed as experimental psychiatric treatments in the 1950s and 1960s, prior to the public controversy surrounding their use by the hippie counterculture. Promising results were reported from this line of research, which was curtailed prematurely due to the crackdown on psychedelics and the subsequent 'War on Drugs'. For decades, virtually no human psychedelic research was conducted.

Since the 1990s, this research has been slowly but steadily resuming, and the results to date are intriguing. Although it is still relatively early days, there is now sufficient evidence to take seriously the claims of earlier researchers. Supervised psychedelic sessions may, after all, have an acceptable safety profile (dos Santos et al. 2018a) coupled with significant and lasting psychological benefits for psychiatric patients (dos Santos and Hallak 2020) and even for healthy volunteers (Gandy 2019). Meanwhile, neuroimaging studies of the psychedelic state are providing tantalising clues about the biological bases of consciousness and self-awareness (dos Santos et al. 2016b). If these preliminary findings are replicated, then psychedelics may well find a place in twenty-first-century psychiatry (Sessa 2005, 2012, 2018). But many questions remain. The transformative mechanisms of psychedelic experience are incompletely understood, and this strikingly novel type of therapeutic intervention raises many fascinating and puzzling issues, both scientific and philosophical.

This book is organised around one specific philosophical question that relates to the role of the mystical experience in psychedelic therapy. Patients and subjects who show the greatest psychological benefit from psychedelic experiences tend to be those who report a mystical experience, as defined by widely used psychometric questionnaires, and often the degree of mystical experience predicts the degree of benefit. A mystical experience is sometimes described as an overwhelmingly powerful apparent encounter with 'ultimate reality'. Space, time, and the sense of individual selfhood fade away, to be replaced by a sense of union with 'another Reality that puts this one in the shade' (Smith 2000, p. 133). In some cases, this Reality is experienced as a divine or cosmic consciousness that underlies and unifies the entire manifest universe, evoking philosophical doctrines such as idealism and pantheism (Shanon 2002, p. 162). The apparent centrality of the mystical experience has led researcher Charles Grob to describe psychedelic therapy as an 'existential medicine' (Grob 2007, p. 213).

But this picture of psychedelic therapy raises an obvious worry: what if the divine universal consciousness is not real? Many philosophers and scientists today subscribe to a broadly naturalist, materialist, or physicalist world view, according to which mind and consciousness are not fundamental in the universe but are relatively recent products of complex evolution. From this perspective, the mystical apprehensions of psychedelic subjects look like 'metaphysical hallucinations' (Flanagan and Graham 2017, p. 294)—subjectively compelling but ultimately misleading by-products of aberrant brain activity, on a par with psychedelic subjects' visions of walls 'breathing' or kaleidoscopic fractals (cf. Roche 2010). And there seems to be something seriously questionable about a treatment or enhancement modality that works by inducing metaphysical hallucinations. The journalist Michael Pollan, discussing the use of psychedelics to treat psychological distress in terminally ill patients, puts the point forcefully: 'Is psychedelic therapy simply foisting a comforting delusion on the sick and dying?' (Pollan 2015). The worry is that psychedelics bring about their salutary psychosocial effects by a deceptive, epistemically (and therefore ethically) bad mechanism.

Call this the 'Comforting Delusion Objection' to psychedelic therapy. There are three popular responses. The first is that there's no problem because the mystical experience is veridical. Far from inducing metaphysical hallucinations, psychedelics afford subjects a direct and transformative apprehension of ultimate reality (Smith 2000, Richards 2015). The second response is that the epistemic status of psychedelic experiences is relatively unimportant: what is more important is that they help people live better lives (Flanagan and Graham 2017). The third response is that the epistemic status of psychedelic experiences is very important, but also poor: we should be wary of permitting or prescribing psychedelic therapy because it does in fact work by the objectionable induction of comforting delusions (Lavazza 2017).

In this book, I present a fourth, relatively unexplored response to the Comforting Delusion Objection. My central thesis is that the Objection fails. My strategy is to start by assuming that (a) the naturalist worldview is true, so no cosmic consciousness exists, and (b) the epistemic status of psychedelic therapy is very important. This is the worst-case scenario for someone seeking to answer this objection. Clearly, if a cosmic consciousness or divine Reality exists, the objection fails (the first response above); and, clearly, if the epistemic status of psychedelic therapy is relatively unimportant, the objection fails (the second response above). Here I aim to show that the objection fails *even if* neither of these conditions holds—and this will show that the objection fails, whatever is the case.

My grounds for concluding that the Comforting Delusion Objection fails, even given assumptions (a) and (b) above, are twofold. First, the epistemic risks of psychedelic therapy, from a naturalistic standpoint, are less than one might suppose. Despite first appearances, psychedelic therapy does not work by instilling comforting metaphysical beliefs in a divine Reality. Such beliefs are sometimes acquired, but they are not necessary for therapeutic benefits, nor do they always accompany such benefits. The construct of a 'mystical-type experience', which mediates clinical outcomes, sometimes reflects experiences as of a cosmic consciousness or divine Reality. However, it sometimes reflects more naturalistic experiences of 'ego dissolution', connectedness, emotional catharsis, and psychological insight. Psychedelics promote well-being by temporarily disrupting the sense of self, allowing patients to access new ways of seeing themselves and their lives. Such existentially significant changes to self-awareness do not depend on changes to metaphysical beliefs about the ultimate nature of reality.

Second, psychedelic therapy is *epistemically innocent*, in the technical sense defined by Lisa Bortolotti (2015). Bortolotti defines epistemically innocent imperfect cognitions as those that have real epistemic flaws but also offer significant epistemic benefits that are unavailable by any other means. This is the status of psychedelic therapy, given naturalism. Psychedelic experiences can lead to knowledge acquisition, both directly and indirectly—*even if* naturalism is true and the cosmic consciousness experience is a metaphysical hallucination. In the course of defending these claims, I will deal with issues concerning the nature of conscious experience, the relations between psychology and neuroscience, and the theory and philosophy of self-awareness. The second main thesis of the book is that a sustained and detailed interaction between philosophy and psychedelic science can be mutually beneficial: I aim to show that psychedelic science reveals phenomena of serious philosophical interest, while philosophy offers valuable tools for clarifying and interpreting results from psychedelic science.

I begin in Chapter 2 by reviewing recent scientific evidence concerning the safety, and therapeutic and transformative efficacy, of carefully controlled psychedelic administration. The recent wave of clinical studies suggests that psychedelics can indeed be given safely and responsibly, without serious adverse effects, to carefully selected and prepared subjects in carefully controlled conditions. These studies also provide evidence for durable psychological benefits following one (or very few) psychedelic sessions conducted in this fashion. But they also provide evidence that these benefits are mediated, at least in part, by mystical experiences, giving rise to the Comforting Delusion Objection. I outline the objection and my proposed response to it in more detail. I suggest that what is needed is a *natural philosophy* of psychedelics: a synthetic, big-picture inquiry integrating multidisciplinary evidence to address philosophical issues in a manner continuous with science and consistent with naturalism.

In the spirit of such a natural philosophy, I begin with detailed attention to the phenomena under investigation. As such, Chapter 3 presents an overview of the phenomenology of psychedelic therapy, including patients' own impressions of the therapeutic mechanisms. Psychedelic experiences are notoriously variable and often held to be ineffable. Nonetheless, significant progress has been made on identifying typical themes from quantitative and qualitative reports. Subjects often describe an expansion of consciousness, a heightening of emotional experience, strange visions and insights, and a blurring of boundaries between self and world. Many subjects interpret these experiences in non-naturalistic terms, but many do not, instead emphasising experiences of psychological insight, emotional catharsis, acceptance, and *connectedness* to various aspects of self and world (Carhart-Harris et al. 2018a, Breeksema et al. 2020). This provides our first major clue that psychedelic therapy is not a simple matter of inducing existentially comforting metaphysical beliefs.

Although they provide suggestive evidence, we cannot assume that subjects' impressions of the therapeutic mechanisms are correct. To determine how psychedelic therapy works, we need to examine a broader range of evidence. In Chapter 4, I survey three different theories of how psychedelics cause lasting psychological benefits. The first ascribes these benefits to psychedelics' direct effects on the molecular-level mechanisms of neuroplasticity. On this view, psychedelic therapy is an experience-independent pharmacotherapy, and the remarkable phenomenology is a mere cluster of therapeutically epiphenomenal 'psychotomimetic' side effects. The second and third theories differ in detail, but both ascribe lasting benefits to non-naturalistic metaphysical ideations—the transcendent vision of a 'Joyous Cosmology' (Watts 1962) supposedly encountered in the mystical experience.

I argue that all three theories are inadequate. The neuroplasticity theory struggles to account for the robust correlation between measures of mystical-type experience and lasting benefits. This correlation suggests that the psychedelic experience itself is causally relevant to those benefits. However, on closer examination, we find that some subjects satisfy psychometric criteria for a 'mystical-type experience' without having a transcendent vision of cosmic consciousness. These criteria are broad enough to capture more naturalistic experiences of 'ego dissolution' and connectedness as well. Not all mystical-type experiences *in the psychometric sense* are non-naturalistic metaphysical hallucinations. The conclusion is that the key causal factor in psychedelic therapy is genuinely psychological—an aspect of the experience itself—but is not essentially tied to non-naturalistic metaphysical ideations.

In Chapter 5, I argue that the relevant psychological factor is change to the sense of self. A few studies pinpoint experiences of psychological insight as strongly linked to lasting benefits, and the relevant insights are often autobiographical in character. Moreover, several studies have shown that psychedelics can induce lasting increases in 'mindfulness-related capacities' for taking an open, non-reactive stance toward one's inner experience—a stance that intrinsically involves changes to the sense of self. These studies constitute an important experimental vindication of the old idea that there are deep commonalities between psychedelic and meditative states (e.g., Huxley 1954, Watts 1962, Leary et al. 1964). Finally, neuroimaging research has consistently implicated certain large-scale brain networks, the Default Mode and Salience networks, in psychedelics' lasting benefits, and both networks are linked to self-representation by considerable independent evidence.

At this point, a question arises: how exactly do neurobiological changes, such as modulation of the Default Mode and Salience networks, relate to psychological changes, such as autobiographical insights and increased mindfulness-related capacities? I propose that *neurocognitive theory*, which attributes computational or information-processing functions to neural structures, provides a vital explanatory bridge between biological and psychological accounts of the psychedelic state (cf. Gerrans 2014). If we can specify the cognitive functions performed by the neural systems that psychedelics target, then this will allow us to explain why modulating those networks should lead to transformative experiences of ego dissolution, connectedness, catharsis, and insight.

In Chapters 6 and 7, I outline such a theory: the *predictive self-binding* account of psychedelic therapy (Letheby and Gerrans 2017). According to this account, one function of the networks targeted by psychedelics is to maintain a hierarchical predictive model of the self. This predictive self-model acts as a 'centre of representational gravity': by parsing information into self-relevant and self-irrelevant, into 'me' and 'not me', it functions as an organising principle that governs and constrains cognitive processing. In pathological conditions, detrimental forms of self-modelling often become rigidly entrenched. By 'unbinding' the self-model, psychedelics facilitate experiences of ego dissolution and psychological insight in which pathological self-models can be revised. On this view, psychedelic therapy has a two-factor structure: it involves (a) the induction of neural and psychological plasticity at multiple levels, and (b) the discovery and consolidation of new forms of self-modelling.

I conclude Chapter 7 with some brief remarks on philosophical questions about self and self-consciousness. I have argued elsewhere that psychedelic evidence supports two controversial philosophical claims: that the self does not exist (Letheby and Gerrans 2017), and that there can be conscious experiences lacking all forms of self-consciousness (Letheby 2020). However, both arguments face serious objections. For present purposes, I content myself with two weaker, but still significant, claims: (i) there can be conscious experiences lacking anything like the *ordinary* sense of self, and (ii) the *kind* of self that we automatically take ourselves to be does not exist. Theoretically and existentially, this is plenty to be getting on with.

The upshot of Chapters 4–7 is that the epistemic risks of psychedelic therapy, given naturalism, are surprisingly small. In Chapter 8, I argue that its epistemic benefits, given naturalism, are surprisingly large. The concept of 'epistemic innocence' (Bortolotti 2015, 2020) encapsulates the overall epistemic status of psychedelic therapy, given naturalism: this intervention carries non-trivial epistemic risks, insofar as some subjects do acquire strong beliefs in a cosmic consciousness or spirit world, but these risks are offset by the fact that it also offers significant, often unique, epistemic *benefits*. I survey the major proposals about psychedelic-induced knowledge gain that are consistent with naturalism, and argue that psychedelics offer what philosophers call 'knowledge by acquaintance' with various often unrevealed aspects of the human mind, including its potential for diverse and beneficial modes of attention and cognition. This has connections with philosophical discussions of Frank Jackson's (1982, 1986) famous thought experiment about Mary the super-neuroscientist. It also justifies the increasing use of the appellation 'psychedelic', meaning 'mind-manifesting' or 'mind-revealing' (Osmond 1957), in preference to the many available alternatives.

At later times, subjects can re-evoke these beneficial modes of attention and cognition, at least to some extent. Therefore, psychedelics also make available ability knowledge, or *knowledge-how*. The question of factual or propositional knowledge is more vexed. It is highly likely that psychedelics facilitate genuine psychodynamic insights into previously unconscious or unattended mental states, but the possibility of 'placebo insights' (Jopling 2001)—spurious apparent insights with real therapeutic benefits—must be kept in mind. The only viable solution is for psychedelic-induced apparent epiphanies to be subjected to sober scrutiny during the post-session integration period. I argue that psychedelic experiences also facilitate the acquisition of *new knowledge of old facts*, allowing subjects to experience existing beliefs in more vivid and motivating ways. Finally, I argue that psychedelic experiences have indirect epistemic benefits consequent on their lasting psychological benefits (Letheby 2016).

In Chapter 9, I turn to the philosophical project of 'naturalising spirituality'. I argue that psychedelic research vindicates the claim that there are transformative experiences and practices that (a) can legitimately be called 'spiritual', and (b) are compatible with adherence to a naturalistic world view. The existential transformation afforded by some psychedelic experiences provides a paradigm for naturalistic spirituality: the temporary suspension of our default, self-referential mode of cognition, making available broader perspectives, experiences of connectedness, and feelings of wonder and awe. This has connections to Iris Murdoch's (1970) notion of 'unselfing' (cf. Kähönen 2020). There is considerable convergence between typical features of psychedelic-induced spiritual experiences and themes common to multiple philosophical accounts of naturalistic spirituality (Stone 2012), which provides further support for the general approach.

Finally, in Chapter 10, I summarise the discussion and make some suggestions for future research. My account makes several testable predictions—for instance, psychedelic-induced changes to the activity of specific brain networks should correlate with distinct types of ego-dissolution experiences, and psychedelic-induced changes to metaphysical beliefs (e.g., about the mind–body relation) should account for relatively little variance in clinical outcomes. In closing, I reflect on the broader significance of my arguments. Psychedelic science is a fast-moving field, and this book will be out of date in some respects before it hits the shelves—which is a good thing. In the coming years, we are set to learn more than ever before about these controversial substances, their risks, benefits, and potential applications, and the mechanisms underlying their remarkable effects. The philosophical discussion of psychedelics, in particular, is in its infancy. But I think it is not premature to bet that, when psychedelics cause lasting therapeutic benefits, these benefits are not brought about mainly by the induction of comforting delusions. Psychedelics can, as many have insisted, facilitate genuine insights and spiritual experiences—and this is a claim that even a philosophical naturalist should endorse.

2
On the need for a natural philosophy of psychedelics

Central to the entire LSD controversy is: 'With how much credence should the chemical experience be accepted?' Should it be totally accepted as the real reality, or is it preferable to attempt to study the state, sorting out the veridical from the illusory? Evidently, a choice must be made. The state must be either taken on faith without examination or it must be subjected to sorting and analysis. The overgullible will be easily persuaded, the overcritical will analyse it out of existence. Perhaps a third approach is possible––an attempt to measure without changing, to evaluate without destroying.

Sidney Cohen, *Drugs of Hallucination.*

2.1 Introduction

In this chapter, I review the history of psychedelics in science and psychiatry, recent evidence for their safety and therapeutic and transformative efficacy, and the facts about them that give rise to the Comforting Delusion Objection. I describe the main extant responses to the Objection, introduce my response, and outline my plan for defending it in the subsequent chapters. Psychedelics have struck many researchers as raising significant philosophical questions (Smythies 1953, Smith 1964, Shanon 2001), yet until recently have been largely ignored in academic philosophy. I propose that what is needed in this age of interdisciplinarity is a *natural philosophy* of psychedelics: a trans-disciplinary synthesis that integrates empirical findings with theoretical and conceptual considerations, to address some of the fascinating and distinctively philosophical questions raised by these controversial substances.

2.2 The psychedelic renaissance

The term 'psychedelic', meaning, roughly, 'mind-manifesting' (Osmond 1957), has been applied to a wide variety of drugs that cause dramatic changes to perception, emotion, and cognition (Sessa 2012). Psychedelics, thus construed, form a pharmacologically heterogeneous class: the Mexican psychoactive sage, Salvia Divinorum (or its active principle, Salvinorin A), acts by agonism of the kappa opioid receptor in the brain, for instance (Roth et al. 2002), while dissociative anaesthetics such as ketamine produce psychedelic effects at low doses by blockade of N-methyl-D-aspartate (NMDA) glutamate receptors (Krystal et al. 1994).

However, the term is sometimes reserved for a more restricted class: the 'classic' psychedelics, such as lysergic acid diethylamide (LSD), psilocybin (found in 'magic' mushrooms), mescaline (found in various cacti), and N,N-dimethyltryptamine (DMT, found in various plants and animals, and a key ingredient in the Amazonian beverage *ayahuasca*; Nichols 2016). These drugs, and others of this class, exert their psychoactive effects primarily by mimicking the action of the neurotransmitter serotonin (5-HT) at a specific receptor subtype: the serotonin-2a (5-HT2A) receptor (Vollenweider et al. 1998, Halberstadt 2015, Carhart-Harris 2019). It is these *serotonergic* (serotonin-acting) psychedelics that are my focus in this book, and I will reserve the word 'psychedelic' for them henceforth.[1]

Naturally occurring psychedelics have been used for religious, spiritual, and medicinal purposes for centuries, if not millennia, by various cultures around the world, especially in the Americas (Grinspoon and Bakalar 1979, Miller et al. 2019). Western scientists and intellectuals showed some interest in mescaline throughout the late nineteenth and early twentieth centuries (e.g., Mitchell 1896, Ellis 1897, Klüver 1926, Guttmann 1936). But the story of modern psychedelic science really begins with the Swiss chemist Albert Hofmann's accidental discovery, in 1943, of the potent psychedelic effects of LSD (Hofmann 1980). Hofmann was originally investigating LSD and related compounds for purely medicinal purposes, but he and his colleagues were struck by the dramatic and bizarre alterations to consciousness that this new molecule produced at utterly minute doses. In subsequent years, the similarity between the effects of LSD and mescaline was recognised. Following this, the amateur mycologist R. Gordon Wasson (1957) confirmed that *Psilocybe* mushrooms were still in regular ceremonial use in Mexico. Hofmann identified psilocybin as the active ingredient and worked out how to synthesise it (Hofmann et al. 1958). Psychedelic science began in earnest.

Throughout the 1950s and 1960s, psychedelics were studied and used in many different ways (Grof 1975, pp. 1–4). Early researchers were impressed by the similarity between some psychedelic experiences and naturally occurring psychoses, leading to a conception of the drugs as 'psychotomimetic' (psychosis-mimicking) or 'psychotogenic' (psychosis-causing). This led to two major applications: the study of psychedelics' mechanisms of action, in the hope of uncovering the biochemical bases of mental illness, and the controlled ingestion of psychedelics by psychiatrists, to increase their empathy with their psychotic patients (Osmond 1957). The discovery of

---

[1] Note that the 'entactogenic' substance 3,4-methylenedioxymethamphetamine (MDMA or 'Ecstasy') does not count as psychedelic on this definition: Although its effects are partly serotonergically mediated, it differs both pharmacologically and phenomenologically from the classic psychedelics (Nichols 1986, Roseman et al. 2014).

LSD's serotonergic action was crucial in confirming that serotonin played a role in emotion and cognition. As such, it contributed to the 'psychopharmacological revolution' and the birth of modern biological psychiatry (Dyck 2010).

But stereotypically psychotic symptoms were not the only mental changes observed after psychedelic administration. Many subjects reported overwhelming experiences of a spiritual or religious nature: ineffable mystic union with the divine, direct experience of the primordial Good in existence, and transcendent visions of a 'Joyous Cosmology' (Watts 1962). Experiences of this type seemed to happen unbidden, even when expectations were quite different (Mangini 1998). Researchers who had thought that psychedelics might scare alcoholics sober by mimicking safely the terrifying symptoms of delirium tremens were surprised when many of their patients were moved to kick the bottle by powerful religious raptures. Experiences of this kind piqued the interest of intellectuals with a prior interest in mysticism, such as Aldous Huxley (1954) and Alan Watts (1960), whose writings laid the groundwork for the psychopharmacological spirituality of the 1960s counterculture.

Thus emerged a second, quite different conception of psychedelics, as agents of spiritual experience. Adherents of this approach looked to the drugs for clues about the nature of naturally occurring mystical states and even about the (pre-) historical genesis of religion. We can (anachronistically) dub this an 'Entheogenic Conception', using the neologism coined by Ruck et al. (1979) to foreground psychedelics' spiritual and religious uses: *generating the divine within*. The most famous academic application of the Entheogenic Conception was Walter Pahnke's (1963) 'Good Friday Experiment', in which psilocybin was administered to divinity students. While listening to a Good Friday service, one group of volunteers received psilocybin, and another an active placebo: those in the psilocybin group reported transcendent mystical experiences. Pahnke's experiment had serious methodological flaws (Doblin 1991) but was nonetheless a milestone in establishing the potential of drugs in the study of religious experiences. A recent, more rigorous replication (Griffiths et al. 2006) is discussed further in section 2.3.3. Recent research has also documented numerous commonalities between psychedelic experiences and meditative states, vindicating the basic intuitions of pioneers such as Huxley and Watts (Millière et al. 2018, Smigielski et al. 2019a, 2019b, Heuschkel and Kuypers 2020).

The third, *psychotherapeutic*, conception of psychedelics is implicit in what I have said about their apparently transformative effects on alcoholics. Startled by the fact that 'psychotomimetic' drugs seemed able to catalyse lasting positive behavioural change, researchers noted that psychedelic subjects often experienced a seeming 'upsurge' (Sandison 1954) of previously unconscious material: repressed memories, desires, and fantasies. In line with the dominant psychoanalytical orientation of the day, some researchers concluded that psychedelics weakened the barriers of repression in a way that could facilitate therapeutic progress, by allowing access to the unconscious and enhancing the therapist–patient bond (Sandison et al. 1954, Eisner and

Cohen 1958). Hence the 'psycholytic' (mind-loosening) form of therapy practiced in Europe: repeated sessions of classical psychoanalysis enhanced by low doses of psychedelics (Leuner 1967).

Psychiatrists in the US tended rather to practice 'psychedelic therapy': the administration of one (or very few) high doses, with considerable preparation and interpersonal support, aimed at facilitating an overwhelming and transformative mystical or 'peak' experience (Faillace 1966). Positive results were reported from this method. Although much of the research was methodologically problematic, with over-reliance on anecdotal evidence and under-reliance on control groups (Smart and Storm 1964, Mangini 1998), a recent meta-analysis of six randomised controlled trials (RCTs) from the 1950s and 1960s found evidence for the efficacy of a single high dose of LSD in the treatment of alcoholism (Krebs and Johansen 2012).

Psychotomimetic, entheogenic, and psychotherapeutic investigations were three prominent strands of psychedelic research, but by no means the only ones. Some researchers were interested in psychedelics' potential to enhance creativity (Harman et al. 1966; cf. Sessa 2008), others in their potential as a research tool for charting the human psyche (Osmond 1957). Aldous Huxley (1954) viewed the 'antipodes of the mind' disclosed in psychedelic experience as a promising region for disciplined scientific exploration. Later, Stanislav Grof famously compared psychedelics' 'potential significance for psychiatry and psychology to that of the microscope for medicine or the telescope for astronomy' (Grof 1975, pp. 32–33). This approach has connections with the recent interdisciplinary enterprise of 'philosophical psychopathology', which uses observations from non-ordinary conditions as a basis for conclusions about the structure and function of the ordinary mind (Graham and Stephens 1994). This 'telescopic' conception has been one of the most prominent rationales for the use of psychedelics in recent cognitive neuroscience (e.g., Carhart-Harris et al. 2014).

In a seminal 1957 article that introduced the term 'psychedelic' to the scientific lexicon, Humphry Osmond summarised these various lines of investigation:

> Nearly everyone who works with [psychedelics] and allied compounds agrees there is something special about them. Such words as 'unforgettable' and 'indescribable' abound in the literature. Few workers, however, have emphasised that the unique qualities of these substances must be investigated in many directions at the same time, a consideration that makes work in this field all the more difficult. I shall try to remedy this deficiency by citing several reasons for ascribing importance to them ...
>
> (1) The primary interest of these drugs for the psychiatrist lies in their capacity to mimic more or less closely some aspects of grave mental illnesses, particularly of schizophrenia. The fact that medical men have been preoccupied with transient states resembling mental illnesses that have been called model psychoses, however, does not mean that the only use for these compounds is in the study of pathological conditions ...

(2) Psychiatrists have found that these agents have a place in psychotherapy. This practice may sound like carrying the idea of 'a hair of the dog that bit you' rather far, but it seems to be justified.

(3) Another potentiality of these substances is their use in training and in educating those who work in psychiatry and psychology, especially in understanding strange ways of the mind.

(4) These drugs are of value in exploring the normal mind under unusual circumstances.

(5) Last, but perhaps most important: there are social, philosophical, and religious implications in the discoveries made by means of these agents.

(Osmond 1957, pp. 419–420).

Despite this wealth of promising research programmes, the heyday of psychedelic science was short-lived. LSD, in particular, became the topic of intense socio-political controversy after its highly publicised adoption by the hippie counterculture, exemplified by Timothy Leary's notorious exhortations to 'turn on, tune in, and drop out' (Pahnke 1967). Psychedelics' real but relatively manageable risks (more on which shortly) were both increased by reckless recreational use and exaggerated by sensationalistic journalism (Masters and Houston 1966), inextricably linking psychedelics in the public imagination to fried brains, damaged chromosomes, and delusional leaps from rooftops (Dyck 2010). The net result was that psychedelics were prohibited and virtually all research into their effects on humans stopped. Funding dried up, and displaying an interest in the topic became tantamount to career suicide for any respectable scientist or psychiatrist (Sessa 2005).

Since the 1990s, in a changed socio-political climate, human research on psychedelics has resumed. This line of research is promising and has been aided by the many methodological, technological, and theoretical developments that have occurred in the mind and brain sciences since the 1970s. It is relatively early days, but the field has matured sufficiently that it is now commonplace to speak of a 'psychedelic renaissance' (Sessa 2018, Kelly et al. 2019, Holoyda 2020). Indeed, in the past few years, the expansion of the field has accelerated dramatically (Aday et al. 2019a, Doblin et al. 2019). A new generation of researchers—and even some first-generation psychedelic scientists (e.g., Richards 2015)—have picked up the loose ends described above: psychotomimetic, entheogenic, psychotherapeutic, and other potential applications of psychedelics are being probed with a multitude of methods. I will now review recent findings about the therapeutic and transformative potential—and, crucially, the safety profile—of carefully controlled psychedelic administration in human volunteers.

2.3 Evidence for safety and efficacy

2.3.1 Safety

One of the main reasons given for the prohibition of psychedelics in the 1960s was that these drugs were just too dangerous to be used safely. Political discourse and media coverage surrounding LSD, in particular, painted an alarming picture of a substance capable of causing instant and permanent insanity, genetic defects, and moral corruption (Masters and Houston 1966, Dyck 2010, Mangini 1998). This broad picture of psychedelics as far too hazardous to contemplate using still holds great sway in the public imagination today. Moreover, in most countries, these drugs are classified in the most restrictive legal categories, due to their having 'high abuse potential' and 'no accepted medical use' (Nutt et al. 2013, Krebs 2015). So how can psychedelic therapy even be a prospect worth discussing?

The fact is that, while they are no more risk-free than any other intervention, the dangers of psychedelics seem to have been greatly exaggerated (cf. dos Santos 2014). In a review of the literature, Rick Strassman (1984) found that adverse psychological reactions to psychedelics were relatively rare and. when they did occur, typically transient and manageable with interpersonal support. In the relatively few cases of prolonged psychosis following exposure to a psychedelic, there is often evidence of a pre-existing latent vulnerability, such as a family history of psychotic illness. The incidence of prolonged psychotic episodes when stringent exclusion criteria are applied seems to be very low.

Strassman's findings have been borne out by the dozens of studies conducted since the early 1990s in which psychedelics have been administered to healthy subjects and to psychiatric patients. Hundreds, if not thousands, of volunteers have now been carefully screened, selected, prepared, dosed, and followed-up, in accordance with strict safety guidelines (dos Santos et al. 2018a). These guidelines recommend, among other things, the exclusion of anyone with a personal or immediate family history of psychotic illness, in order to minimise the probability of serious adverse effects (Johnson et al. 2008). Subjects receive the drug in a comfortable, quiet setting, with therapists present to provide reassurance. Often they are given a carefully curated playlist of music to guide the experience (Kaelen et al. 2018). Typically, there are several preparation sessions before the first drug session in which subjects can develop rapport and trust with the supervising therapists, and be educated about the range of possible drug effects and how best to handle these psychologically (e.g., with an attitude of openness and curiosity).

The results by now are clear: when such guidelines are followed, psychedelics have an excellent physiological and psychological safety profile (Nichols 2016, Sessa 2018, dos Santos et al. 2018a.) These substances are physically non-toxic and non-addictive[2]

---

[2] Modak et al. (2019) provide an extremely rare, possibly unique, case report of apparent physical dependence on LSD. Stone et al. (2006) report findings concerning the existence of a 'hallucinogen

at standard therapeutic and transformative doses. Human fatalities attributable to their direct action are virtually unknown, at least in the cases of LSD, psilocybin, mescaline, and DMT—barring a few massive overdoses at several hundred times the standard therapeutic dosage (Nichols and Grob 2018). They can acutely elevate heartrate and blood pressure, and thus are contraindicated for those with certain health conditions. Moreover, subjects sometimes report headaches in the days after the dosing session, but these are transient and relatively mild (Johnson et al. 2012). In a seminal paper that outlines safety guidelines for human psychedelic research, Johnson et al. summarise the drugs' physiological safety profile as follows:

> Hallucinogens generally possess relatively low physiological toxicity, and have not been shown to result in organ damage or neuropsychological deficits... Nonhuman animal studies have shown MDMA (structurally similar to some classical hallucinogens, but with a substantially different pharmacological mechanism of action) to have neurotoxic effects at high doses, although MDMA has been judged to be safe for human administration in the context of several therapeutic and basic human research studies. In contrast, there is no evidence of such potential neurotoxic effects with the prototypical classical hallucinogens (i.e., LSD, mescaline and psilocybin). Some physiological symptoms may occur during hallucinogen action, such as dizziness, weakness, tremors, nausea, drowsiness, paraesthesia, blurred vision, dilated pupils and increased tendon reflexes ... In addition, hallucinogens can moderately increase pulse and both systolic and diastolic blood pressure ... However, these somatic effects vary and are relatively unimpressive even at doses yielding powerful psychological effects...
>
> The physical adverse effects of these agents observed in cancer patients were manageable and similar to effects observed in physically healthy individuals. These researchers noted that any other symptoms experienced during sessions with cancer patients were symptoms already associated with their existing illness ... Early clinical research also safely administered LSD to chronic alcoholics and cancer patients with considerable liver damage, suggesting hepatic concerns are 'negligible unless the dysfunction is of a critical degree' (Grof 1980, p. 164).
>
> Participants and review committees may be concerned that LSD or other hallucinogens are associated with chromosomal damage. These concerns stem from an anti-LSD media campaign by the USA government in the late 1960s ... However, many follow-up investigations soon squarely refuted the hypothesis that LSD use in humans was a significant risk for chromosomal damage or carcinogenic, mutagenic or teratogenic effects...
>
> **(Johnson et al. 2008, pp. 606–607).**

---

dependence syndrome', in which physical dependence is not at issue, but rather problematic patterns of compulsive use. However, their definition of 'hallucinogen' includes substances other than classic psychedelics, such as MDMA and phencyclidine (PCP).

On the psychological front, subjects receiving high doses often experience considerable fear or anxiety during the dosing session (Griffiths et al. 2008), but this is managed with interpersonal support, and follow-ups in these studies have found no serious, lasting adverse effects (Garcia-Romeu et al. 2016). A recent study found that even quite high doses of psilocybin can be tolerated well by healthy volunteers (Nicholas et al. 2018). Writing in 2016, Ross et al. noted that over 2,000 doses of psilocybin had been administered in rigorous research trials during a 25-year period, with 'no reports of any medical or psychiatric serious [adverse events], including no reported cases of prolonged psychosis or HPPD [hallucinogen persisting perception disorder]' (Ross et al. 2016, p. 1176). In a more recent systematic review of psychedelics' long-term effects, Aday et al. noted that 'few subjects reported lasting negative side effects', citing the finding of Studerus et al. (2011) that:

> 1/110 participants who received psilocybin reported experiences of anxiety and depression in the weeks following administration which warranted treatment. Additionally, 'a few' noted less severe emotional instability—but all adverse effects were resolved within a month.
>
> **(Aday et al. 2020, p. 184).**

Aday et al. conclude:

> All in all, limited harm has been reported in the new era of research which utilizes extensive safety protocols ... and the drugs' potential for dependency is low ... In subjective accounts, [patients] with depression ... and addiction ... have noted the lack of long-term adverse side effects as being a considerable benefit over previous treatments they had attempted (e.g., antidepressants).
>
> **(Aday et al. 2020, p. 184).**

In non-clinical settings, the risks are no doubt greater, but there is still evidence that they have been exaggerated. An oft-cited multicriteria decision analysis rated LSD and psilocybin among the least harmful of 20 commonly used recreational drugs, taking into account multiple types and dimensions of harm (Nutt et al. 2010). Researchers have extensively studied members of religious organisations, such as the Native American Church and Santo Daime, that routinely use psychedelics such as peyote and ayahuasca in their rituals. There is now a large body of evidence that members of these communities have good mental and physical health relative to the broader population (Halpern et al. 2005, 2008, Bouso et al. 2012, 2013, Barbosa et al. 2009, 2012, 2016, Ona et al. 2019; cf. Jiménez-Garrido et al. 2020).

Religious contexts aside, population-level studies have found lifetime use of psychedelics to be either un-associated or *negatively* correlated with various mental health problems such as psychosis, psychological distress, and suicidality (Hendricks et al. 2014, 2015a, 2015b, Krebs and Johansen 2013, Johansen and Krebs 2015, Rougemont-Bücking et al. 2019). Similar studies have found psychedelic use to be associated with lower levels of criminal behaviour (Hendricks et al. 2014, 2018), lower levels of opioid use (Pisano et al. 2017), decreased suicide risk among marginalised women who use prescription opioids (Argento et al. 2018), and decreased perpetration of intimate partner violence by men (Walsh et al. 2016, Thiessen et al. 2018). Correlations have also been found with higher levels of pro-environmental behaviour (Forstmann and Sagioglou 2017) and higher levels of liberal political beliefs (Nour et al. 2017; for a review of epidemiological studies, see Johnson et al. 2019).

On the other hand, one recent study found that psychedelic use was positively correlated with mental health and behavioural problems in a sample of university students (Grant et al. 2019). Furthermore, Shalit et al. (2019) found significant correlations between 'hallucinogen' use and various mental health problems, although their definition of 'hallucinogen' was not limited to classic psychedelics but included other substances such as PCP (an NMDA-antagonist dissociative) and Salvia divinorum. Like the above associational studies, these findings do not speak directly to questions of causality, but they do underscore the fact that uncontrolled use of psychedelics may have a poorer safety profile than controlled use.

One must also consider the ill-understood phenomenon of HPPD: the reoccurrence of psychedelic effects at some point after the acute experience has subsided (Halpern and Pope 2003, Skryabin et al. 2018, Nutting et al. 2020). The prevalence of HPPD is unknown but it seems to be more common in uncontrolled settings: no cases resulting from supervised clinical use have been documented in recent research (Ross et al. 2016, Aday et al. 2020). Clearly these drugs are not risk-free: their use, especially in uncontrolled settings, can sometimes have seriously adverse consequences (cf. Bienemann et al. 2020). Johnstad (2020) gives a historical description of harms that can result, even in clinical settings, when appropriate care is not taken. But the evidence suggests that psychedelic administration, especially of the careful and controlled variety, is far less hazardous than received wisdom and international drug policy would have it.

An important note on scope: the topic of this book is the phenomenon of rapid and lasting psychological transformation that seems often to occur when psychedelics are taken in moderate-to-high doses in structured and controlled environments, such as clinical trials and religious rituals. Henceforth, everything that I say about psychedelic use and its effects should be understood as referring to this specific phenomenon, unless otherwise indicated.

2.3.2 Therapeutic efficacy

Besides evidence for its safety, there is mounting evidence that supervised clinical use of psychedelics can have lasting psychological benefits (for comprehensive reviews, see dos Santos and Hallak 2020, Aday et al. 2020, Wheeler and Dyer 2020). I do not engage here with the emerging literature on 'microdosing'—the practice of taking minute doses of psychedelics, insufficient to induce an altered state of consciousness, for putative therapeutic or enhancement benefits (e.g., Johnstad 2018, Polito and Stevenson 2019, Fadiman and Korb 2019, Lea et al. 2020). Nor do I engage with proposals to examine psychedelics' effects on such conditions as age-related changes in cognition and affect (Aday et al. 2019b), cluster headaches (Sewell et al. 2006), and disorders of consciousness such as vegetative and minimally conscious states (Scott and Carhart-Harris 2019). My sole concern, as noted above, is the supervised administration of moderate-to-high, *consciousness-altering* doses for psychologically therapeutic or transformative purposes.

Moreno et al. (2006) conducted a small, open-label trial of psilocybin for obsessive-compulsive disorder (OCD). Nine patients with OCD, all of whom had failed to respond to standard treatments, each received four psilocybin sessions a week or more apart: a low, medium, and high dose, with a very low dose inserted randomly as a comparator. The psilocybin sessions were well tolerated, and every patient showed significant symptom reductions, lasting 24 hours or more, in at least one dosing session. So far, this is the only published clinical research on psychedelics for OCD. In this study, clinical outcomes were not significantly correlated either with drug dose or with qualitative aspects of the psychedelic experience. This finding can fairly be regarded as an anomaly. The study's open-label design and small sample size limit its evidential value and, as we will see, many other studies have found strong associations between qualitative aspects of the psychedelic experience and various lasting psychological benefits.

A somewhat better-studied indication is the treatment of addiction (Bogenschutz and Johnson 2016). As we saw in section 2.2, a meta-analysis of RCTs from the 1950s and 1960s found that a single high dose of LSD significantly outperformed placebo in the treatment of alcoholism (Krebs and Johansen 2012). It should always be borne in mind that effective double-blinding is a serious methodological challenge in psychedelic research, where the effects of the active treatment are usually (un-)blindingly obvious to the patient. This is one issue in psychedelic research that could usefully be analysed from a philosophy of science perspective.

Two recent open-label pilot studies have addressed the potential of psilocybin to treat alcohol and tobacco addiction, respectively. Bogenschutz et al. (2015) administered one or two doses of psilocybin in conjunction with Motivational Enhancement Therapy to 10 volunteers diagnosed with alcohol dependence. During the first four weeks of the programme, while the patients were only receiving therapy, there were no significant changes to drinking behaviour, but the first psilocybin session, at four weeks, was followed by significant improvements in drinking behaviour, as well as reduced craving and increased motivation to quit. In this instance, the clinical outcomes were correlated with psychometric ratings of mystical experience, as well as with the overall intensity of the drug experience. Remarkably, the changes were largely maintained at follow-ups 36 weeks after the psilocybin sessions.

Meanwhile, Johnson et al. (2014) administered psilocybin to 15 addicted cigarette smokers, with mean smoking rates of 19 cigarettes per day and a mean duration of 31 years' smoking. Each subject had previously made multiple failed quit attempts.

Six months after receiving a moderate and a high dose of psilocybin in the context of a structured smoking cessation intervention, 12 of the 15 (80%) were verified nicotine-abstinent by biomarkers. One year after the sessions, 10 subjects remained abstinent; more than 16 months after, 9 did (Johnson et al. 2017). Like the alcoholism trial, this open-label study requires replication in larger samples with placebo controls before firm conclusions can be drawn. Nonetheless, 80% is a remarkable six-month abstinence rate, far superior to current gold-standard treatments for tobacco addiction (West et al. 2015). In this study, those who responded to the treatment showed much higher rates of mystical experience than non-responders, independently of the overall intensity of psychedelic effects, suggesting that mystical experiences specifically were involved in causing clinical outcomes (Garcia-Romeu et al. 2014). One participant in this study commented:

> It felt like I'd died as a smoker and was resurrected as a nonsmoker. Because it's my perception of myself, and that's how I felt. So I jumped up and I said 'I'm not a smoker anymore, it's all done.'
>
> **(Noorani et al. 2018, p. 759).**

Psychedelics have also been studied for the treatment of depression (reviewed by Muttoni et al. 2019, Goldberg et al. 2020, Romeo et al. 2020). In an open-label pilot study, 17 patients with major depressive disorder received a single dose of ayahuasca and showed significant reductions in depressive symptoms lasting three weeks (Osório et al. 2015, Sanches et al. 2016). Eight patients participated in a follow-up interview, four to seven years later. Six of these ranked their ayahuasca session among the 10 most important experiences of their life (dos Santos et al. 2018b). Meanwhile, in a double-blind RCT involving 35 patients with treatment-resistant depression, half of the patients showed significant antidepressant effects lasting up to a week after a single dose of ayahuasca (Palhano-Fontes et al. 2019).

In another open-label study, 12 patients with treatment-resistant depression each received a moderate and a high dose of psilocybin with non-directive psychological support. Patients showed significant reductions in depressive symptoms (Carhart-Harris et al. 2016b), which were largely maintained six months after dosing (Carhart-Harris et al. 2018b). The magnitude of clinical improvement was correlated with distinctive changes to brain activity, discussed further in Chapter 5 (Carhart-Harris et al. 2017). One participant in this study commented:

> [Through the psilocybin experience] I got a wider perspective, I stepped back. It helped me appreciate that the world is a big place [and] that there's a lot more going on than just the minor things that were going on in my head.
>
> **(Watts et al. 2017, p. 534).**

Thus, there is preliminary evidence that one or two controlled psychedelic experiences can durably reduce depressive symptoms. Indeed, the U.S. Food and

Drug Administration (FDA) has granted 'Breakthrough Therapy' designation to psilocybin-assisted treatment of depression, lending its assistance to fast-track Phase 3 clinical trials that will rigorously test the treatment's efficacy in hundreds of subjects across multiple study sites (Meikle et al. 2020).

The best-studied therapeutic application in the psychedelic renaissance has been the amelioration of psychosocial distress in terminally ill patients (reviewed by Reiche et al. 2018, Muttoni et al. 2019, Goldberg et al. 2020). Those with a terminal diagnosis undergo many forms of suffering, not least of which is considerable anxiety, depression, and existential distress relating to their illness and impending death. Effective ways of dealing with this distress are badly needed. In the 1960s and 1970s, psychedelics were used to ease the psychological suffering of terminally ill patients (Dyck 2019). Clinicians and patients alike reported that the treatment was extremely helpful (Pahnke and Richards 1966, Richards 2015):

> One patient, after his LSD experience, wondered how he could have been so worried about death, which now seemed to be just another step in the life process. Others frankly and calmly stated that they would be 'ready to go' when the time to die came. This degree of acceptance and willingness to face the unknown was in strong contrast to the atmosphere of fear among the family and patient before psychedelic psychotherapy was started.
>
> **(Pahnke 1969, pp. 15–16).**

Several clinical trials from this era are reviewed by Reiche et al. (2018). All studies reported positive results. In some, lasting benefits correlated with ratings of mystical or 'peak' experience. More recently, Grob et al. (2011) reported a pilot study in which 12 patients with anxiety relating to a terminal diagnosis each received one placebo session and one moderate-dose psilocybin session in double-blind fashion. Psilocybin sessions were followed by significant reductions in anxiety lasting three months and reductions in depressive symptoms that reached significance six months after dosing. Similar results were found in a study of LSD in 12 patients with terminal illness, with reductions in anxiety lasting 12 months. This was the first clinical trial of LSD-assisted psychotherapy in over 40 years (Gasser et al. 2014).

These findings have since been replicated in two larger, double-blind RCTs—one at New York University (NYU) and one at Johns Hopkins University. These are the 'most rigorous controlled trials to date' of psilocybin, perhaps of any psychedelic, for a therapeutic application (Nutt 2016, p. 1163). Between the two studies, a total of 80 terminal patients with clinically significant anxiety and depression received psilocybin and placebo sessions. High-dose psilocybin sessions led to significant decreases in anxiety and depression that were sustained six months after treatment, with the degree of mystical experience a strong predictor of clinical improvement (Griffiths et al. 2016, Ross et al. 2016). A long-term follow-up was conducted in the NYU study. Over half of the surviving patients who participated in the follow-up still showed significant anxiolytic and antidepressant effects, three to four years post-treatment

(Agin-Liebes et al. 2020). One patient in the NYU trial described the lasting effects of the treatment as follows:

> I feel like a whole bunch of crap has been dumped off the surface. This stuff that made my world shut down so much and made me look at the ground and watch the clock numbers clicking by. There's life and so many things going on, just watching that tree over there blowing in the breeze, seeing people in the street, and all the different people in vehicles rushing by! I just feel good about being alive … It's always there; we just don't notice, and I'm trying to notice and not forget that I can see it at any time. I can hear it any time. It's like waking up in the most profound way, that this is really what life is, it's really like this. We're just not noticing.
>
> **(Belser et al. 2017, p. 375).**

The success of these studies strengthens the basis for the Phase 3 studies described above. If these studies find compelling evidence of safety and efficacy, this will raise the possibility of psilocybin being approved for medicinal use by the FDA. Although there are significant financial, logistical, and cultural obstacles, psilocybin may well become a legal medicine within the next decade (Rucker et al. 2017, Nutt 2019). This lends further urgency to the issues I am discussing in this book. A coherent philosophical conception of what exactly these strange and controversial drugs offer could be extremely useful, if they are to be incorporated smoothly into mainstream psychiatry and society.

2.3.3 Transformative efficacy in healthy subjects

As we have seen, there is considerable preliminary evidence for the therapeutic efficacy of psychedelics in anxiety, depression, and addiction. Another set of studies suggests that controlled psychedelic use can have lasting psychological benefits for mentally healthy volunteers (reviewed by Elsey 2017, Gandy 2019; cf. Bouso et al. 2018). This builds on earlier claims that psychedelic experiences can be enriching and valuable for subjects who do not have a psychiatric diagnosis, but nonetheless may be seeking personal growth or have existential concerns regarding mortality, spirituality, and meaning in life (Masters and Houston 1966).

In a seminal study, Griffiths et al. (2006) administered high doses of psilocybin to 36 mentally healthy, psychedelic-naïve subjects, all of whom reported regular or semi-regular participation in religious or spiritual activities. The vast majority of these subjects were highly educated and gainfully employed. This study was an attempt to replicate more rigorously Pahnke's Marsh Chapel experiment mentioned in Section 2.2.

Approximately two-thirds of the subjects studied by Griffiths et al. had a 'complete' mystical experience, according to standard psychometric scales. Of those who did have such experiences, a clear majority rated their psilocybin session among the top five most personally meaningful, or the top five most spiritually significant, events of their lives. Some even rated their session as the *single* most personally meaningful or spiritually significant event of their life. In written comments, reflecting on the meaningfulness and significance they ascribed to the psilocybin experience, volunteers made comparisons to such events as the birth of a child or the death of a parent. Subjects' impressions of the value of the experiences were maintained 14 months later (Griffiths et al. 2008). One subject described gaining:

> [the] understanding that in the eyes of God—all people … were all equally important and equally loved by God. I have had other transcendent experiences, however, this one was important because it reminded and comforted me that God is truly and unconditionally loving and present.
>
> **(Griffiths et al. 2008, p. 629).**

Similar results were found in another study of 18 mentally healthy, mostly psychedelic-naïve participants administered multiple doses of psilocybin (Griffiths et al. 2011).

Remarkably, a pooled analysis of data from these two trials found that subjects who had a 'complete' mystical experience showed significant increases in Openness to Experience, one of the 'Big Five' personality domains in psychology (Digman 1990). These increases remained significant 14 months after the dosing session (MacLean et al. 2011).[3] Subjects themselves, as well as community observers, reported improvements in well-being and interpersonal relationships that they attributed to the psilocybin sessions.

More recently, Griffiths et al. (2017) tested the combined effects of psilocybin and spiritual practices, such as meditation, on various measures of well-being in healthy subjects. There were three groups in this study. One group received a very low, essentially inactive, dose of psilocybin, plus a 'standard' (moderate) level of support and encouragement to engage in spiritual practices. A second group received a high dose of psilocybin and the same standard level of spiritual practice support. A third group received a high dose of psilocybin and a high level of spiritual practice support. At six-month follow-up, both high-dose psilocybin groups showed far greater improvements than the low-dose group on various positive outcome measures, such as self-reported increases in well-being and gratitude. The high-dose high-support group showed even larger improvements than the high-dose low-support group, suggesting that spiritual practices contributed somewhat to the outcomes. But the outcome differences between groups 1 and 2 were far greater than those between 2 and 3, suggesting that the psilocybin experience accounted for most of the difference. Persisting positive effects were correlated with both degree of engagement in spiritual practices

---

[3] A recent correlational study found that recreational users of psychedelics showed higher levels of Openness to Experience than controls who used no drugs or preferred other drugs (Erritzoe et al. 2019), although of course this does not speak to questions of causality.

and psychometric ratings of mystical experiences under psilocybin, but more strongly with the latter.

Interestingly, Griffiths et al. reported that several subjective effects of psilocybin were rated more strongly by those in the high-dose high-support group than by those in the high-dose standard-support group, suggesting that engagement in spiritual practices affects the kinds of experiences one has when administered psychedelics. This hypothesis has received further support from a remarkable study conducted by Smigielski et al. (2019a). These researchers administered psilocybin or placebo to experienced practitioners of mindfulness meditation (in the Zen tradition) on the fourth day of a five-day silent group retreat. Subjects who received psilocybin underwent mystical-type experiences of 'oceanic boundlessness', with unusually low levels of anxiety. These researchers concluded that proficiency in meditation practice:

> seems to enhance psilocybin's positive effects while counteracting possible dysphoric responses ... [highlighting] the interactions between non-pharmacological and pharmacological factors, and the role of emotion/attention regulation in shaping the experiential quality of psychedelic states.
>
> **(Smigielski et al. 2019a, p. 1).**

Immediately before and after the retreat, subjects completed a mindfulness questionnaire. Unsurprisingly, all subjects showed an increase in trait mindfulness from pre- to post-retreat. However, as the researchers had hypothesised, the increase was larger in the psilocybin than the placebo group. At four-month follow-up, those in the psilocybin group showed increases in psychological constructs such as 'appreciation for life' and 'self-acceptance'. These increases correlated with the degree of oceanic boundlessness experienced under psilocybin.

The findings of Griffiths et al. (2017) and Smigielski et al. (2019a) suggest that psychedelic administration can enhance the beneficial effects of spiritual practices such as meditation, and vice versa. Other studies have found that psychedelic administration *alone* can promote some of the psychological capacities cultivated in such practices. For example, Madsen et al. (2020) found that capacities for mindful awareness, as well as the personality trait Openness to Experience, were significantly elevated in healthy, psychedelic-naïve participants three months after a single experience with psilocybin. Several other studies have found evidence of increased mindfulness-related capacities during and after a psychedelic experience (Soler et al. 2016, 2018, Sampedro et al. 2017, Mian et al. 2020, Uthaug et al. 2019, 2020); I discuss these in more detail in section 5.2.2. The commonalities between meditative and psychedelic states offer intriguing clues about the nature and consequences of the latter (Millière et al. 2018, Heuschkel and Kuypers 2020). I will return to this connection repeatedly in the later chapters of the book.

In another study, Carhart-Harris et al. (2012a) administered intravenous psilocybin or placebo to healthy volunteers. After administration, these subjects were prompted to recall autobiographical memories, while undergoing a brain scan with functional magnetic resonance imaging (fMRI). Self-reported ratings of well-being were increased at two-week follow-up, and these increases correlated with enhanced vividness of memory recall under psilocybin. Memory recall under psilocybin also produced different patterns of neural response than recall under placebo, with increased activation in sensory, including visual, areas of the cortex.

At least one study has provided evidence that even quite high doses of psilocybin can lead to experiences that are positively valued by subjects and that have lasting beneficial effects. Nicholas et al. (2018) recruited volunteers with prior psychedelic experience and administered an escalating series of doses, with the highest being 0.6 mg per kg of body weight—a nearly 50% increase on the dose administered by Griffiths et al. (2006). Psilocybin sessions led to an increase in self-reported well-being and life satisfaction 30 days later, correlating with ratings of mystical experience during the session.

A couple of studies have also shown lasting psychological benefits of a single LSD session in healthy volunteers. Lebedev et al. (2016) reported that 19 subjects showed significant increases in Openness to Experience, and in measures of optimism, two weeks after a supervised LSD session. The extent of these increases was strongly correlated with an increase in the unpredictability or 'entropy' of brain activity during the drug experience. Meanwhile, Schmid and Liechti (2018) administered LSD to healthy volunteers who reported increases in well-being, life satisfaction, and other positive psychological effects at both 1- and 12-month follow-ups. These increases correlated with ratings of mystical experience while under LSD.

Many questions remain, and many findings require replication. But researchers have already amassed an impressive body of evidence that psychedelics can be administered safely in clinical settings, and reliably cause states of consciousness that are rated as highly valuable and meaningful, leading to lasting, positive psychological and behavioural changes in both psychiatric patients and healthy volunteers. A certain caution about these findings is warranted, given the general methodological difficulties of psychedelic research and the specific methodological limitations of several studies (Aday et al. 2020). However, for the purposes of this book, I will assume that the picture emerging from these studies with respect to safety, and therapeutic and transformative efficacy, is essentially accurate.

A second assumption of the book is that the therapeutic use of psychedelics for psychiatric symptom reduction, and their use by healthy subjects for positive psychological transformation, constitutes a single, more-or-less unified phenomenon, with common causal mechanisms. This is a substantive assumption, but it is one I hope to vindicate by the arguments that follow. I will typically use the term 'psychedelic therapy' rather than the umbrella term 'psychedelic transformation' (Letheby 2015), and will focus mainly on clinical applications, but my intention is that much of what I say will apply, *mutatis mutandis*, to transformative use by healthy subjects. As such, I will draw liberally on studies of healthy volunteers, as well as psychiatric patients, in developing my account of psychedelic therapy.

The question now becomes: what follows, philosophically, if this picture is accurate?

2.4 An existential medicine?

It should be clear that psychedelic therapy is an unusual psychopharmacological intervention, in a number of ways. One of the most obvious is the apparent causal role of the mystical experience in mediating positive results.

In several of the studies I have discussed, psychometric ratings of the degree of mystical experience predict clinical and behavioural outcomes. For example, such ratings correlated with increases in Openness to Experience in Griffiths et al.'s (2006, 2008) seminal studies of mystical experience (MacLean et al. 2011), and with various positive outcome measures in two studies of psilocybin and spiritual practices (Griffiths et al. 2017, Smigielski et al. 2019a). They also correlated with lasting psychological benefits in the studies of healthy volunteers carried out by Nicholas et al. (2018) and Schmid and Liechti (2018).

Granted, Lebedev et al. (2016) did not report rates of mystical experience in their LSD study of healthy volunteers. And, in the Moreno et al. (2006) study of psilocybin for OCD, outcomes seemed independent of specific experiential variables. But Bogenschutz et al. (2015) found that mystical experience was a key predictor of improvements in drinking behaviour—albeit so was the overall intensity of the psychedelic experience. Johnson et al. (2014) found that mystical experience predicted improvements in tobacco addiction independently of overall experience intensity (Garcia-Romeu et al. 2014). In the study of psilocybin for treatment-resistant depression, ratings both of mystical experience and of 'insightfulness' predicted positive outcomes (Roseman et al. 2018a, Carhart-Harris et al. 2018b). And in the two RCTs of psilocybin for psychological distress in terminal illness, mystical experience was strongly associated with reductions in anxiety and depression (Griffiths et al. 2016, Ross et al. 2016).

As well as such quantitative data, clinical wisdom among experienced psychedelic therapists suggests that psycho-spiritual or existential epiphanies are crucial in overcoming anxiety, depression, substance abuse, and other psychological maladies—consistent with the emphasis on spirituality in recovery programmes such as Alcoholics Anonymous (Pahnke and Richards 1966, Grof 1975, Kelly et al. 2011).

This is a far cry from standard psychiatric treatments, to say the least. The seemingly central role of the mystical experience has led Charles Grob to describe psychedelic therapy as an 'existential medicine'. Referring specifically to its use in terminal illness, he writes:

> Under the influence of hallucinogens, individuals transcend their primary identification with their bodies and experience ego-free states before the time of their actual physical demise, and return with a new perspective and profound acceptance of the life constant, change.
>
> (Grob 2007, p. 213).

To examine this issue more closely, we need to be clear about what exactly constitutes a 'mystical experience'. Clearly, the term is vacuous if it simply refers to any experience that subjects feel moved to describe as 'religious' or 'mystical' (Masters and Houston 1966, p. 256). But in the psychology of religion and clinical psychedelic research, the term has a much more specific, standardised meaning. It refers to a distinct type of experience that has been reported by contemplative practitioners and religious devotees throughout the ages, and is often reported by those who take psychedelics in conducive settings.

The notion of mystical experience used in much psychedelic research derives from the work of W.T. Stace (1960), who conducted a thorough survey of the mystical literature of the world's religions. The current definition is based on Stace's analyses and operationalised in such instruments as the Pahnke-Richards Mystical Experience Questionnaire (MEQ) and the Hood Mysticism Scale (Griffiths et al. 2008, 2011, 2017, MacLean et al. 2012). According to this definition, there are seven phenomenological components of a mystical experience proper—as distinct from 'visionary' experiences and other related phenomena (Richards 2015, p. 78). These are internal and external unity, noetic quality, transcendence of time and space, ineffability, paradoxicality, sense of sacredness, and deeply felt positive mood.

Internal and external unity refers to the sense of 'oneness' or 'interconnectedness': either a 'pure consciousness event' (Forman 1998) allegedly lacking mental contents altogether, or a sense of profound union with the entire manifest universe. *Noetic quality* refers to a strong sense of gaining a genuine and unmediated insight, or of encountering ultimate reality; the mystical experience, by definition, is felt to be 'more real than real'. *Transcendence of time and space* is fairly self-explanatory, if not easy to grasp intellectually: subjects of mystical experience report a sense that time had slowed dramatically or stopped completely (an experience as of eternity or atemporality; being 'outside time'), and that normal spatial awareness was gone (either because there was no space, as in a pure consciousness event, or because they felt 'externally unified' with everything and thus not located in any specific spatial position).

Mystical experiences are described by subjects as being *ineffable*, in that existing language—perhaps any possible language—is utterly inadequate to their description. When attempts at description are nonetheless made, they typically feature *paradoxicality* of some kind, often reporting the simultaneous experience of apparently opposing or contradictory qualities: for example, the experience of an '*empty* unity which is at the same time *full* and complete' (Pahnke 1963, p. 70; emphasis original.) The *sense of sacredness* is a feeling that whatever reality is encountered in the mystical experience is highly, perhaps ultimately, valuable and worthy of reverence. Finally, *deeply felt positive mood* refers to the joy and rapture that accompany such revelations (albeit often preceded by, or intermingled with, awe and fear; cf. Wasson 1957). Despite the alleged futility of verbal description, first-person accounts offer the clearest illustrations of these seven features:

During this stage … comes that experience called by the mystics 'the realization of the God within us'. This comes to many under these drugs, and is an indescribable, piercing, beautiful knowledge and knowing, which goes beyond the body, the mind, the reason, the intellect, to an area of pure knowing … There is no sensation of time. God is no longer only 'out there' somewhere, but He is within you, and you are one with Him. No doubt of it even crosses one's awareness at this stage. You are beyond the knower and the known, where there is no duality, but only oneness and unity, and great love. You not only see Truth, but you are truth. You are Love. You are all things! It is not an ego-inflating experience, but on the contrary, one which can help one to dissolve the ego. It gives one a splendid flash of what can be, and what one must surely aim for. It resolves the goal, and the goal is found worthy of pursuit. The consciousness or awareness is expanded far beyond that of the normal state. And this level of consciousness, which actually is available to us at all times, is found to be that part of us which, for want of a better way to express it, might be called the 'God-ness' of us. And we find that this God-ness is unchangeable and indestructible, and that its foundation is Love in its purest form …

(John W. Aiken 1962, quoted in Harman 1963).

I was plunged into ecstasy—an ecstasy infinitely exceeding anything describable … There was awareness of undifferentiated unity, embracing the perfect identity of subject and object, of singleness and plurality, of the One and the Many. Thus I found myself (if indeed the words 'I' and 'myself' have any meaning in such a context) at once the audience, the actors and the play! Logically, the One can give birth to the Many and the Many can merge into the One or be fundamentally but not apparently identical with it; they cannot be *in all respects* one and many simultaneously. But now logic was transcended. I beheld (and myself was) a whirling mass of brilliant colors and forms which, being several colors and several forms, were different from one another—and yet altogether the *same* at the very moment of being different! I doubt if this statement can be made to seem meaningful at the ordinary level of consciousness. No wonder the mystics of all faiths teach that understanding comes only when logic and intellect are transcended! In any case, this truth, even if at an ordinary level of consciousness it cannot be *understood*, can, in a higher state of consciousness, be directly *experienced* as self-evident. Logic also boggles at trying to explain how I could at once *perceive* and yet *be* those colors and those forms, how the *seer*, the *seeing* and the *seen*, the *feeler*, the *feeling* and the *felt* could all be one; but, to me, all this was so clearly self-evident as to suggest the words 'childishly simple!' … there was awareness of unutterable bliss, coupled with the conviction that this was the *only* real and eternal state of being, all others (including our entire experience in the day-to-day world) being no more than passing dreams. This bliss, I am convinced, awaits all beings when the last vestiges of their selfhood have been destroyed—or, as in this case, temporarily discarded.

(Blofeld 1966, pp. 28–30).

This is the type of experience that seems to be crucially involved in psychedelics' mechanism of therapeutic and transformative action. It is also the kind of experience that led intellectuals such as Aldous Huxley, Alan Watts, and Timothy Leary to connect psychedelics with the consciousness alterations aimed at by the meditative disciplines of Hinduism and Buddhism (Huxley 1954, Watts 1962, Leary et al. 1964). Detailed descriptions of psychedelic-induced mystical experiences are available elsewhere (e.g., Masters and Houston 1966, Shanon 2002, Estevez 2013) and I will discuss their phenomenology more in Chapter 3. For now, suffice it to say that, despite considerable debate, these drug-induced experiences seem to be very similar to prototypical mystical experiences that occur spontaneously or are occasioned by non-pharmacological methods. Not only are blind raters unable to distinguish reports of psychedelic and non-psychedelic mystical experiences (Smith 1964) but the former are experienced by those who undergo them as *more* intensely mystical and beneficially transformative than the latter (Yaden et al. 2017). It is the apparent centrality of such experiences to psychedelic therapy that invites the worry I am exploring in this book.

2.5 The Comforting Delusion Objection

There is no denying that many psychedelic experiences, especially overwhelming and transformative ones, involve subjectively compelling experiences of an apparently supernatural or transcendent dimension to existence. It is not for nothing that many traditional cultures view ritual psychedelic use as a method for communicating with deities or the spirit world (Metzner 1998, Shanon 2002). And such beliefs are not confined to participants in traditional rituals. In the clinical study of psilocybin for OCD mentioned earlier, nearly half of the subjects reported experiences such as 'exploration of other planets, visiting past-life reincarnations, and interacting with deities' (Moreno et al. 2006, p. 1739). It is unclear whether these subjects believed that their experiences were veridical or not. But some subjects do adopt metaphysical beliefs on the basis of psychedelic experiences. Consider the following report from a patient treated in the 1970s with the classic psychedelic dipropyltryptamine (DPT):

> I seemed to transcend time and space and I lost complete identification with the 'real' world. The experience seemed to me to be as if I was going from this world back to another world before this life had occurred ... I felt that I had been in that mass of energy at one time before. When I was there everything seemed to make sense ... It was a very beautiful world, one in which love was very much a part ... The basic theme that I perceived ... was that life continues to go on and we are basically some form of essence from a Supreme Being and we are part of that Supreme Being ... The results of the use of the hallucinogenic drug on my life have been very profound. I seem to have a much deeper understanding of life and death. I don't have the fear of death that I once had ... I have found that everyday living

seems to be much more enjoyable ... I am a much more content individual, having had the great opportunity to just glimpse for a very short moment the overall thinking of God ... to be reassured that there is a very beautiful, loving masterful plan in this Universe for all of us.

(Richards 1978, p. 124; my emphasis).

According to the eminent religious scholar Huston Smith, the 'basic message of the entheogens [is] that there is another Reality that puts this one in the shade' (Smith 2000, p. 133). We have already seen evidence that the mystical experience is a key part of psychedelics' transformative mechanism, and a defining element of the mystical experience is the noetic quality: the powerful sense of direct, undeniable knowledge—the compelling feeling that the transcendent Reality encountered is 'more real than real'.

But what if there is *not* 'another Reality that puts this one in the shade'? In that case, the mystical experience would seem to be nothing more than a 'metaphysical hallucination' (Flanagan and Graham 2017): an intense and vivid conscious experience that misrepresents the metaphysical nature of reality. This possibility raises disquieting questions about the use of psychedelics in psychiatry, including the one posed forcefully by Michael Pollan (2015): 'Is psychedelic therapy simply foisting a comforting delusion on the sick and dying?'

Call this the Comforting Delusion Objection to psychedelic therapy.[4] The Objection is simple: it says that psychedelics induce their salutary psychological effects mainly by inducing metaphysical beliefs that are comforting but probably false, and we should therefore hesitate to use these substances for therapeutic or transformative purposes. The Objection gains much force from the intellectual and cultural dominance of philosophical naturalism: roughly, the view that there is no other Reality that puts this one in the shade; that the natural world is the only reality there is. Naturalism is difficult to define in a precise and uncontroversial manner, but it is typically taken to entail at least the rejection of non-natural or supernatural entities and forces, and the acceptance that the universe is populated solely by the kinds of in-principle-detectable entities, processes, properties, and forces studied by the natural sciences. Naturalism of one kind or another is the dominant view in the philosophy of mind today (Papineau 2016). And differences of detail aside, card-carrying naturalists share a commitment to rejecting the literal existence of disembodied minds, spirits, and transcendent forms of consciousness not dependent on any specific brain or other material cognitive system.

There are three common responses to the Comforting Delusion Objection. One is to say that there is no problem, because the transcendent dimensions seemingly accessed in psychedelic experience are in fact real—at least when it comes to the

---

[4] I am using Pollan's phrase because it vividly and memorably evokes the relevant concern, not because I think that all non-naturalistic metaphysical beliefs qualify as delusions in a clinical sense (although this position might find sympathy in some philosophical quarters!)

Ultimate Reality or Ground of Being, often described as a cosmic consciousness that underlies, gives rise to, or is identical with the entire manifest universe. This quint-essentially psychedelic metaphysic has been described as 'idealistic monism with pantheistic overtones' (Shanon 2002, p. 163)—the view that reality is, despite appearances, entirely constituted by a single, unitary mind or consciousness, and that this consciousness is in some sense divine or sacred. After interviewing hundreds of ayahuasca users, Benny Shanon reported that most of them believed 'truly existing other realities [were] being revealed' in their psychedelic experiences (Shanon 2002, p. 165). The popularity of this kind of position among psychedelic researchers over the years attests to the fact that many people really do have psychedelic experiences with compelling apparent metaphysical implications, and do take these experiences to disclose genuine truths about the nature of reality. Explicit endorsements of something like this view can be found in the writings of (inter alia) William Richards (2015), Huston Smith (2000), Aldous Huxley (1954), Alan Watts (1962), Stanislav Grof (1975), and Frances Vaughan (1983). These scholars and others like them believe that psychedelic mysticism discloses objectively real transcendent dimensions or levels of existence, including forms of consciousness or intelligence that are ontologically (not just phenomenologically) outside time, prior to evolution, and independent of any material substrate As such, they reject naturalism, at least in the way that I have characterised it.

A second common response is to say that, ultimately, it is not so important whether psychedelic-induced mystical experiences are veridical or not. Instead, we should judge these experiences by their fruits: whether they produce good results in people's lives by making them happier, more altruistic, less fearful of death, and so forth. This kind of response can be found among those who are highly sceptical of mystical metaphysics, such as Owen Flanagan (2018), and among those who are highly sympathetic to it, such as William Richards (quoted in Pollan 2015).[5] Flanagan describes the psychedelic mystical vision as 'existentially meaningful, morally motivating and also likely to be false' (2018, p. 1). He nonetheless argues that the existential meaning and moral motivation outweigh the falsity: in this case, at least, the Good and the Beautiful outweigh the True. This is part of his broader project of protesting the pathologisation of various mental states on solely epistemic grounds. On this view, what is most important is not whether the mystical experience is veridical (which cannot be established with certainty, as advocates of this position stress) but whether it benefits people who undergo it and those around them. Many psychedelic researchers take this view. One of the scientists interviewed by Michael Pollan quipped that the question of whether the mystical experience is veridical was 'above [his] pay grade' (Pollan 2015).

---

[5] Shortly before this book went to press, Greif and Šurkala (2020) published a thoughtful article about the compassionate use of psychedelics in which they respond to the Comforting Delusion Objection. Their response is not readily classified by the schema I am using here. I will discuss it briefly in section 10.2, Chapter 10.

For better or worse, as a philosopher, this question is not above my pay grade: it is right there in the job description. And I agree with Flanagan, as well as with proponents of the third response such as Andrea Lavazza (2017) that, insofar as it represents reality as grounded in a transcendent universal consciousness, the mystical experience is probably not veridical. What distinguishes Lavazza's response is that he thinks the epistemic status of the experience is indeed important. Contrasting 'realistic' forms of well-being, based on accurate understanding of reality, with 'unrealistic' ones based on misrepresentation, Lavazza argues that the former are preferable, but that psychedelic experience belongs to the latter kind. Thus, he takes a naturalistic view according to which the epistemic credentials of psychedelic therapy are (a) important and (b) poor; thus, he concludes that we should be wary of this particular path to well-being. Something like this view has been defended by others (e.g., Roche 2010) and continues a philosophically influential tradition of scepticism about altered states of consciousness and their epistemic credentials (cf. Windt 2011).

At a first pass, one might formulate the Comforting Delusion Objection as follows:

1. Naturalism is true.
2. If the epistemic status of psychedelic therapy is poor, then we should hesitate to recommend or prescribe it.
3. Therefore, we should hesitate to recommend or prescribe psychedelic therapy.

On this way of construing the argument, the various responses canvassed thus far would amount to rejecting premise one (Richards, Smith, Huxley et al.); rejecting premise two (Flanagan et al.); or accepting the conclusion (Lavazza, Roche et al.).

However, it should be apparent that the argument, as I have just formulated it, is an *enthymeme*: it has a hidden or suppressed premise, without which it is invalid. When this premise is made explicit, the argument goes like this:

1. Naturalism is true
2. If the epistemic status of psychedelic therapy is poor, then we should hesitate to recommend or prescribe it
3. If naturalism is true, then the epistemic status of psychedelic therapy is poor
4. Therefore, we should hesitate to recommend or prescribe psychedelic therapy

In my opinion, the weakest link in this reformulated argument is premise three. My strategy will be to try to undermine this claim. As such, the fourth response to the Comforting Delusion Objection—the response that I plan to defend—involves accepting premises one and two: that (a) naturalism is true, so pantheistic idealism and other 'cosmic consciousness'-type views (e.g., Shani 2015, Albahari 2019a) are false, and (b) the epistemic credentials of psychedelic therapy are indeed important. However, I contend that, *even if* naturalism is true, psychedelic therapy still has significant epistemic benefits, and can even accurately be described as involving authentic spiritual experience.

Specifically, I will argue for three claims:

(i) Psychedelic therapy, given naturalism, involves *less epistemic risk* than one might suppose: its mechanism of action, despite first appearances, does not constitutively involve the promotion of non-naturalistic metaphysical beliefs, nor is such promotion an inevitable side effect.

(ii) Psychedelic therapy, given naturalism, is 'epistemically innocent' (Bortolotti 2015), meaning that, despite its real epistemic risks, it nonetheless has *significant epistemic benefits* that are often unavailable by any alternative means.

(iii) Some of the key components of psychedelic therapy are elements of a viable *naturalistic spirituality*.

To argue for these claims, I will be using conceptual and methodological tools from philosophy and the cognitive sciences to attempt a speculative synthesis of evidence concerning the nature and mechanisms of psychedelic transformation. This synthesis will reveal that the prima facie picture of psychedelic therapy I have painted in this chapter is misleading in important respects. It is true that psychometric constructs such as 'mystical-type experience' strongly predict beneficial outcomes from psychedelic therapy. But it will turn out that not every experience captured by these constructs is a non-naturalistic metaphysical hallucination. Some transformative psychedelic experiences feature apparent encounters with a cosmic consciousness or divine Reality, but others do not.

Thus, I will argue that the picture of psychedelic therapy underlying the Comforting Delusion Objection is empirically implausible. It is simply false that the central mechanism of this treatment is the induction or strengthening of non-naturalistic metaphysical beliefs. The induction or strengthening of such beliefs sometimes accompanies the process, but not always. The common factor that unites these therapeutically valuable experiences is profound changes to the sense of self. These changes enable subjects to access new perspectives on themselves and their lives, new ways of seeing themselves and experiencing their worlds.

Before getting underway, however, there is an obvious question to be addressed: why accept premises one and two of the Comforting Delusion Objection? That is, why accept that naturalism is true, and that the epistemic status of psychedelic transformation is important? Why not simply accept the claim, which seems plausible to many psychedelic subjects and researchers, that the cosmic consciousness is real—that mystical states of consciousness reveal genuine truths about the metaphysical nature of reality? Or why not follow others in holding that that the epistemic status of psychedelic experience is relatively unimportant?

Taking these questions in reverse order, I cannot hope to *demonstrate* that we should care about epistemic status in our evaluation of treatment and enhancement modalities. The most I can do, without delving into foundational debates on value theory, is to gesture at the sorts of considerations that I find persuasive, and hope that others share my intuitions to some extent. There is a famous thought experiment that aims to demonstrate the importance of epistemic factors in paths to well-being. This is Robert Nozick's (1974) Experience Machine. The hypothetical Machine provides users with a lifelong stream of virtual reality experiences as pleasurable and varied as one can wish for. Moreover, one can remain ignorant of the virtual status of these experiences, so that one's life in the Machine is subjectively indistinguishable from a maximally rich and excellent life in the real world. Should one plug in?

A common intuition, which Nozick invites us to share, is that plugging in would be a mistake: despite its hedonic excellence, there is something inferior about life in the Machine. An obvious candidate, of course, is that life in the Machine is not *real*: it is merely a subjectively satisfying hallucination. The thought experiment is meant to show that the hedonic quality of our experiences is not all that we value, or ought to: it also matters that our experiences are real, and that we engage in genuine relationships with an actual external world and real, autonomous others. Truth, knowledge, and reality are important in their own right. Indeed, Nozick, writing in the early 1970s, explicitly relates the Machine to the ongoing debate about 'psychoactive drugs'—by which I believe he means psychedelics, specifically:

> ... plugging into an experience machine limits us to a man-made reality, to a world no deeper or more important than that which people can construct. There is no *actual* contact with any deeper reality, though the experience of it can be simulated. Many persons desire to leave themselves open to such contact and to a plumbing of deeper significance. This clarifies the intensity of the conflict over psychoactive drugs, which some view as mere local experience machines, and others view as avenues to a deeper reality; what some view as equivalent to surrender to the experience machine, others view as following one of the reasons *not* to surrender!
>
> **(Nozick 1974, p. 49; emphasis original).**

This sums up a long-running tension between two distinct conceptions of psychedelics, as epistemically detrimental agents of hallucination ('mere local experience machines') and as agents of knowledge, insight, and spirituality ('avenues to a deeper reality'). We will return to this tension momentarily. My position is this: I agree with Nozick that it *matters* whether psychedelics are mere local experience machines or avenues to a deeper reality. Ultimately, I will argue that each of these conceptions has some of the truth, but the latter has enough of it to carry the day. However, the question must be posed.

The intuition that epistemic factors matter can be pumped further. One way is to consider hypothetical treatments that caricature the apparent features of psychedelic therapy that underlie the Comforting Delusion Objection. Imagine, for instance, a pill that causes immediate, dramatic, and lasting reductions in symptoms of anxiety, depression, and addiction, as well as positive personality change in healthy subjects. However, this pill also has the ineliminable side effect of inducing a deep and unshakeable conviction in conspiracy theories about the Illuminati, or flat-earthism, or any epistemically poor belief you care to name. Should we really simply *disregard* the distinctively epistemic harms of this treatment in our overall evaluation of its costs and benefits? In my view, we should not. My point is not that we could never be justified in recommending or prescribing such a treatment. We might conclude, on balance, that its benefits outweigh its costs. My point is simply that we should do the calculation, and factor its epistemic costs and benefits into our overall deliberations, rather than simply deeming its epistemic profile unimportant and unworthy of consideration.

What, then, of the first premise of the Objection? This is not the place to mount a full exposition and defence of philosophical naturalism. Much ink has been spilled on that project, which requires at least a book of its own. However, I will indicate briefly how I understand 'naturalism' in the present context, and some of the main reasons why I find it more plausible than alternative views. I invite any readers who are unpersuaded to treat this book as a conditional exercise in seeing how much sense can be made of psychedelic phenomena within naturalistic constraints. I suggest that the answer is: a surprising amount. We can do justice not only to the body of scientific evidence, but also to much of what seems important to psychedelic subjects—including the epistemic and spiritual dimensions of psychedelic experience—without invoking non-naturalistic posits. My contention that the Comforting Delusion Objection fails is unaffected even if *all* the premises of the Objection turn out to be false. I am simply taking a relatively untrodden path to the conclusion that the Objection fails: trying to reconcile psychedelic therapy with (a) a naturalistic outlook and (b) a concern for epistemic responsibility, or intellectual honesty (cf. Metzinger 2013a).

2.6 Naturalising the Entheogenic Conception

'Naturalism' is a notoriously ambiguous term in contemporary philosophy. Many philosophers describe themselves as naturalists, but there is considerable disagreement about the core commitments of the doctrine (Horst 2009). All versions have in common some kind of endorsement of the natural sciences as an especially effective means of acquiring knowledge of the world, and some kind of disavowal of supernatural entities or forces—which of course raises the question of what counts as 'natural' or 'supernatural', and on what principled criteria a theory or view could be deemed non-naturalistic.

We can start with the common distinction between metaphysical and methodological naturalism. Methodological naturalists believe that philosophy is, or ought to be, continuous with the natural sciences, and they reject the idea of a 'first philosophy' that could support an a priori critique of scientific method. Adherents of this view criticise armchair reasoning and pure conceptual analysis, insisting that philosophical conclusions must be not only consistent with, but based upon and integrated with, the best-supported theories in the sciences. The overwhelming success of natural science in describing the detailed structure of the external world, easily taken for granted but evidenced by the stunning technological and medical achievements of the past few centuries, suggests that scientific methods are getting something very right about how to investigate reality—and a key aspect of scientific method is the attempt to subordinate a priori intuitions to the evidence of observation and experiment. Methodological naturalists recommend that we take this epistemological lesson seriously and treat the deliverances of the sciences as our starting point and best guide to what the world is really like. One way to cash this out is to view philosophy as a limiting case of theorising, perhaps a type of 'metatheory' at one end of a continuum of abstraction, with observation and experiment at the other (Audi 2000, Forrest 2000).

Metaphysical naturalism, on the other hand, also known as 'ontological' or 'philosophical' naturalism, is not a claim about how we should do philosophy but a claim about what exists. This is where the rejection of non-natural or supernatural entities comes in. As I have said, it is difficult to make this rejection both precise and principled. But one common form that metaphysical naturalism takes in the philosophy of mind is adherence to some species of materialism or physicalism: the claim that paradigmatically mental phenomena such as thought, perception, and consciousness are wholly material or physical in character (Horst 2009). Of course, this raises the question of what it is to be 'material' or 'physical', which hardly seems easier than what it is to be natural (cf. Hempel 1980).

Fortunately, we do not need precise definitions of these terms to give a suitable working characterisation of naturalism. According to Steven Horst, the broad view that travels by this name in current philosophy of mind is that 'all mental phenomena are to be accommodated within the framework of nature as it is understood by the natural sciences' (2009, p. 225). Further, according to Horst, naturalistic philosophical accounts of the mind do not '(a) [allow] the existence of paradigmatically non-natural *entities* such as God, angels or Cartesian souls or non-natural *properties*, or (b) [treat] the world of nature as understood within the sciences as non-fundamental' (Horst 2009, p. 225; emphasis original).

This is the type of view that I have in mind when I speak of a *naturalistic* account of psychedelic transformation. It is condition (b) that makes this view incompatible with mystical metaphysical views such as the pantheistic idealism of Shanon's ayahuasca subjects.[6] An adherent of idealism or related views can allow that the natural sciences describe the manifest world accurately, but nonetheless maintain that the world of nature as understood *within the sciences* is non-fundamental. Science describes and treats various entities, properties, and forces—such as quarks, electrons, gravity, and galaxies—as merely physical, in the sense of lacking mental properties. But idealists claim that such things are, in some sense, ultimately or essentially mental. The view that I will assume also includes the premise that phenomenal consciousness specifically—the famous 'what-it-is-likeness' of subjective experience (Nagel 1974)—is an evolved, natural, intracranial phenomenon (Revonsuo 2006). Conscious

---

[6] Of course, a pantheistic cosmic consciousness of the kind that Shanon's subjects describe probably runs afoul of condition (a) too; it is hard to imagine a more paradigmatically non-natural entity.

experiences are simply identical, in some sense, to states or processes occurring entirely within the brain (Smart 1959, Bechtel and McCauley 1999)—even if the relevant states or processes are better characterised in functional than chemical or physiological terms (Putnam 1967).

Since the metaphysical content of my view is that conscious experiences are in some sense brain processes of some kind, why use the label 'naturalism' rather than terms such as 'physicalism' and 'materialism', which refer more specifically to metaphysical theses about the mind? One reason is that I want to situate my account of psychedelic transformation in the context of the broader *naturalising* programme in recent philosophy. For the past few decades, philosophers have been examining various phenomena that initially seem like poor fits for a naturalistic worldview, such as morality (Sturgeon 2006), free will (Dennett 1984), and mental representation or 'intentionality' (Dretske 1995). The project is to develop thoroughly naturalistic theories of these phenomena. The aim is thereby to show that certain familiar or important features of our lives and the world do not require us to believe in anything non-natural or supernatural, but are ultimately unmysterious parts of the one closed causal system described by the natural sciences.

This is the project that I am attempting in relation to psychedelics. The history of psychedelic research has seen many different conceptions of these substances, involving different beliefs about their essential nature, their most significant effects, and so forth. In particular, there has been a long-running tension between an Entheogenic Conception of psychedelics as agents of knowledge, insight, and spirituality—typically packaged with non-naturalistic metaphysical claims—and a *psychotomimetic* (or 'hallucinogenic') conception, bound up with naturalism and a scientific approach, that views psychedelics primarily as agents of cognitive distortion and hallucination: in short, as epistemically harmful by definition (Langlitz 2013). My project here is to *naturalise* the Entheogenic Conception: to show that a conception of psychedelics as agents of knowledge, insight, and spirituality is, despite first appearances, perfectly compatible with a naturalistic worldview and a scientific outlook.

This is intended as a contribution to the 'progressive initiative to demystify the psychedelic experience' being pursued explicitly by some researchers in the area (Carhart-Harris et al. 2018a, p. 549). It can also be seen, philosophically, in terms of the clash between Wilfrid Sellars' (1963) 'manifest' and 'scientific' images of humankind: our reflective everyday conception of ourselves and the world, and the worldview disclosed by the sciences, respectively. The Entheogenic Conception, as I have described it, is part of the *manifest image* of psychedelic transformation: it is part of the reflective but pre-scientific picture of this phenomenon endorsed and expressed by many who are familiar with it. I will try to show that it need not conflict, and can indeed be integrated, with the scientific image of this phenomenon. So in my attempt to answer the Comforting Delusion Objection, I will be developing an account of psychedelics as agents of knowledge gain and spiritual experience in a wholly naturalistic world. In so doing, I aim to provide a conceptual framework for thinking about psychedelics' putative epistemic and spiritual benefits that can interface with scientific research on these topics and that does not depend on a metaphysical commitment to anything non-natural or supernatural.

I am also using the term 'naturalism' to signal the methodological orientation, not just the metaphysical constraints, of my project. Here I am following the kind of methodological naturalism mentioned earlier, which sees philosophy as continuous with the natural sciences. On one version of this approach, philosophy has three key functions:

> (1) Philosophy's most basic task is to reflect upon, and integrate, the results of investigations in the particular sciences to form a coherent overall view of the universe and our place in it.
>
> (2) Philosophy is concerned with certain problems in particular sciences, for example, in physics, biology, psychology, and mathematics. These problems arise in the most speculative and conceptually difficult parts of the sciences.
>
> (3) Some sciences, or areas of sciences, are traditionally done in philosophy, in some cases, but certainly not all, because they are not mature enough to go out on their own: epistemology, logic, morals, politics and aesthetics.
>
> **(Devitt and Sterelny 1999, pp. 275–276).**

All of these are relevant to my purposes. What I am attempting is, to my knowledge, a novel project: a *natural philosophy* of psychedelics (cf. Thagard 2019), by which I mean an overarching, big-picture synthesis that integrates findings from various scientific disciplines in order to answer quintessentially philosophical questions about psychedelics. These questions, involving such concepts as *self*, *knowledge*, and *spirituality*, are either not addressed explicitly or not (yet) answerable fully by empirical investigations. This kind of synthetic exercise (Schliesser 2019) in natural philosophy, similar in spirit to the movement known as 'neurophilosophy' (Churchland 1989), has been pursued fruitfully in relation to the emotions (Prinz 2004), self-awareness (Metzinger 2003), morality (Churchland 2011), and clinical delusions (Gerrans 2014), to name just a few. Psychedelic experience is an obvious subject for such an inquiry, given the Big Questions that it raises and the complex nature of the research, which spans disciplines and levels of scale and explanation.

There remains the question: Why metaphysical naturalism about the mind? Why prefer the view that conscious experiences are brain processes to mystical idealism? One answer comes by way of methodological naturalism. Natural science has proven itself over the past few centuries to be our most reliable way of finding out about reality, and our current best science of consciousness, cognitive neuroscience, overwhelmingly endorses the claim that consciousness is a phenomenon that occurs solely within the brain. Cognitive neuroscience is based on the 'heuristic identity theory', the assumption that mind and brain are in some sense identical, and the remarkable and rapid success of this research programme constitutes a prima facie vindication of this foundational postulate (Bechtel and McCauley 1999).

Moreover, there are positive discoveries within cognitive neuroscience that support more directly an identification of consciousness with brain activity. All the instances of phenomenal experience in which we have compelling reason to believe (from introspection, others' verbal reports, or behavioural and physiological analogies) are intimately correlated with specific types of brain activity. Phenomena such as phantom limbs and dreaming suggest that brain activity is sufficient for consciousness: the usual external triggers of certain experiences are not required for experiences to occur. And cases of deafferented limbs and cortical lesions suggest that brain activity is necessary for consciousness: even if all the right extracranial events occur, the relevant signals must be processed in the brain for experience to eventuate (Revonsuo 2006).

Not only are conscious experiences intimately correlated with specific intracranial processes that seem to be both necessary and sufficient for them: they are also intimately correlated with specific cognitive functions that evolved to enable the adaptive success of the organism. This is most simply explained by the assumption that consciousness either contributes something itself to adaptive success, or is an unavoidable concomitant of cognitive adaptations. Consciousness is a 'biological data format' (Metzinger 2009, p. 8).

Nonetheless, non-physicalist views are making a comeback in philosophy. More and more thinkers are turning to such views as idealism, panpsychism, and variants thereof (e.g., Shani 2015, Albahari 2019a, Goff 2019). One of the key motivations is the perceived inability of physicalism to solve the Hard Problem of Consciousness. It cannot be denied that consciousness, as experienced from the inside, and brain activity, as viewed from the outside, seem about as different as two things could possibly be. Explaining how the former could possibly 'emerge from', or be identical with, the latter is rightly viewed as one of the great intellectual challenges of our age. The perceived failure of physicalism to provide anything approaching a plausible solution leads some to conclude that the problem is insoluble and so consciousness must not emerge from, or be identical to, complex brain activity: it must somehow be fundamental and ubiquitous in the universe, as idealists and panpsychists claim.

I think that this inference is premature. Unlike some naturalists (e.g., Dennett 1991, Churchland 1996, Seth 2016, Carruthers and Schier 2017) I think that the Hard Problem is very real, very Hard, and very much unsolved. But this does not mean that it can never be solved within physicalist constraints. The modern sciences of mind and brain are young: scientific psychology little more than a century old, cognitive science about 60 years, cognitive neuroscience about 40. Perhaps the conceptual breakthrough or revolution that will allow us to comprehend how the trick is done is decades or centuries away. Less than a century ago, vitalists were still maintaining that organic life could never be explained in chemical terms—a prediction that now looks short-sighted (Dennett 1991). As Thomas Nagel (1974) has pointed out, we may have good reason to believe that physicalism is true even if we cannot yet understand how it *could* be true. This is roughly the position that I think we are in. The fact that nobody can yet imagine what kind of conceptual revolution could solve the Hard Problem is no conclusive reason for pessimism: such is simply the nature of conceptual revolutions.

Importantly, even if the Hard Problem is never solved, the falsity of physicalism does not follow. In the philosophy of mind, *Mysterianism* is the position that human beings are too cognitively limited to solve the mind–body problem. We are very smart, but not infinitely so—and consciousness, according to Mysterians, is where we meet our limit (McGinn 1989). What the possibility of Mysterianism shows is this: even strong pessimism about the prospects for an intellectually satisfying resolution of the Hard Problem does not constitute strong grounds for rejecting physicalism in favour of non-physicalist views (cf. Prinz 2003). Such pessimism is an epistemological stance with no direct consequences for metaphysics (Cummins et al. 2014).

In my view, we have sufficient grounds to tentatively accept physicalism about the mind, and the Hard Problem is not reason enough to reject it. Of course, a very common view in psychedelic circles is that the nature of psychedelic experience, mystical or otherwise, *is* reason enough. These experiences render many who undergo them incredulous that consciousness could be 'mere' neural information processing. But undermining this inference is one of the central burdens of this book. I intend to show that a naturalistic view of the mind has ample resources to explain the many strange and striking phenomena encountered in psychedelic experience—including those that most readily evoke non-naturalistic interpretations.

The task of a natural philosophy of psychedelic therapy is to answer the question *Are psychedelic experiences an existential medicine, metaphysical hallucinations, both, or neither?* on the basis of an interdisciplinary synthesis integrating our best current evidence and theory concerning these experiences and their causes and consequences. In the spirit of such a natural philosophy, let us begin with close attention to the phenomena: in this case, the psychedelic experience itself.

3
The phenomenology
of psychedelic therapy

The colossal egotism of anyone who thinks he can write an LSD report! It
can't be done, not with all the languages in the world!
Jane Dunlap, *Exploring Inner Space: Personal Experiences under LSD-25.*

3.1 Introduction

The most basic implication of psychedelic research is that there is far more in the
human mind than is dreamt of in much of our philosophy (Sjöstedt-H 2015).
Psychedelic experiences, by many accounts, can be among the most remarkable and
meaningful available to human beings (Huxley 1954, Shanon 2002, Griffiths et al.
2006, Yaden et al. 2017). Unfortunately, there are two major obstacles to describing
such experiences. The first is that the effects of psychedelics are far more variable
than those of other drugs, being strongly influenced by 'set and setting': the psychological state of the person taking the drug and the environment in which they take
it (Johnson et al. 2008, Studerus et al. 2012, Haijen et al. 2018). The second reason is
that psychedelic experiences are commonly held to be ineffable: many subjects say the
state is unlike anything in their prior experience and words cannot do it justice.

Nonetheless, there are certain themes that occur frequently in both quantitative
and qualitative studies of psychedelic phenomenology. In this chapter, I will survey
some of the most common alterations of consciousness reported by subjects who
take moderate-to-high doses of psychedelics in structured, controlled settings such
as clinical trials or religious rituals. I make no attempt at an exhaustive or systematic
survey. First, I describe various typical features of the experience relatively briefly, before focusing in more detail on patients' experiences of the therapeutic process: their
impressions of how the experience benefited them psychologically. Of course, subjective impressions of transformative mechanisms may be mistaken, but they provide intriguing prima facie evidence, especially when there is considerable unanimity.
In any case, they form part of the *explanandum*: subjects' verbal narratives require
explanation as much as any behavioral or clinical change. I focus here on attempts
in recent qualitative studies to probe subjects' impressions of the therapeutic process
directly (reviewed by Breeksema et al. 2020). The findings of these studies will play an

important evidential role in Chapter 4, where we consider multiple theories of how psychedelic therapy works.

As I have noted, the topic of this book is the type of transformative process that often occurs when psychedelics are administered in structured clinical or religious settings. Therefore, I largely neglect some of the more exotic effects that may result from different dosages and routes of administration, or in different contexts. For instance, high-dose intravenous or smoked N,N-dimethyltryptamine (DMT) is reputed to have a distinctive phenomenology (Strassman 2001, Tramacchi 2006) but may be less therapeutically useful because of its brevity and overwhelming intensity.[1]

I will use direct quotation liberally, for the obvious reason that those who have undergone psychedelic experiences are best qualified to describe them. It bears emphasising that detailed narrative accounts come closest to conveying a real sense of what psychedelic experience is like. Anyone interested in a detailed appreciation of psychedelic phenomenology should consult the classic sources such as Huxley (1954), Dunlap (1961), Watts (1962), Masters and Houston (1966), Cohen (1970), Grof (1975), Strassman (2001), Shanon (2002), and Pollan (2018), as well as online repositories such as Erowid (www.erowid.org), which contain many thousands of experience reports by users of legal and illegal drugs.

3.2 Perception

Unusual perceptual experiences, especially in the visual modality, are the most famous effect of psychedelics; think of the colourful, swirling, tie-dye psychedelic aesthetic of the 1960s. Visual effects can be grouped loosely into three categories: intensification, alteration, and novelty. Subjects often report a general intensification of their visual experience: colours appear brighter and more vivid; lines, edges, and depths clearer and sharper than usual. Aldous Huxley describes the intensification of colour in his famous account of mescaline experience: 'Mescalin [*sic*] raises all colours to a higher power and makes the percipient aware of innumerable fine shades of difference, to which, at ordinary times, he is completely blind' (Huxley 1954, p. 27). Often attention to visual detail is described as being greatly enhanced. Looking at a simple natural object such as a leaf, or a mundane artificial object such as a pair of trousers, a subject may marvel at hitherto unnoticed features and patterns, registering all manner of fine detail and gestalt structure that ordinarily would be completely overlooked:

> . . . the depth of light and structure in a bursting bud go on forever. There is time to see them, time for the whole intricacy of veins and capillaries to develop in consciousness, time to see down and down into the shape of greenness, which is not green at all, but a whole spectrum generalising itself as green—purple, gold, the

---

[1] Although some recent evidence hints at therapeutic utility for the at least equally brief and intense experiences occasioned by smoked 5-MeO-DMT (Davis et al. 2019, Uthaug et al. 2019, 2020).

sunlit turquoise of the ocean, the intense luminescence of the emerald. I cannot decide where shape ends and color begins. The bud has opened and the fresh leaves fan out and curve back with a gesture which is unmistakably communicative but does not say anything except, 'Thus!' And somehow that is quite satisfactory, even startlingly clear.

(Watts 1962, p. 27).

Mention of gestalt structure brings us to the borderline between intensification and alteration. Pareidolia—the perception of patterns in ambiguous stimuli—is common: subjects may experience the phenomenon of seeing faces in clouds, for instance, in a much more vivid and realistic fashion than usual. I call this 'alteration' because real aspects of the external environment are being perceived, but the perception is not merely more intense than usual: its contents are qualitatively different. Other types of alteration include seeing stationary objects as morphing or moving, as in the common experience of 'walls breathing', and seeing objects overlain with simple or complex geometric patterns (perhaps a borderline case between alteration and novelty). One fascinating species of alteration occurs when subjects see other people, or their own reflections, in various guises: for instance, they may see the supervising therapist, or themselves, in the visual guise of mythical or archetypal figures, or with features emphasised and altered to present the appearance of belonging to a particular culture or time period (Masters and Houston 1996, Shanon 2002).

The most common type of visual novelty, or stimulus-independent imagery, consists of 'closed-eye visuals', which often take the form of elementary or complex geometric patterns, usually coloured and dynamic, seen with the eyes closed:

I soon discovered in my visual field the emergence of an exquisitely beautiful, multidimensional network of intricate, neon-like geometric patterns, drawing my attention ever more deeply within. I could see this display with open eyes, but found that when I closed my eyes it was even more vivid and sharply focused. I recognised life within the undulating designs and began to feel as though I somehow could enter into the energy flowing within them. Soon, I felt immersed in incredibly detailed imagery best described as Islamic architecture and Arabic script, about which I knew nothing.

(Richards 2015, p. xix).

Sometimes completely novel percepts are seen with the eyes open, integrated with the rest of the environment. This is a peyote subject describing a fireball that he saw in the room during the onset of the drug effects:

It drifted, swaying a little from side to side, while moving toward me ... when the ball of fire had come close enough I poked at its centre with my finger. It then exploded, a lavish shower of multicoloured sparks cascading and dropping on the rug at my feet.

(Masters and Houston 1966, pp. 7–8).

This fireball and its behaviour were part of the subject's visual experience, but had no obvious basis in the actual objects and events of his physical environment.

The following report exemplifies many typical changes to visual perception:

> I lay on my stomach and closed my eyes and brilliantly colored geometrical patterns of fantastic beauty collided, exploded, raced by. Other things too: teeth and pearls and precious stones and lips and eyes. Outside of the window the branches of the tree were gigantic arms with transparent muscles, now threatening, now embracing. Glasses started rolling on the table, the bookcase was full of swimming books, the door bulged like a balloon, the carpet in the other room was full of thousands of little green snakes. The dial on the telephone was a huge pearl-studded wheel. The shapes and colors of objects got more and more intense, the outlines etched with luminous clarity and depth. Anything with a polished metal surface turned into gleaming gold or silver ... The faces of other people became clear and beautiful and open. At one point all faces were colored green.
>
> **(Pahnke and Richards 1966, pp. 185–186).**

More elaborate stimulus-independent imagery is also common. With the eyes closed, subjects may see remarkable things: vivid and intense visions of ancient civilisations or alien landscapes, animals, deities, and natural scenes:

> I became the joyous white Pegasus accompanied by my beloved stallion. Together we galloped through the exquisite golden light of space while celestial music of inexpressible beauty seemed to make the rhythm of the universe, of its melody and of our movements one. We crossed one and then another and another of the millions of Milky Ways which fill infinity.
>
> **(Dunlap 1961, p. 76.)**

> When the [ayahuasca] had its effect, I found myself presented with pure enchantment. The forest was full of animals—both natural and phantasmagoric; notably there were dragons, felines, and big birds. The dominant colours were green and blue. I was sitting viewing the forest as if it were a stage. It was as if a screen were raised and another world made its appearance. At moments, however, it seemed to me that even though I was sitting here on the bench, my own self was over there in the forest and I was dancing with the various creatures in it. It was all blissful, and very real. And I saw it all with open eyes.
>
> With the second cup I was offered, the scene changed. What now presented itself to me was an enchanted city, a city of gold and precious stones. It was of indescribable beauty. And again, so very real.
>
> **(Shanon 2002, pp. 6–7).**

Sometimes subjects behold, and may become participatively immersed in, visionary sequences presenting parables or metaphors for specific situations in their own life or general themes in human life:

> I opened my eyes and there was a picture over the mantle
>   ... There seemed to be in front of this picture many veils hanging and I pushed each veil aside one by one, knowing that as I got the last veil aside I would finally see God ... Finally the last veil was to be removed. I knew it was the last veil and tried to prepare myself for the great experience of seeing God. I raised my hand over my head and then leaned backwards to make myself more receptive in order to feel the full force of God. And finally the last veil was pulled aside and there were my three children crying for their father ... Before me was going all the selfish feelings—all the selfish attitudes that I had had throughout my entire married life.
>
> **(Pahnke and Richards 1966, p. 187).**

The phenomenon of parable illustrates the artificiality of analysing psychedelic experience into a list of ostensibly distinct phenomenological components. Visual parables and metaphors constitute an alteration to perceptual experience, but also an experience of apparent *insight* (a phenomenon we will return to shortly): they engender novel understanding or comprehension, or at least feelings thereof. Indeed, the blurring of boundaries between normally distinct experiential modalities is a general and distinctive feature of the psychedelic state. The most obvious example is synaesthetic-like interactions between sensory modalities, to which I return shortly. But the vivid perceptual representation of abstract concepts and psychodynamic insights, as in the preceding quotation, could also be seen as a quasi-synaesthetic phenomenon.

While visual effects are most common, auditory perception can also be a significant locus of unusual experience. Intensification is common: subjects report that they appreciate music more intensely than usual, apprehending details and patterns to which they would normally be oblivious, and responding emotionally to the music very strongly:

> The various pieces of music were wonderful, because they were multi-dimensional. I could hear tiny variations and subtle changes and shadings in the voices and instruments, as if I were inside the mind of the composer as HE heard it. There was the sense of the composer touching the divine and channeling its perfection down to the human level, so that other people could be aware of it and uplifted, too, but simultaneous awareness of the impossibility of the task, as imperfect human beings, imperfect instruments, and imperfect voices are involved. Somehow all of that imperfection was also woven into the perfection the music was channeling. I was inside the music, the composer, the players, the singers, the shaft of the woodwind, the metal keys of the woodwinds, and the finger pressing the keys.
>
> **(Richards 2015, pp. 66–67).**

Music plays a key role in structured psychedelic sessions: it is an important part of traditional psychedelic rituals and of modern clinical trials (see O'Callaghan et al. 2020 for a review). In many trials, subjects are asked to lie on a comfortable couch, wear eyeshades to block external distraction, and listen through headphones to a selection of music intended to enhance the experience and mirror its natural dynamics. The standard instruction is to 'let go', listen to the music, and open to inner experience. Subjects have stronger emotional responses to music while on psychedelics (Kaelen et al. 2015) and most report that the music played a central role in their experience (Kaelen et al. 2018). Moreover, subjects' self-reported emotional response to the music correlates with the degree of both mystical-type and insightful experiences (Kaelen et al. 2018).

This emphasis on the importance of music may seem in tension with the idea that psychedelics sometimes induce 'introvertive' mystical experiences of pure being or consciousness, in which all perceptual experience is absent.[2] However, the apparent tension dissolves when we note that psychedelic experiences have distinct temporal phases. A typical psilocybin experience, for example, might last for 4–6 hours. It would be possible for a subject to enjoy a period of apparently pure or contentless awareness during this time, while the 'ascent to' and 'descent from' this peak of the experience involved intense perceptions of music, visual imagery, emotional and insightful experiences, and gradual alterations to the sense of self.

In the auditory modality, the line between intensification and alteration blurs. One psilocybin subject, for example, described hearing his own breathing as though it were the sound of a waterfall (Malitz et al. 1960, p. 10). Straightforward novelty is fairly common too. The peyote subject quoted earlier heard music that was being played by characters in a vision he observed (Masters and Houston 1966, p. 9). Hearing 'celestial music' or 'music of the spheres' is sometimes reported on ayahuasca (Shanon 2002, p. 153). Auditory verbal hallucinations, or hearing voices, can also occur at high doses (Masters and Houston 1966).

Synaesthetic-like interactions between sensory modalities are commonly reported. However, it is questionable whether these constitute genuine synaesthesia: some studies suggest that they fail to meet established criteria (Luke and Terhune 2013, Terhune et al. 2016). Auditory-visual interactions are especially common, with subjects reporting that their closed-eye visual imagery changes in time with the rhythm of the music, and that its content is significantly affected by the emotional tone of the music and the associations evoked (Kaelen et al. 2018):

Music had become something much greater and more profound than mere sound. Freely trespassing the borders of the other senses, it was palpable enough to touch, forming three-dimensional spaces I could move through ... the music formed a vertical architecture of wooden timbers, horizontals and verticals and diagonals

---

[2] I am grateful to Miri Albahari for pointing out this apparent tension.

that were being magically craned into place, forming levels that rose one on top of the other, ever higher into the sky like a multistoried tree house under construction … So it went, song by song, for hours.

(Pollan 2018, pp. 247–248).

Tactile, gustatory, and olfactory perception are perhaps less notable sites of perceptual changes than vision and audition, but dramatic intensification in these modalities is very common:

Sensations were acute. I heard, saw, felt, smelled and tasted more fully than ever before (or since). A peanut butter sandwich was a delicacy not even a god could deserve … To touch a fabric with one's fingertip was … to experience intense touch-pleasure.

(Masters and Houston 1966, p. 10).

Reports of perceptual distortion or novelty in these three modalities are relatively rare. Intensification and apparent enhancement seem to be the main effects of psychedelics on touch, taste, and smell (Cohen 1970, p. 49).

Changes to spatial and temporal experience are common in the psychedelic state. We can group these, loosely, with 'perceptual changes'. Changes to spatial perception, in particular, often play out in the visual modality. Perceptions of distances can be greatly distorted: objects may seem closer or farther away than they really are, and relative proportions of objects may be altered. Sometimes subjects feel as though their own body has expanded or diminished, resulting in Alice in Wonderland-type experiences:

S-1, a twenty-six-year-old male … ingested about 80 micrograms of LSD. He … reported that he felt himself to be six inches in height. Curiously, the objects in the room underwent a similar and proportionate transformation, while the guide and another observer retained their normal dimensions, appearing to him to be giants. Although an inch taller than the guide, S tilted his head back to look up at her, stating that he felt as David must have felt looking up at Goliath. He also compared himself to Alice after she had taken a drink from the bottle. At one point S was given a box filled with many miniature Japanese figures. He greeted these with expressions of delight announcing that they were more his own size. Then he clutched the figures to him as if they might help to protect him from the onslaughts of the giants.

(Masters and Houston 1966, pp. 70–71).

Alan Watts went so far as to single out time dilation and ego dissolution as the two definitive effects of psychedelics: 'there are certain types of change which are usual enough to be considered characteristic of psychedelics: the sense of slowed or arrested time, and the alteration of "ego boundary"' (Watts 1964). An example of time dilation is provided by the British MP Christopher Mayhew, who took mescaline on live television:

> At regular intervals, about twice every five minutes at the peak of the experience, I would become unaware of my surroundings, and enjoy... a state of complete bliss, for a period of time which, for me, did not end at all... I would be aware of a pervasive, bright, pure light, like a kind of invisible sun snow. For several days afterward I remembered the afternoon not as so many hours spent in my drawing room interrupted by these kinds of excursions, but as countless years of complete bliss interrupted by short spells in my drawing room. But to the film team, and to Dr Osmond [the supervising psychiatrist], the excursions lasted no time at all.
>
> **(quoted in Durr 1970, p. 54).**

Another subject describes an experience of extreme time dilation:

> Time. Each second separated by infinity. The Camera has stopped, and the world is caught in a silly snapshot pose. To see it so is enough to make one burst into laughter...
>
> **(Cohen 1970, p. 124).**

Although time may seem to move more quickly or more slowly than normal, the latter is much more common. The peyote subject quoted earlier described feeling as though he had been smoking a cigarette for hours, then looking down to see that the first ash was still on it, implying that he had been smoking it for less than a minute (Masters and Houston 1966, p. 9). As with many phenomenological features, the experiences of time dilation and spatial alteration reach their apex in the 'transcendence of time and space' that is definitive of the mystical state.

3.3 The sense of self

Despite the salience of perceptual changes, the popular conception of psychedelic experience as primarily perceptual, associated with the term 'hallucinogen', is an oversimplification at best. Perceptual effects may predominate at low doses, but at moderate-to-high therapeutic or transformative doses, many of the more salient effects involve changes to emotion, thinking (including feelings of creativity and insightfulness, altered perspectives, and religious or philosophical ideations), attention, salience, meaningfulness, and the quality of consciousness itself (Shanon 2002).[3]

---

[3] This may seem in tension with my insistence on the importance of music in the previous section, but again this tension is merely apparent. My point is this: Often, what subjects emphasise most is not perceptual changes in and of themselves as purely aesthetic phenomena. Rather, they tend to emphasise profound emotional, existential, and noetic changes. In such accounts, perceptual experiences such as listening to music or visual imagery assume importance insofar as they act as a vehicle for experiences of this kind.

Of course, as we have noted, these other changes are often deeply intertwined with perceptual alterations. Some of these other changes figure centrally in patients' retrospective accounts of psychedelic therapy, which I will examine in the next section. First, however, let us consider that quintessential, philosophically provocative effect of psychedelics: alterations in the sense of self.

Here is a fairly representative example from a 22-year-old psychology student who volunteered for an LSD study in the 1960s, out of curiosity about the drug's famous *visual* effects:

> The strangest thing happened on the way to me this day. I met myself and found that I'm really not me after all. Or perhaps I should say that I have found out what it is like to exist. For that's all there was left that instant ... when feeling, thinking, being, all were caught up into one ebbing unity; a unity which was me, but not me, too. A me-not me which stood there nakedly and pointed back at itself in a sorrowful joy, and asked 'Why?' ... But then the 'why' didn't matter and it just *was* ... Have you ever felt like all that existed was you, and that suddenly the reason for your 'you-ness' was knocked out from underneath you? ... from now on I'm going to feel a little different about the kind of language we use to describe psychotics and their 'little worlds'. I'm going to look a little closer at what the mystics are trying to tell us; at what the philosophers have to say about this ... I think others feel the same way, with or without the damned drug, and I think maybe they've struggled with what to do with it all and what to make out of it all ... The world looked to me like it must to a little child, all big and beautiful. And I was experiencing it without the imposed controls that we have to slap on the world in order to become adults ... I was, literally, experiencing the world as a child would ... I was almost drunk with rapture and I felt like bursting ... I notice the physical boundaries of my body coming back and the same thing is happening to my mind. But does it have to be this way? Do we have to live alone?
>
> **(Cohen 1970, pp. 18–19).**

For this subject, as for many others, the importance of perceptual changes (at least in a narrowly aesthetic sense) was eclipsed by dramatic, existentially significant changes to the sense of self, as well as to thinking, attention, and emotion.

The psychedelic-induced experience of an absent or diminished sense of self has gone by many names. In the recent literature, it is usually called 'ego dissolution' (Nour et al. 2016). Ego dissolution is standardly understood to be a central component of the mystical-type experience, a corollary of the sense of profound unity that is definitive of this state:

Thus, although perceptual and emotional/existential/noetic changes are intertwined, the importance of the former often derives greatly from their intertwinement with the latter.

Although consciousness of self seemed extinguished, I knew that the boundaries of my being now had been dissolved and that all other boundaries also were dissolving. All, including what had been myself, was an ever more rapid molecular whirling that then became something else, a pure and seething energy that was the whole of Being. This energy, neither hot nor cold, was experienced as a white and radiant fire. There seemed no direction to this whirling, only an acceleration of speed, yet one knew that along this dynamic continuum the flux of Being streamed inexorably, unswervingly toward the One.

At what I can only call the 'core' of this flux was God, and I cannot explain how it was that I, who seemed to have no identity at all, yet experienced myself as *filled with God*, and then as (whatever this may mean) *passing through God* and into a Oneness wherein it seemed God, Being, and a mysterious unnameable One constituted together what I can only designate the ALL. What 'I' experienced in this ALL so far transcends my powers of description that to speak, as I must, of an ineffably rapturous Sweetness is an approximation not less feeble than if I were to describe a candle and so hope to capture with my words all of the blazing glory of the sun.

(Masters and Houston 1966, p. 308).

There were profound feelings of unity, first with a red tulip, and then with a rose of the same color. When looking at the rose as an object, it seemed to come alive before my eyes. Its petals seemed to breathe as, slowly and gracefully, they unfolded, seeming to express the ultimate in beauty. Fascinated, I watched these movements of cosmic gentleness until, suddenly, I *knew* the rose; that is to say, I somehow became One with the rose, no longer existing as an ego passively viewing an object in its environment. Although in the objectivity of my critical mind I knew there were no physical changes in the flower, subjectively I seemed to see it in a totally new perspective, one which elicited tears and deep feelings of reverence. The rose seemed to stand out in naked beauty, as though it were the only thing existing in the world. Supporting the ancient monistic school of thought, I expressed the philosophical insight that 'we are all the same thing'. Once I sought to express my experience by speaking of 'becoming one with the very essence of Roseness.' Another time I commented that, 'There is more to beauty than we know.'

(Richards 2015, pp. 65–66).

There are two points worth making here. The first is that 'ego dissolution' and 'mystical experience' are not synonymous. There are many types of psychedelic alterations to the sense of self, some of which involve no sense of unity or religious/spiritual content. Benny Shanon describes some varieties of altered self-experience under ayahuasca:

The first phenomenon is a dissociation between the self and the mental material that one experiences. Content is passing through my mind, but I am not experiencing myself as being the source that generates it. Instead of being the generator of the thoughts that I am entertaining, I feel that I am a channel that receives them. The source of the mental material may or may not be given a particular identity . . .

The second phenomenon has to do with control. Experientially, the feeling is that one is no longer in full control of the thoughts one entertains. Rather, one feels that other people or agents are controlling one's thoughts.

(2002, pp. 198–199).

In the parlance of recent philosophical psychopathology, Shanon is describing a loss of the *sense of agency* over thoughts (Graham and Stephens 1994, Gallagher 2000).

The second point is that ego dissolution is not always welcomed as pleasant or desirable. Even when the experience is ultimately positively valenced overall, the loss of the sense of self may be preceded or accompanied by fear (Griffiths et al. 2011). And if the subject is unprepared or attempts to resist the experience, it can become a dysphoric 'bad trip'. Indeed, one of the most commonly used psychometric scales in psychedelic research has three main factors, one tracking perceptual changes ('Visionary Restructuralisation'), another tracking positively valenced ego dissolution, including unitive and mystical experiences ('Oceanic Boundlessness'), and another tracking negatively valenced, stereotypically psychotic ego dissolution ('Anxious Ego Dissolution'; Dittrich 1998). Here is an example of the latter:

I had an excited feeling in the pit of my stomach ... However, soon I had the feeling of being choked from inside. I had difficulty breathing. Then I began to feel nauseated and restless. I said to the psychologist, 'I don't feel good at all.' Suddenly the tightness in my throat increased and I began to feel as if my body were on fire both inside and outside. My neck and back felt very tense. I became very frightened and had the feeling of acute panic. I was being swirled and sucked down, down, down, into oblivion ... I fearfully cried out, 'How long will this last? Will this go on all the time? I don't like this. I want out!' The fear was overwhelming me as I was thrust down into blackness. My body was burning up and I began to sweat ...

The indescribable feeling of being swirled and thrust into some place else was easing somewhat. It seemed that I had been in this torment for weeks. After it had eased up, I knew beyond a doubt that I was in another world. I felt it was no use telling the psychologist about it because he wouldn't understand. I remember thinking, 'This is what the psychotic feels like.' That feeling of panic and terror had left me tremulous and weak.

(Cohen 1970, p. 99).

One of the most philosophically controversial issues is whether there can be conscious states, induced by psychedelics or otherwise, that completely lack any sense of self (Millière 2017, Millière et al. 2018, Henriksen and Parnas 2019, Millière and Metzinger 2020, Letheby 2020, Millière 2020, Sebastián 2020, Fink 2020). Most experience reports are somewhat ambiguous on this point. However, some reports seem to describe a total loss of self-consciousness. These often come from users of the short-acting psychedelic 5-MeO-DMT (Millière et al. 2018). The following example from Pollan also exemplifies the dysphoric variety of ego dissolution:

I felt a tremendous rush of energy fill my head ... Terror seized me—and then, like one of those flimsy wooden houses erected on Bikini Atoll to be blown up in the nuclear tests, 'I' was no more, blasted to a confetti cloud by an explosive force. I could no longer locate [myself] in my head, because it had exploded that too, expanding to become all that there was. Whatever this was, it was not a hallucination. A hallucination implies a reality and a point of reference and an entity to have it. None of those things remained.

(Pollan 2018, pp. 276–277).

A happier account is provided by a research subject administered intravenous DMT:

I immediately saw a bright yellow-white light directly in front of me ... I was consumed by it and became part of it. There were no distinctions—no figures or lines, shadows or outlines. There was no body or anything inside or outside. I was devoid of self, of thought, of time, of space, of a sense of separateness or ego, or of anything but the white light. There are no symbols in my language that can begin to describe that sense of pure being, oneness, and ecstasy. There was a great sense of stillness and ecstasy.

(Strassman 2001, pp. 244–245.)

Taken at face value, such reports seem to demonstrate clearly that there can, indeed, be 'totally selfless' states of consciousness (Millière 2020)—that is, phenomenally conscious mental states that completely lack any sense of self. However, the interpretation of such reports is controversial. I will return to these issues in Chapter 7.

Another important point is that ego dissolution is not a monolithic affair, because self-consciousness is not monolithic. On a broad level, recent theoretical discussions recognise a distinction between 'narrative' and 'minimal' forms of self-awareness (Gallagher 2000, Lou et al. 2017). Narrative self-awareness refers to the autobiographical sense of being a temporally extended entity with a specific history and personality, whereas minimal self-awareness refers to the bare feeling of being a subject of experience at a moment in time. On some accounts, minimal self-awareness arises from basic sensorimotor processes, particularly *interoceptive* processes that represent the internal condition of the body (Damasio 1999, Seth 2013).

Early clinical accounts of psychedelic states recognised this distinction, distinguishing the loss of 'bodily ego feeling' from the loss of 'mental ego feeling' under LSD (Savage 1955). More recently, Girn and Christoff (2018) have offered a more fine-grained (but non-exhaustive) taxonomy of aspects of self-consciousness affected by psychedelics. They include (i) the sense of ownership over the body and thoughts (feeling that *this is my body* or *this is my thought*), (ii) the sense of agency over actions and thoughts (feeling like the one who has initiated or authored the action or thought), (iii) the sense of self-location (the feeling of 'being located at a particular point in space'), (iv) the minimal self (the bare feeling of being a subject of experience),

(v) autobiographical or narrative self-awareness, (vi) body image and body representation, and (vii) the sense of bodily boundaries (Girn and Christoff 2018p. 133; cf. Millière 2020).

Psychedelics can affect all of these aspects of self-consciousness. Indeed, so can meditative practices such as 'mindfulness' or *Vipassana*, drawn from the Buddhist tradition. One traditional aim of this practice is to radically alter the sense of self (Goleman 1972, Albahari 2014). As such, changes to self-awareness are the most obvious point of phenomenological overlap between psychedelic experiences and meditative states (Millière et al. 2018). But it is less often appreciated that meditation practice, especially under intensive retreat conditions, can induce many other stereotypically psychedelic changes to consciousness. Indeed, Jack Kornfield's (1979) phenomenological study of intensive Vipassana meditation reads like a compendium of psychedelic phenomena. Here are the categories of unusual experiences reported by Kornfield's informants:

CATEGORIES OF UNUSUAL EXPERIENCES REPORTED
Somatic experiences
1. Spontaneous movement
2. Alterations in body image
3. 'Energy' flow experiences
4. Other proprioceptive changes such as temperature, weight, etc.
5. Unusual breathing patterns
6. Unusual experiences during walking
7. Changes in perception of pain
Visual experiences
8. Eyes open
9. Eyes closed
10. Auditory experiences
11. Gustatory and olfactory experiences
Mental experiences
12. Strong emotions and mood swings
13. Rapture and bliss
14. Psychological insights
15. Equanimity
16. Insights into basic mental and physical life processes
17. Dream changes
18. Time changes
19. Concentration changes
20. Effortless awareness
21. 'Out-of-the-body experiences'
22. Other general perception changes including creativity and psychic phenomena

(Kornfield 1979, pp. 44–45).

Some examples include feeling one's body divided in half or one's torso expanding; feeling one's body 'heavily pulled in all directions', or feeling as though floating when one was really 'stone still'; experiencing one's body growing 'huge, then tiny, tiny'; seeing 'still objects moving', 'colours more intense', 'hallucinations while walking', and 'LSD melting-like visions'; and seeing 'camera-like flashes of light', '[visions] of Buddha', and 'images of body cells [and] organs' (Kornfield 1979, pp. 46–47). In addition to such 'unusual' experiences, practitioners also routinely reported:

> visual thoughts, dream-like images, mental pictures—moving and still—and patterns of colours and visions, from simple subjects to complex visual mandalas. Also, it is commonly reported that certain visual themes appear regularly in meditators' minds, such as visions of Buddha or Christ or various religious imagery, or for some, visions of bodies and corpses and death. For others, spontaneous visions of violence or of lustful scenes and other vivid visual material is often reported as associated with strong emotional discharges.
>
> **(Kornfield 1979, p. 47).**

Clearly, none of these phenomena would be out of place in a psychedelic experience report. As Kornfield emphasises, to speak of a 'meditative state' is, strictly speaking, a misnomer: meditation amounts to a body of practices or techniques, which can induce many different states of consciousness. However, there is an undeniable overlap between these states and those that psychedelics typically induce in controlled conditions.

Returning now to psychedelics' effects on self-consciousness: in this book, for the sake of simplicity, I will operate mainly with a coarse-grained distinction between minimal self and narrative self. By the former, I mean synchronic aspects of self-consciousness that do not involve any autobiographical information: most notably, the sense of being an experiencing subject at a point in time, an entity who *owns* or *undergoes* occurrent perceptual, bodily, and affective experiences. This is sometimes referred to as the 'mineness' of experience (Guillot 2017). By the latter, I mean diachronic aspects of self-consciousness that involve autobiographical information: the sense of being a specific individual who was present in past experience and who may be present in future experience, who has a distinctive personality and trajectory through life. Simplifying, we could think of the minimal self as the immediate pre-reflective feeling of subjectivity, and the narrative self as a richer self-*conception*. Note that I am using the terms 'minimal self' and 'narrative self' in purely phenomenological senses, to refer to experiences *as of* having or being a self. I remain neutral for now on the ontological question as to whether any selves or subjects actually exist. (I will also use the terms 'self-consciousness' and 'self-awareness' interchangeably—again, in a purely phenomenological sense).

Users of psychedelics often report altered bodily experience, including the dissolution of bodily boundaries and feelings of disembodiment. One cancer patient administered psilocybin reported: 'I didn't have a body ... I was just like this soul, this entity' (Belser et al. 2017, p. 368). Another patient in the same study said: 'my consciousness, or my soul, or whatever, was flying out of my body' (Belser et al. 2017, p. 368). This might seem to suggest that the experience of 'ego dissolution' is primarily a disruption to the minimal or embodied self (Millière 2017).

However, some subjects distinguish, without prompting, between the narrative self and the minimal self, and describe a specific, liberating type of experience in which the former is absent while the latter remains:

> Two related feelings were present. One was a tremendous freedom to experience, to be I. It became very important to distinguish between 'I' and 'Me,' the latter being an object defined by patterns and structures and responsibilities—*all of which had vanished*—and the former being the subject experiencing and feeling. My normal life seemed to be all Me, all demands and responsibilities, a rushing burden which destroyed the pleasure and freedom of being 'I'. Later in the evening the question of how to fit back into my normal life without becoming a slave of its patterns and demands became paramount.
>
> **(Durr 1970, p. 79; my emphasis).**

A separate report, by a different subject:

> Although I *lost all sense of 'me-ness'*, the sense of 'I-ness' was intensified unbelievably … It was simply a sense of 'is-ness' or 'am-ness'. *I wasn't anything—I simply was*. And at these moments of really ecstatic clarity there was such a peace and rest and at the same time such exuberance and wildest joy.
>
> **(Durr 1970, p. 80; my emphasis).**

Taken at face value, these reports describe experiences in which the narrative self is lost completely, while the minimal self remains. Experiences of this kind are sometimes reported, and described as therapeutically beneficial, by patients in clinical trials. It seems that the temporary absence of the ordinary autobiographical self-concept allows subjects to appreciate its contingency and mutability—to see that they can reframe their self-image in a seemingly open-ended way. We turn now to these reports.

3.4 The transformative process

Recent qualitative research has examined patient perceptions of the process of psychedelic therapy, investigating which factors are most salient and which are felt to be therapeutically relevant. The results are interesting. In some respects, these studies seem to confirm suspicions that the acquisition of non-naturalistic metaphysical beliefs is crucial to the process. However, they ultimately reveal a more nuanced picture.

3.4.1 Non-naturalistic themes

In a recent study, 13 cancer patients were interviewed about their experiences of psilocybin-assisted therapy, and every single one described 'gaining transpersonal insights into the nature of the universe or existence' (Belser et al. 2017, p. 18) during their psilocybin experience. Seven patients mentioned experiencing 'guiding spirits', that often took the form of loved ones, helping them through the experience. Further, seven patients described 'directly experiencing a state of being or … a realm that was felt to exist at the time of or after death', leading to feelings of 'relief and comfort' (Swift et al. 2017, p. 498). Patients who received psilocybin-assisted therapy for alcoholism also described mystical-type experiences, in some cases of 'connection with God' or 'being in the presence of God' (Nielson et al. 2018, p. 7).

On the other hand, we do not know what epistemic attitudes subjects took towards these visions: no published research to date has rigorously examined psychedelic effects on metaphysical beliefs in clinical populations. It is possible that some of these subjects adopted similar attitudes to Benny Shanon, who takes a skeptical stance toward the remarkable phenomena he personally experienced in over 130 ayahuasca sessions. Attempting to reconcile these powerful subjective impressions with his academic training in philosophy and psychology, Shanon professes agnosticism about the ontological status of his visionary and mystical experiences, respecting and appreciating their wondrous and meaningful qualities in a poetic and pragmatic spirit, without uncritically accepting their literal reality (Shanon 2010, p. 270). Perhaps some of these subjects do likewise.

Furthermore, the phrase 'transpersonal insights' is ambiguous, and need not denote *non-naturalistic* metaphysical epiphanies. The unitive insight that 'all is one' or 'everything is interconnected' could reasonably be described as 'transpersonal', but is arguably consistent with naturalism, bearing on its own no necessary connection to pantheistic idealism or a universal consciousness (Angel 2002, Simpson 2014). The Buddhist doctrine of radical interdependence, with its anti-substantialist metaphysics (at least on some readings; Thakchoe 2019), has parallels in naturalistic metaphysical programmes such as 'ontic structural realism' (Ainsworth 2010) and forms of process philosophy (Seibt 2020), which hold, roughly, that relations or processes, rather than substantial entities, are the fundamental stuff of reality. There are potential 'transpersonal' insights consistent with naturalism in this vicinity (cf. Watts 1964). Moreover, many patients emphasise the ineffability of the 'wisdom lessons' they received, which makes identifying specific metaphysical belief changes problematic.

3.4.2 Psychological insight

Notably, in these and other studies, several less metaphysically loaded themes are often mentioned by patients. For instance, every single patient interviewed by Belser et al. described 'remarkable insights or transformations involving a significant personal relationship' (2017, p. 361). Patients describe 'seeing their loved ones in a new way', leading to a sense of understanding, acceptance, and, in some cases, forgiveness. One patient reported:

> Bit by bit, my daughters were turning into these radiant beings, cleansed of all these fears. It was incredibly emotional, because it was something I have, as their father, long known, but it's a very great pain when you see your children being victimised by fears... to see these beautiful beings not realising their essence.
>
> **(Belser et al. 2017, p. 363).**

Clearly there is a strong emotional component to these experiences. However, gaining new perspectives and understanding of loved ones and relationships can usefully be grouped under the heading of *psychological insight*, which is one of the strongest themes to emerge from recent research on psychedelic therapy (Garcia-Romeu et al. 2019, 2020, Davis et al. 2020). Psychological insight can take many forms, but invariably involves some sense of gaining a new perspective: some sense of realisation, understanding, or clarity—whether it concerns one's life, personality, and values, other people, or important relationships.

The patients interviewed by Belser et al. reported lasting changes to their sense of identity following their psilocybin sessions. Some described realisations concerning their values, needs, and priorities:

> [The psilocybin experience] has made me more aware that... I cannot just live for material stuff and success... I have to satisfy my emotional side as well, which now I am trying to slowly, slowly do. I am trying to do things and live experiences that would make me happy internally. I am not stopping... following my goals, but I realised that being so intense about getting what I want does not have a point...
>
> **(Swift et al. 2017, p. 506; a different paper, reporting on the same cohort of patients).**

In some cases, psychological insight involves a vivid reliving of autobiographical memories, sometimes traumatic, leading to an empowering sense of understanding the causes of psychological problems and grasping possible solutions.

In studies of both alcohol and tobacco addiction, patients reported that the experience of ego dissolution enabled them to revise their self-conception beneficially:

> There was a part there where I felt gone ... it wasn't like [the last psilocybin session] where I always remembered I was Adam. There was a part there where I was gone ... I would come back and you know, I remember telling myself you took this [the psilocybin] to try and help. And it is helping... There's the old Adam, then the new Adam without alcohol.
>
> **(Nielson et al. 2018, p. 8).**

> For a few seconds, it was just like 'I'm me, and there are no defining characteristics!' ... that made me realise that I'm not a 'smoker'.
>
> **(Noorani et al. 2018, p. 759).**

A different patient from the same cohort:

> It felt like I'd died as a smoker and was resurrected as a nonsmoker. Because it's my perception of myself, and that's how I felt. So I jumped up and I said 'I'm not a smoker anymore, it's all done.'
>
> **(Noorani et al. 2018, p. 759)**

These reports clearly resonate with the descriptions we saw earlier (in section 3.3) of liberating experiences of being 'I' in the absence of 'Me'—of minimal selfhood persisting while narrative selfhood dissolves.

Patients in the study by Noorani et al. also described changes in values and priorities, and insights into the causes and consequences of their smoking behaviour. This coheres with an observational study of ayahuasca-assisted therapy for addiction in which patients described identifying 'negative thought patterns and barriers related to their addiction' (Argento et al. 2019, p. 781). Patients receiving psilocybin-assisted therapy for alcoholism reported similar insights:

> [Mark] was confronted by the harmful effects that his drinking had on himself and others. He stated that 'at one point, I felt I could have cried for joy', when realising that he was being given 'a new slate'. In the following weeks, he reported increased motivation and drive as well as a strong desire to contribute to the world in a meaningful way. He said, 'I feel like I'm maturing. Maybe a part of me died when I gave up alcohol.' ...
>
> He opted to have the third open-label [psilocybin] session ... He described the experience as 'a crash course' in dealing with feelings of disappointment, regret, shame, and unworthiness. He also reported 'a couple of eureka moments', and said that the session ended with 'calmness, comfort, and reassurance'. He said, 'I wouldn't be surprised if I never drank again' and added, 'I got exactly what I need out of the experience.' ... Two years from his initial intake, Mark contacted the study team to report that he continued to remain abstinent.
>
> **(Bogenschutz et al. 2018, p. 3).**

Terminal patients who received LSD-assisted treatment for anxiety and depression emphasised experiences of reframing or perspective-shifting during the drug session, reporting that the psychedelic state allowed them to see various situations in their life—including their illness and imminent death—in new and different ways, and to realise that the ways they had been conceptualising these situations were not necessarily the best or only perspectives available:

It was less about my illness. I was able to put it into perspective.... Not to see one-self with one's sickness as centre. There are more important things in life ... The evolution of humankind for example ... Your Inner Ego gets diminished, I believe, and you are looking at the whole ... you are indeed starting to build relations with plants or with the entire living world around. You think less about yourself, you are thinking—across borders.

(Gasser et al. 2015, p. 62).

This also falls under the broad rubric of psychological insight (Davis et al. 2020). Similarly, smokers treated with psilocybin reported that they accessed a broader perspective during their experience which made quitting addiction seem much more manageable:

... smoking just seemed like this miniscule flick of the—pshh, like that, it was nothing compared to everything that I was feeling and thinking, and it was all coming together in this holistic picture of everything, past, present and future. And smoking—whatever!—like just so pointless, it's just nothing to do with anything. Like a little pebble in your shoe—just brush it off and then you ... you know, the world is so much bigger!

(Noorani et al. 2018, p. 760).

Thus, we can see that insights into one's own identity, values, motivations, and relationships, psychological epiphanies and accessing broader perspectives, are highlighted repeatedly by patients as important parts of the process of psychedelic therapy.

3.4.3 Connectedness and acceptance

The two reports we have just examined both describe a sense of increased *connectedness*, an experience that has been highlighted repeatedly in qualitative research A shift from feelings of disconnection to feelings of connection emerged as central in a study of psilocybin therapy for treatment-resistant depression (TRD). Watts et al. (2017) interviewed twenty patients six months after they had participated in an open-label trial of psilocybin therapy for TRD. Thematic analysis of the interviews identified two themes that the vast majority of patients, without prompting, described as central to the therapeutic process: a shift from feelings of disconnection pre-treatment to feelings of greater connection post-treatment, and a shift from the avoidance of emotion to its acceptance.

Talk of connectedness invites the question: connected to what? Subjects described a newfound or regained connection to their senses, to the world around them, to themselves (including forgotten or neglected aspects of their personalities and lives), to other people, and to a 'spiritual principle' of some kind. After the treatment, one patient said: 'I would look at people on the street and think "how interesting we are"—I felt connected to them all' (Watts et al. 2017, p. 534). Another commented: 'Before I enjoyed nature, now I feel part of it. Before I was looking at it as a thing, like TV or a painting. You're part of it, there's no separation or distinction, you *are* it' (Watts et al. 2017, p. 534). Interestingly, connection to a spiritual principle was the *least* common response, being endorsed by only 9 of 20 patients, while connection to self, others, and world were each endorsed by 16 out of 20.

The theme of connectedness has been identified in several other qualitative studies. Feelings of greater connectedness to aspects of self, others, nature, and the world were reported by patients receiving psychedelic therapy for cancer-related distress (Swift et al. 2017, Malone et al. 2018, Gasser et al. 2015) and various forms of addiction (Argento et al. 2019, Bogenschutz et al. 2018, Noorani et al. 2018). During the psilocybin session, one cancer patient experienced feelings of 'being connected to everything, I mean, everything in nature . . . and it wasn't like talking about it, which makes it an idea. It was experiential' (Swift et al. 2017, p. 497). A patient who attended an ayahuasca retreat for the treatment of addiction reported:

> A week or two after [the retreat] I was just waking up every morning at like five, six in the morning and going outside and . . . I just sat and stared at the trees and the wind for like two hours, I would sit outside and it was just beautiful. I've never noticed it that much ever in my life. And after I had the ayahuasca it was just amazing, the connection with nature.
>
> (Thomas et al. 2013, p. 38).

The other main factor identified in the study of psilocybin for TRD was a shift from avoidance of emotion to its acceptance. Patients described their pre-treatment depression as characterised by the avoidance and repression of emotion. They reported that during the psilocybin session both the range and intensity of their emotional experience were vastly increased, such that they had no choice but to 'give in' or 'let go' and open up to the feelings they had been avoiding:

> The beauty and the sadness, I was terrified by the depth of emotions. [Patient 7]

> The hardest thing is to give in to what you're experiencing, it's as if you're in a car heading for the edge of the cliff, and you have to try not to turn the steering wheel. [Patient 14]

> Excursions into grief, loneliness and rage, abandonment. Once I went into the anger it went 'pouf' and evaporated. I got the lesson that you need to go into the scary basement, once you get into it, there is no scary basement to go into [anymore]. [Patient 3]
>
> (Watts et al. 2017, p. 538).

Expanded emotional range and intensified emotional experience are key features of the psychedelic state which have been described as therapeutically relevant by patients receiving psychedelic therapy for many conditions (Belser et al. 2017, Gasser et al. 2015, Bogenschutz et al. 2018, Malone et al. 2018, Noorani et al. 2018). Intense emotional experiences in the psychedelic state are often described as cathartic, or as leading to a process of acceptance and 'letting go'. Often a confrontation with, and subsequent acceptance of, difficult or painful emotions is involved. But profoundly positive emotions such as forgiveness, peace, joy, and love can feature centrally too, and often follow the acceptance of difficult or painful feelings. One cancer patient reported feeling:

> overcome with love and all the love that I have for my family and my friends. I felt that it was coming from them; also I felt that I was bathed in it. And if I were religious it definitely would have been a religious experience, I would have said bathed in God's love. And I don't think English really has a way to say this without using that word 'God', um maybe bathed in transcendent love. Bathed in universal love. It was such a strong feeling.
>
> **(Swift et al. 2017, p. 504).**

Many patients report that the expansion of their emotional range and intensification of their emotional feelings outlasts the acute experience to some extent.

Incidentally, the meditators interviewed by Kornfield were no strangers to experiences of this kind. These subjects reported experiences of 'heavy sadness', 'huge [releases] of anger', 'highs of bliss and very depressed lows', and 'doubts, bliss, pain, boredom, serenity, joy, aversion, pain, serenity'. As one put it: 'intense emotions of anger, fear, sadness, and joy—the roller coaster ride—oh, my mind' (Kornfield 1979, p. 48). Kornfield comments:

> In deeper levels of practice ... meditators often experience periods of strong fear and insecurity. These are usually resolved by surrender, by fully experiencing them, leading to a greater development of equanimity ... Some of the most important learning reported ... [takes] place in relation to such intense negative states as rage or terror.
>
> **(Kornfield 1979, p. 54).**

Opening to, and accepting, an expanded and intensified range of emotional experience is another factor common to intensive meditation practice and controlled psychedelic ingestion.

In psychedelic therapy, as in meditation, the theme of acceptance goes beyond acceptance of emotion. Participants also report transformative experiences of coming to accept themselves (Bogenschutz et al. 2018), their bodies (Malone et al. 2018), and aspects of their life, such as cancer (Swift et al. 2017). As with the phenomenological features discussed earlier in the chapter, it is worth emphasising that the analytical separation of these features is somewhat artificial and misleading. For instance, while we could treat changes to emotional experience as a conceptually distinct category, they form part and parcel of virtually every feature that patients identify as therapeutically relevant. (This is why I have not given them a separate sub-section of their own.) Illustrating the same principle, processes of acceptance can overlap strongly with the kinds of psychological insight experiences described in the preceding section (cf. Breeksema et al. 2020, p. 936):

> Lisa ... experienced an amplification of thought moving her into a confused and chaotic state. Underneath the chaotic thinking, she identified a deep well of overwhelming sadness. She was able to eventually surrender control over her thoughts and entered into a state of peacefulness, until her thoughts quieted completely. She heard her own inner voice rupturing the quiet, whispering into her ear: 'I'm going to tell you a secret. It's the worst-kept secret in the universe because everyone knows it but you. You are a perfect creation of the universe.' At that moment she felt that everything in existence was unified and was made of love, though a part of her remained reluctant to fully believe this to be true. The voice repeatedly presented her with this reality, asking 'do you believe this?' over and over until each one of her objections had been addressed and dismissed. She examined herself and found that she finally did accept this to be true, which propelled her into a state of profound self-acceptance and wellbeing. She later said, 'All there is love, this is all that you are, this is all that matters.'
>
> **(Bogenschutz et al. 2018, p. 5).**

Clearly, en route to her ultimate state of 'profound self-acceptance', Lisa was revising deep-seated negative beliefs about herself, and thereby coming to see herself differently.

So here we find significant clues that the therapeutic and transformative effects of psychedelics may not be due entirely to metaphysical visions of another Reality that puts this one in the shade. Even though many patients describe 'transpersonal' experiences of one kind or another, the exact metaphysical content and import of these experiences is not entirely clear. And subjects more commonly emphasise psychological insights, intense emotional experiences, and profound feelings of connectedness and acceptance. This suggests several hypotheses about possible therapeutic mechanisms.

The authors of one qualitative study concluded:

> The participants ... experienced acute and lasting alterations in their perceptions of self, in the quality of their baseline consciousness, and in their relationship with alcohol and drinking. In these cases, experiences of catharsis, forgiveness, self-compassion, and love were *at least as salient as classic mystical content* ... feelings

of increased 'spaciousness' or mindfulness, and increased control over choices and behaviour were reported following the drug administration sessions.

(Bogenschutz et al. 2018, p. 1; my emphasis).

Just before this book went to press, Breeksema et al. published a systematic review of qualitative studies of psychedelic therapy. These authors identified five themes that participants often nominate as therapeutically important: '(1) insights; (2) altered self-perception; (3) feelings of connectedness; (4) transcendental experiences; and (5) expanded emotional spectrum' (Breeksema et al. 2020, p. 936). Their review was not limited to studies of classic psychedelics, but also included studies of other drugs such as ketamine and 3,4-methylenedioxymethamphetamine (MDMA, or 'Ecstasy'). However, there is obvious convergence between their findings and the themes I have emphasised here.

3.5 Conclusion

Psychedelics can cause dramatic changes to perception, emotion, thinking, the experience of reality, and the sense of self. When we ask which changes seem therapeutically important to patients, recent qualitative research paints a nuanced picture. Interviews with successfully treated patients find some mention of non-naturalistic metaphysics and classically religious content. But more commonly emphasised are: (i) intense *emotional experiences*, sometimes felt to be cathartic, that patients believed durably expand their emotional repertoires, allowing a shift from avoidance to acceptance; (ii) *psychological insight* leading to new perspectives and self-perceptions, sometimes facilitated by dissolution of the narrative self; and (iii) experiences of increased *connectedness* to self, body, others, and world.

Of course, patients' impressions of the therapeutic process may be inaccurate. We can be fairly confident that they indeed had the kinds of experiences they describe. But it is another question whether they are correct that these experiences were causally responsible for the lasting psychological benefits. These patients, like most psychedelic clinicians, ascribe those benefits to the psychedelic *experience* itself—the altered state of consciousness induced by the drug. But some theorists have entertained the possibility that psychedelic therapy works by a *non*-experiential, low-level molecular mechanism. On this view, the remarkable phenomenology that we have been examining is actually therapeutically epiphenomenal (Heifets and Malenka 2019)—an 'irrelevant side effect' (Goodwin 2016, p.1201).

In order to reach a verdict on the success or failure of the Comforting Delusion Objection, we need to examine the mechanisms of psychedelic therapy in light of a broader range of evidence. We begin this task in Chapter 4.

4
The mechanisms of psychedelic therapy

The unique promise of psychedelic drugs in psychotherapy—and their dangers if misused—lies in their potency in reliably engendering radically altered states of consciousness...

William A. Richards, 'Mystical and archetypal experiences of terminal patients in DPT[1]-assisted psychotherapy'.

4.1 Introduction

The Comforting Delusion Objection to psychedelic therapy stems from an empirical assumption: that this treatment works by inducing beneficial non-naturalistic beliefs in a Joyous Cosmology. We can call this the Metaphysical Belief Theory (MBT) of psychedelic therapy. The related, but distinct, Metaphysical Alief[2] Theory (MAT), which I outline below, ascribes lasting benefits to the psychedelic-induced *vision* of a Joyous Cosmology—that is, to the metaphysical hallucination itself and to memories of it, irrespective of whether the subject believes it is veridical. Despite their differences, both theories hold that psychedelics' therapeutic effects depend on the *non-naturalistic metaphysical content* of the mystical experience.

These theories also share an even more basic assumption: that the psychedelic experience itself is causally involved in producing beneficial outcomes. This is not uncontroversial. On some views, psychedelic therapy is a pure pharmacotherapy that operates via a low-level molecular mechanism. The remarkable consciousness alterations would then be inconvenient 'psychotomimetic' side effects—epiphenomenal, from a therapeutic standpoint. We can call this the Molecular Neuroplasticity Theory of psychedelic therapy.

In this chapter, I subject these three theories to critical scrutiny. I begin, in section 4.2, by considering evidence for and against the Molecular Neuroplasticity Theory. Psychedelics have been shown to stimulate the molecular mechanisms of neuroplasticity directly in cultured mammalian neurons (Ly et al. 2018), and this effect may contribute to their therapeutic benefits. But a Pure Nneuroplasticity Theory struggles to account for the correlation between mystical-type experience and beneficial outcomes. It is unclear why this correlation should exist if the causal mechanism were experience-independent. The conclusion is inescapable: the central causal

---

[1] Dipropyltryptamine.
[2] This term is defined in section 4.3 below.

factors are cognitive and phenomenological. It is the psychedelic experience itself, and the underlying changes to neurally realised information processing, that do the heavy lifting. In philosophical terms, psychedelic therapy is a 'personal-level' process, which ineliminably involves meaningful conscious experiences (Letheby 2015).

This raises the question: which specific cognitive and phenomenological factors are involved? An obvious candidate is the non-naturalistic metaphysical ideations highlighted by the MBT and MAT. I consider these theories in sections 4.3 and 4.4, respectively. Here, the qualitative evidence surveyed in Chapter 3 plays an important role. It shows that many patients successfully treated by psychedelic therapy do not emphasise non-naturalistic metaphysics in their retrospective accounts. The MBT and the MAT both struggle to account for this fact. My argument here is simple: if these patients had undergone vivid metaphysical hallucinations of a spirit realm or divine Reality, then they would be talking about those hallucinations, whether or not they believed them to be veridical. They are not talking about such hallucinations; therefore, they did not undergo them.

However, this conclusion creates a puzzle. Given the correlation between mystical-type experience and beneficial outcomes, how can there be patients who were successfully treated by psychedelics but did not have a metaphysical hallucination of cosmic consciousness? My answer is that the construct of 'mystical-type experience', as operationalised by standard psychometric instruments, is not equivalent to 'non-naturalistic metaphysical-type experience'. There are experiences that satisfy psychometric criteria for a 'complete' mystical-type experience but do not involve any non-naturalistic metaphysical ideations. Some mystical-type experiences, in the psychometric sense, are not non-naturalistic metaphysical hallucinations: the psychometric instruments cast a broad net. This has implications for the interpretation of studies employing these instruments. It also undermines the intuitive idea that psychedelic therapy is all about transformative metaphysical visions of a Joyous Cosmology.

The ultimate conclusion of this chapter is twofold: psychedelics' lasting psychological benefits (a) do *not* depend on their capacity to induce such metaphysical visions, but (b) *do* depend on some aspect of the psychedelic experience—some aspect, moreover, that correlates fairly reliably with psychometric ratings of mystical-type experience. In Chapter 5, I argue that the relevant factor is the disruption and subsequent revision of mental representations of the self. Changes to the sense of self are the hallmark of mystical-type experience that is common to transcendent visions of cosmic consciousness and more naturalistic experiences of ego dissolution, psychological insight, and connectedness.

4.2 Neuroplasticity theories

When we ask how psychedelic therapy works, a natural place to look is the direct pharmacological action of LSD, psilocin[3], and so forth. After all, this is ostensibly a drug therapy, so it makes sense to seek a pharmacological mechanism. Moreover, attractive candidates exist. It has long been theorised that psychedelics may stimulate the molecular mechanisms of neuroplasticity—the brain's ability to alter its structure and function. In this section, I consider the hypothesis that this is the central mechanism underlying psychedelics' therapeutic potential. Several pieces of evidence, mostly from animal models, support this hypothesis. In humans, Almeida et al. (2019) found that a single dose of ayahuasca increased levels of brain-derived neurotrophic factor (BDNF), a protein involved in neuroplasticity whose expression is reduced in depressed patients, and that this increase correlated with antidepressant effects. But this does not rule out the possibility that the increase in BDNF expression was an effect, rather than a cause, of the observed psychological changes.

More to the point, Ly et al. (2018) reported that classic psychedelics promote the growth of dendritic spines and increase the density of dendritic arbours in cultured mammalian neurons. Clearly, there are pathways whereby psychedelics stimulate neuroplasticity independently of any of their specific, variable effects on cognition and consciousness. (I will assume that this finding generalises to humans, although to my knowledge this has not been established). This *neuroplasticity hypothesis* coheres with the fact that other drugs used to treat some of the same conditions as psychedelics, such as selective serotonin reuptake inhibitor (SSRI) antidepressants, stimulate the molecular mechanisms of neuroplasticity via multiple pathways, and this is thought to be relevant to their therapeutic effects (Rantamäki and Yalcin 2016).

Vollenweider and Kometer (2010) note that there are two ways of interpreting the neuroplasticity theory of psychedelic therapy. One way is to see it as a modern, 'implementation-level' version of the traditional view that psychedelics cause psychological change by inducing transformative peak or mystical experiences. According to this *Implementational* Neuroplasticity Theory, the psychedelic experience itself is the catalyst for neuroplastic changes—just as non-drug-induced experiences can catalyse such changes—and the various molecular events, such as increased synthesis of BDNF and activation of its target TrkB receptor, simply *implement* or realise the very same processes that have traditionally been described in 'higher-level' (psychological) vocabulary as 'insight', 'learning', 'personal growth', and so forth. This complementarity approach fits with the remarks of Bogenschutz and Pommy (2012, p. 551) that psychological models may be 'at least as useful' as lower-level (i.e., biological) models in explaining psychedelic therapy.

---

[3] The biologically active dephosphorylated metabolite of psilocybin (Passie et al. 2002).

On the other hand, it is possible to formulate a non-implementational version of the neuroplasticity theory that genuinely conflicts with traditional psychological accounts. On this *Pure* Neuroplasticity Theory, psychedelic therapy operates via an experience-independent mechanism. Psychedelics cause multiple effects in the human brain downstream from their agonist actions at various neurotransmitter receptors. On this view, one group of effects includes transient and variable alterations to conscious experience, realised by brain-wide changes to information processing in neural networks—the psychedelic experience itself. Another, *distinct* group of effects includes promotion of neuroplasticity at the molecular level—the effects observed by Ly et al. These two categories of effects are in principle separable and, on this hypothesis, it is the latter that mediates clinical benefits—perhaps by enhancing the efficacy of psychotherapy standardly delivered before and after psychedelic sessions, or simply by re-opening a 'critical period' of plasticity in which it is easier to change entrenched, deleterious patterns of thought and behaviour.

This is the sort of view that underlies the search for molecular variants of classic psychedelics capable of delivering their therapeutic benefits without the inconvenient 'psychotomimetic side effects' (Yang et al. 2015, Anderson 2012, DARPA 2019). If this view is correct, then there is no important connection between psychedelics' ability to alleviate psychiatric distress and their ability to induce the kinds of experiences that we surveyed in Chapter 3: their mysticogenic and visionary properties are unrelated to their therapeutic potential. This possibility has been suggested by some commentators on recent clinical trials (e.g., Goodwin 2016).

The problem is that this pure version of the Molecular Neuroplasticity Theory seems straightforwardly empirically inadequate. If psychedelics' therapeutic effects depend on an experience-independent process of plasticity catalysed at the molecular level, then those therapeutic effects should be independent of specific experiential variables (except insofar as the latter correlate strictly with dosage). It should be the dose of the drug, or perhaps some other low-level neurobiological factor, that predicts how well a patient responds to psychedelic therapy—not the specific set of 'psychotomimetic side effects' that a given administration happens to induce.

But the most robust predictor of responses to psychedelic therapy is not dosage, or any other such factor: it is ratings of mystical-type experience. Across multiple studies and multiple conditions, what predicts good clinical outcomes is the extent to which a patient has a complete mystical-type experience, as defined by psychometric scales. Positively valenced experiences of ego dissolution are associated with lasting benefits, whereas emotionally challenging, unpleasant, or merely non-mystical experiences are associated with fewer benefits. Such findings are readily explicable if the mechanism is experiential, but quite mysterious if we suppose that the real mechanistic action is happening at the cellular and molecular level, independent of the specific contents of the altered state of consciousness (ASC).

From one perspective, this is unsurprising. After all, neuroplasticity is simply the brain's capacity to change its structure and function, for better or worse. Why suppose that merely enhancing neuroplasticity should reliably have a beneficial, rather than a neutral or detrimental, effect? Rantamäki and Yalcin (2016) make this point in relation to evolving theories of the therapeutic mechanisms of SSRIs. Discussing the limitations of a pure neuroplasticity theory of SSRIs' clinical effects, they write:

> It is important to note that the behavioural outcome of increased BDNF signaling critically depends on specific brain area and neurocircuit ... BDNF-TrkB signaling importantly regulates synaptic plasticity and connectivity in many, if not most, neuronal networks but *the network function itself and plasticity within the network determines the ultimate outcome*. Therefore, direct activation of essentially all TrkB receptors (i.e., using TrkB specific agonists) within the brain may not be therapeutically rational ...
>
> **(Rantamäki and Yalcin 2016, p. 286; my emphasis).**

In other words, whether increased neuroplasticity leads to a beneficial outcome or not will depend on the specific neural networks in which plasticity is enhanced, and the specific information that those networks process—i.e., how the window of plasticity is used to 're-wire' the networks. We will return to this point in Chapter 6.

Rantamäki and Yalcin relate this point to the striking finding that SSRI administration plus physical rehabilitation completely reverses developmental amblyopia ('lazy eye syndrome') in rats—an outcome produced by neither treatment alone. It also relates to the finding that SSRI administration plus psychotherapy often outperforms either treatment alone (Craighead and Dunlop 2014, Cuijpers et al. 2020), and to the fact that SSRIs do not just enhance neuroplasticity but also induce therapeutically relevant changes to emotional processing via their effects on serotonergic neurotransmission (Harmer and Cowen 2013). When SSRIs alone do have a therapeutic effect, this may result from a combination of (a) their pro-plasticity effects and (b) specific content-related factors, such as the changes to emotional processing biases and/or the presence of a supportive social environment (cf. Gerrans and Scherer 2013).

None of this is to suggest that psychedelics' apparent experience-independent effects on neuroplasticity are totally irrelevant to their therapeutic benefits. It is possible that these effects contribute to the short-term 'afterglow' that seems sometimes to follow even unpleasant or dysphoric experiences (Hofmann 1980, Majić et al. 2015). And when truly lasting benefits do result, it seems plausible that pro-plasticity effects at the molecular level make a causal contribution, as they surely must with SSRIs. However, while such effects may contribute, the dose-independent correlation between mystical-type experience and beneficial outcomes shows that they are not sufficient for lasting change. To identify the missing factor, we need to look to the content of the psychedelic experience itself.

4.3 The Metaphysical Belief Theory

The robust correlation between mystical experience and clinical outcomes suggests that it is these sorts of experiences, specifically, that cause lasting reductions in symptoms of anxiety, depression, and addiction, as well as positive personality change in healthy volunteers. On this view, psychedelics don't heal or transform people: mystical experiences do. Controlled psychedelic administration is just one (quite powerful and reliable) way to induce a transformative mystical experience (Richards 2008).

This hypothesis receives further support from the observation that there are non-pharmacologically-induced ASCs, such as near-death experiences, some meditative states, and spontaneously occurring mystical experiences, that (a) are widely reputed to have lasting psychological benefits, sometimes profoundly transforming personality and behaviour at a single stroke—the so-called 'quantum change' phenomenon (Miller 2004)—and (b) share overlapping phenomenological features and, in some cases, neural correlates with the psychedelic state (Millière et al. 2018, Timmermann et al. 2018; see Letheby 2015 for discussion). To take just one example, in Chapter 3, we saw considerable phenomenological overlap between psychedelic experience and mindfulness meditation, and mindfulness-based interventions, like psychedelic therapy, have shown promise in the treatment of anxiety, depression, and addiction (Goldberg et al. 2018). It seems likely that the pharmacological action of psychedelics is first and foremost a catalyst for beneficial *psychological* processes.

If this is correct, then how exactly do mystical experiences produce lasting psychological benefits across such a wide range of conditions? A simple and appealing answer runs as follows: a mystical experience, by definition, constitutes an overwhelmingly vivid and realistic, apparently direct apprehension of the ultimate metaphysical nature of reality (noetic quality), in which this nature, while strictly ineffable, is experienced as being profoundly unified (internal and external unity), worthy of reverence (sense of sacredness) and such as to evoke an extremely joyful response (deeply felt positive mood). In short, a mystical experience is a totally compelling, apparently direct experience of the truth of a Joyous Cosmology–as Huxley put it, 'insight into the nature of things accompanied by the realization that, in spite of pain and tragedy, the universe is all right, in other words that God is Love' (Huxley 1969, quoted in Gill 1981, p. 606). The experience is so vivid and realistic that its contents cannot but be believed, and those contents are so reassuring and comforting on a deep, existential level that such a belief cannot but have profound, far-reaching psychological benefits.

Of course, coming to believe in a Joyous Cosmology on the basis of mere rational arguments or intellectual considerations will rarely have such dramatic effects. However, the suggestion here is that when such a belief is backed by the authority of utterly intense, apparently direct experience, its psychological impact can be enormous. According to this *Metaphysical Belief Theory* (MBT), psychedelics cause lasting benefits by (a) inducing mystical experiences as of a Joyous Cosmology, which in turn (b) induce strong *beliefs* in a Joyous Cosmology, and the latter do the bulk of the therapeutic work. This, of course, is the core empirical assumption underlying the Comforting Delusion Objection.

The MBT is intuitive, and it is not new. Willis Harman attributes the lasting psychological benefits of supervised LSD sessions to drug-facilitated mystical insights at odds with 'the belief-and-value system implicit in our 'scientific' culture', and claims specifically that belief in the objective accuracy of these insights is necessary for therapeutic outcomes: 'it is only when the subject does take [the mystical experience] to be valid that there result any significant changes in his personality or behavior patterns' (Harman 1963). He cites results from a study, then in progress, in which the degree of self-reported psychological benefits from a single LSD session correlated with increased assent to such statements as these:

'I believe that I exist not only in the familiar world of space and time, but also in a realm having a timeless, eternal quality.'

'Behind the apparent multiplicity of things in the world of science and common sense there is a single reality in which all things are united.'

'It is quite possible for people to communicate telepathically, without any use of sight or hearing, since deep down our minds are all connected.'

'Of course the real self exists on after the death of the body.'

'When one turns his attention inward, he discovers a world of 'inner space' which is as vast and as real as the external, physical world.'

'Man is, in essence, eternal and infinite.'

'Somehow, I feel I have always existed and always will.'

'Although this may sound absurd, I have the feeling that somehow I have participated in the creation of everything around me.'

'I feel that the mountains and the Sea and the stars are all part of me, and my soul is in touch with the souls of all creatures.'

'Each of us potentially has access to vast realms of knowledge through his own mind, including secrets of the universe known so far only to a very few.'

(Harman 1963).

I have not been able to determine whether this study was ever completed, or its results published. However, such findings would constitute prima facie support for the MBT, as do the results of another study in which 'increased awareness of an Ultimate Reality' correlated with self-reported benefits from a single LSD session (Savage et al. 1964).

A *pure* metaphysical belief theory would maintain that metaphysical beliefs consequent on psychedelic mystical experience are the sole causal factor mediating therapeutic outcomes. Perhaps very few people have ever held this view: most would allow at least some role for non-experiential, pharmacological factors, or psychological processes other than metaphysical belief change. But the idea that metaphysical belief change is the central therapeutic mechanism has obvious appeal, especially when considering the treatment of existential distress in terminal illness. One terminal patient said of his psilocybin experience: 'I am convinced beyond any doubt that there is a spiritual realm ... The spirit guide showed me a world that I believe to be very, very real' (Malone et al. 2018, p. 3). Perhaps psychedelics alleviate the anxiety and depression of cancer patients by giving them a conviction in 'the world's fundamental All Rightness, in spite of pain, death and bereavement' based on 'the direct total awareness, from the inside, so to say, of Love as the primary and fundamental cosmic fact' (Huxley 1965, quoted in Beauchamp 1990, p. 60). Perhaps the patients who respond to the treatment are precisely those who become convinced by it that there is another Reality that puts this one in the shade, and perhaps the acquisition of this conviction is the mechanism underlying their clinical response.

Suggestive comments can also be found in reflections by healthy volunteers on their transformative psilocybin-induced mystical experiences:

> The understanding that in the eyes of God—all people ... were all equally important and equally loved by God. I have had other transcendent experiences, however, this one was important because it reminded and comforted me that God is truly and unconditionally loving and present.

> The sense that all is One, that I experienced the essence of the Universe and the knowing that God asks nothing of us except to receive love.

> The complete and utter loss of self ... The sense of unity was awesome ... I now truly do believe in God as an ultimate reality.

> My conversation with God (golden streams of light) assuring me that everything on this plane is perfect; but I do not have the physical body/mind to fully understand.
> **(Griffiths et al. 2008, p. 629).**

These descriptions fit well with the idea that changes to metaphysical beliefs play a central role in causing lasting psychological benefits—not just in patients, but in healthy volunteers, too.

The study described by Harman highlights the empirical consequences of the MBT. According to this theory, the psychedelic mystical experience itself is not the direct cause of clinical improvement: it is an ineliminable part of the process, but the crucial variable is what patients believe *about* the experience. On this view, mystical experiences cause psychological benefits indirectly, by causing psychologically beneficial metaphysical beliefs. Accordingly, if mystical experience and metaphysical belief change vary independently, then the MBT entails that the latter should account for more variance in clinical outcomes.

To expand on the prediction: suppose that a therapeutic trial of psychedelics were conducted that quantified (a) rates of mystical experience and (b) changes in non-naturalistic metaphysical beliefs (e.g., increased or decreased assent to the existence of a cosmic consciousness or spirit world.) Suppose further that (a) and (b) varied somewhat independently—i.e., there were not a perfect correlation between mystical experience and increased assent to non-naturalistic beliefs. There is anecdotal evidence for such a dissociation: some people such as Benny Shanon (2002) seem to retain a cautious agnosticism about the veracity of their psychedelic-induced metaphysical epiphanies. The MBT would predict that, in such a trial, increased non-naturalistic belief would predict clinical outcomes more strongly than would mystical experience per se. According to this theory, what causes lasting change is not *experiences* as of another Reality, but acquired or strengthened *belief* in such a Reality.

The study described by Harman provides prima facie evidence for the MBT. But there is evidence against it too. This evidence comes from qualitative studies of cohorts treated in recent clinical trials. We saw in Chapter 3 that many patients, when asked about their impressions of the therapeutic process, make little mention, if any, of a cosmic consciousness or spirit world, emphasising instead such factors as acceptance and connectedness, psychological insight, powerful emotional experiences, and altered self-perceptions. Assuming that such patients as these were indeed treated successfully by psychedelic therapy, it seems unlikely that the primary mechanism of change is the induction of compelling non-naturalistic metaphysical beliefs:

> I feel like a whole bunch of crap has been dumped off the surface. This stuff that made my world shut down so much and made me look at the ground and watch the clock numbers clicking by. There's life and so many things going on, just watching that tree over there blowing in the breeze, seeing people in the street, and all the different people in vehicles rushing by! I just feel good about being alive ... It's always there; we just don't notice, and I'm trying to notice and not forget that I can see it at any time. I can hear it any time. It's like waking up in the most profound way, that this is really what life is, it's really like this. We're just not noticing.
>
> (Belser et al. 2017, p. 22).

> It was less about my illness. I was able to put it into perspective ... Not to see oneself with one's sickness as centre. There are more important things in life ... The evolution of humankind for example ... Your Inner Ego gets diminished, I believe, and you are looking at the whole ... you are indeed starting to build relations with plants or with the entire living world around. You think less about yourself, you are thinking—across borders.
>
> (Gasser et al. 2015, p. 62).

> It was like when you defrag the hard drive on your computer, I experienced blocks going into place, things being rearranged in my mind, I visualized as it was all put into order, a beautiful experience with these gold blocks going into black drawers that would illuminate and I thought: 'My brain is bring defragged, how brilliant is that!'
>
> (Watts et al. 2017, p. 10).

These patients do not sound like people deriving emotional comfort from their newly acquired or strengthened belief in transcendent metaphysical dimensions of reality. Some psychedelically treated patients clearly do acquire or strengthen non-naturalistic metaphysical beliefs, and emphasise this in their accounts—but others do not. Such belief changes, while they may contribute to benefits in some cases, cannot be the *primary* mechanism underlying the rapid, durable, transdiagnostic efficacy of psychedelic therapy.

As Bogenschutz et al. put it, their alcoholic patients treated with psilocybin 'experienced acute and lasting alterations in their perceptions of self, in the quality of their baseline consciousness, and in their relationship with alcohol ... experiences of catharsis, forgiveness, self-compassion, and love were at least as salient as classic mystical content' (Bogenschutz et al. 2018, p. 1). In a related vein, discussing a cohort of terminal patients treated for anxiety and depression with LSD, Gasser et al. propose 'facilitated access to emotions, confrontation of previously unknown anxieties, worries, resources and intense emotional peak experiences' (Gasser et al. 2015, p. 57) as candidate mechanisms of psychological change.

Similar points can be made regarding the 2016 studies of psilocybin therapy for cancer-related psychosocial distress. These are the largest, most rigorous studies of psychedelic therapy published to date, and they describe its application to the condition for which the MBT seems most plausible: existential distress accompanying terminal illness. As mentioned in Chapter 3, all the cancer patients interviewed by Belser et al. (2017) reported gaining 'transpersonal wisdom lessons' in their psychedelic experiences, but the exact nature and content of these lessons are unclear. Moreover, emotional catharsis, expanded emotional range, and changed perceptions of interpersonal relationships were also reported by all participants. Another analysis of interview data with the same patients found that *emotional shifts* and *experiences of reconnection to aliveness and belonging* were the most commonly reported themes (Swift et al. 2017). Belser et al. conclude that:

[while] the construct of a 'complete mystical experience', ... has been shown to be one mediator of positive outcomes in randomized controlled trials ... the findings of this study suggest a more complex topography... there are important relational, bodily, affective, and other aspects of participant experiences that may play critical roles ... Participants described powerful and healing catharses suggesting an emotional trajectory ... many participants 'remembered' aspects of themselves that had been forgotten. They recovered a sense of what is most important and vital in their lives, such as being present in the moment or being kind to other people. Participants described feeling 'reborn', more expansive, more confident, more connected, and more alive. They described a feeling of empowerment and being 'unstuck', with resulting healthier behaviors.

(Belser et al. 2017, pp. 26–27).

Thus, the results of recent qualitative research sit uneasily with the MBT. While newly acquired or strengthened belief in a Joyous Cosmology doubtless contributes to therapeutic benefits in some cases, it seems unlikely to be the core mechanism whereby psychedelics induce lasting psychological benefits. If it were, we would expect most successfully treated patients to offer clear and emphatic reports similar to that of the DPT subject quoted in Chapter 2:

> I am a much more content individual, having had the great opportunity to just glimpse for a very short moment the overall thinking of God ... to be reassured that there is a very beautiful, loving masterful plan in this Universe for all of us.
>
> **(Richards 1978, p. 124).**

Instead, many patients emphasise 'relational, bodily, affective, and other aspects of [their] experiences'—*even* those treated for existential distress in an end-of-life context.

One possible objection to my arguments runs as follows: perhaps all successfully treated psychedelic patients do, in fact, come to believe in a non-naturalistic metaphysical realm, but some of them downplay or conceal this fact due to embarrassment or discomfort about endorsing such views on the basis of a drug-induced experience. This certainly seems possible. Indeed, Michael Pollan attaches disclaimers in this spirit to descriptions of his own psychedelic experiences: 'As I read those words now, doubt returns in full force: "Fool, you were on drugs!"' (2018, p. 269). It may be that many psychedelic patients are reluctant to talk about their apparent metaphysical revelations due to similar scruples.

However, I know of no positive evidence for this view. We should hesitate to conclude that many patients and subjects are omitting to mention the single most significant and psychologically transformative aspect of their psychedelic experience without some definite reason to think that they are. This alternative hypothesis seems especially unlikely given the supportive environment fostered by psychedelic clinicians, and the open, anxiety-free mindset that is reputed to characterise the psychedelic afterglow (Majić et al. 2015). In my view, if these patients had undergone non-naturalistic metaphysical-type experiences, then they would be talking about them (due to the supportive environment, the nature of the afterglow, and the highly salient character of such experiences). They are not talking about such experiences (according to the qualitative evidence); therefore, they did not undergo them.

The only specific reason that I am aware of to favour the alternative hypothesis is a prior conviction that the mechanism of change *must* be the induction or strengthening of non-naturalistic metaphysical beliefs. The main ground, in turn, for such a conviction is the robust correlation between mystical experience and clinical outcomes. However, it is important to realise that, even if mystical experiences mediate clinical outcomes, this does not necessarily entail that non-naturalistic metaphysical beliefs do. The reason is simple: not all 'mystical experiences', in the relevant, operational sense, are experiences as of non-naturalistic metaphysical realities. There are states of consciousness that (a) satisfy standard psychometric criteria for a 'complete' mystical-type experience, but (b) are *not* experiences as of 'another [metaphysical] Reality that puts this one in the shade'.

This point is made very clearly by Pollan in his reflections on a psilocybin-induced experience in which he underwent a complete sense of ego dissolution, a merging of his sense of individuality into a Bach cello suite, and a visionary confrontation with, and acceptance of, the reality of death. Subsequently, he filled out the Mystical Experience Questionnaire (MEQ) used in much contemporary psychedelic research and found that his experience satisfied the criteria for a 'complete' mystical experience. Yet nothing he had experienced tempted Pollan, the avowed naturalist, to believe in another Reality, a cosmic consciousness, or a spirit world:

> I could easily confirm the 'fusion of [my] personal self into a larger whole', as well as the 'feeling that [I] experienced something profoundly sacred and holy' and 'of being at a spiritual height' and even the 'experience of unity with ultimate reality'. Yes, yes, yes, and yes—provided, that is, my endorsement of those loaded adjectives doesn't imply any belief in a supernatural reality ... It had been my objective to have [a mystical experience], and *at least according to the scientists* a mystical experience I had had. Yet it had brought me no closer to a belief in God or in a cosmic form of consciousness or in anything magical at all ...
>
> **(Pollan 2018, p. 284; my emphasis).**

This is an important result. It shows that, from the fact that a subject's psychedelic experience satisfies psychometric criteria for a 'complete' mystical experience (i.e., was a mystical experience 'according to the scientists'), it does not follow that their experience involved the apparent apprehension of a non-natural or supernatural Reality; of a cosmic consciousness, spirit world, or divine Ground of Being. There are experiences that do not depict realities inconsistent with naturalism, that nonetheless prompt subjects to give high scores to items on the MEQ and related questionnaires.

Henceforth, I will make a terminological distinction in recognition of this fact. I will use the term 'mystical-type experience' for experiences that attain high scores on standard psychometric measures of mystical experience, such as the MEQ and the Unity, Spiritual Experience, and Blissful State subscales of the 11D-ASC (11 Dimensions of Altered States of Consciousness) scale (cf. Carhart-Harris et al. 2018b). I will use the term 'metaphysical hallucination' for experiences that vividly and realistically represent apparent non-naturalistic realities,[4] such as a cosmic consciousness or an objectively existing realm of disembodied spirits. Using this terminology,

---

[4] Of course, on a literal construal of the phrase, there can be metaphysical hallucinations that are consistent with naturalism, because there are false metaphysical claims that are consistent with naturalism. In reserving this term for *non-naturalistic* metaphysical hallucinations, I am making a pragmatic terminological stipulation in the interests of convenience and brevity.

we can put the essential point very simply: some mystical-type experiences are not metaphysical hallucinations. Thus, the finding that mystical-type experiences are important for positive effects does not entail that non-naturalistic metaphysical ideations are.

Another illustrative example is provided by a philosophy student who took LSD under supervision in a 1960s study. His experience contained no apparent insights into the metaphysical nature of reality. Instead, it was centred around a recognition of the constructed nature of the ordinary sense of self, as well as a heightened sense of aesthetic appreciation and connectedness to other people. Nonetheless, the subject had this to say:

> The entire experience seemed to be charged with value and significance; the world and its occupants seemed enormously beautiful, delightful and harmonious and I was included within that general harmony ... Emotionally and aesthetically and *religiously* the experience was the most intense, impressive and valuable day I have ever experienced.
>
> **(Cohen 1970, pp. 102–103; my emphasis).**

We cannot know for sure, but it seems likely that this subject would have given high scores to many items on the MEQ.

I will return to the idea of naturalistically acceptable but 'religiously ... valuable' experiences, or something near enough, in Chapter 9. For now, the important point is this: there is no reason to think that patients are downplaying the apparent metaphysical contents of their transformative psychedelic experiences. A more plausible view is that (a) while some mystical-type experiences feature non-naturalistic metaphysical ideations, others do not, and (b) there is some more basic, universal feature of the mystical-type experience, common to both categories, which explains its propensity to cause lasting psychological benefits.

In fact, recent quantitative findings speak to this point. Roseman et al. (2019) found that scores on their new 'Emotional Breakthrough Inventory' predicted self-reported psychological benefit following a psychedelic experience. High scores on both the Emotional Breakthrough Inventory and the MEQ, as well as low scores on the 'Challenging Experience Questionnaire' (Barrett et al. 2016), predicted lasting benefits. Similarly, in a retrospective survey study, Garcia-Romeu et al. (2019) found that scores of mystical-type experience and of psychological insight predicted reductions in problematic alcohol use following a psychedelic experience.

In another survey study, Davis et al. (2020) reported that ratings of mystical-type experience and of psychological insight predicted lasting benefits following a psychedelic experience. Importantly, they found that ratings of psychological insight were a *stronger predictor* of benefits than ratings of mystical-type experience. This mirrors the earlier findings of Carhart-Harris et al. (2016b, 2018b) in their open-label study of psilocybin therapy for treatment-resistant depression. While these researchers found the usual correlation between mystical-type experience and lasting benefits, they found that reductions in depressive symptoms and positive personality change (Erritzoe et al. 2018) were both more strongly predicted by acute experiences of 'insightfulness'. I will discuss these findings further in Chapter 5. In short, preliminary but intriguing evidence fits well with the idea that ratings of 'mystical-type experience' are a proxy for some beneficial psychological process that is distinct from, but sometimes co-occurs with, metaphysical hallucinations.

A possible objection relates to the findings of Griffiths et al. (2019) that 'God encounter' experiences induced by psychedelics lead to strong increases in self-reported well-being, and also lead many people to cease identifying as atheists. However, the relevant survey was only taken by those who reported having a God encounter experience (drug-induced or otherwise), so this sample is not representative of (a) those who have transformative psychedelic experiences or even of (b) those who have psychedelic-induced mystical-type experiences. Indeed, only half of the God encounter experiences satisfied criteria for being a complete mystical-type experience. Thus, we have evidence for a double dissociation between God encounter experience and mystical-type experience: there are God encounter experiences that are not mystical-type (according to the findings of Griffiths et al.), and vice versa (according to the arguments I have given above). This fits well with a long-standing distinction between mystical and other religious experiences, where the dissolution of the ego and concomitant feelings of unity are understood as a necessary condition of the former but not the latter (Stace 1960). Therefore, the findings about God encounter experiences do not undermine my conjecture that psychedelic-induced *mystical-type* experiences exert psychological benefits through some primary mechanism other than metaphysical belief change.[5]

My conjecture yields a further testable prediction, directly contradictory to that derived above from the MBT: if we were to test both (a) rates of mystical-type experience and (b) increases in non-naturalistic metaphysical beliefs in trials of psychedelic therapy, these should dissociate to an extent—i.e., they should not be perfectly correlated—and, of the two, rates of mystical-type experience should be a stronger predictor of clinical outcomes.

Research into this prediction is underway. The Metaphysical Belief Questionnaire (MBQ) introduced by Timmermann et al. (in preparation) provides an initial means for quantifying psychedelic-induced changes in metaphysical beliefs about the nature of reality. It is to be hoped that this new psychometric instrument will provide rigorous quantitative evidence that allows firmer conclusions to be drawn concerning the truth or falsity of the MBT.

---

[5] These findings do suggest that increased non-naturalistic metaphysical belief can have psychological benefits—but this is not something I wish to deny. In cases where such belief change occurs, I have no doubt that it contributes to beneficial outcomes. I am simply denying that it is the main driver of change: My contention is that there is a more fundamental causal mechanism that unifies both naturalistic and non-naturalistic transformative experiences induced by psychedelics.

4.4　The Metaphysical Alief Theory

Suppose I am correct that changes in metaphysical beliefs do not do the heavy lifting in psychedelic therapy. There is a related alternative that may occur to philosophically informed readers: perhaps it is changes in metaphysical *aliefs*. 'Alief' is a philosophical term of art introduced by Tamar Gendler (2008). It refers to a mental representation of the world that is not reflectively endorsed or believed, but nonetheless influences thought, emotion, and action. The classic example is a person with fear of heights walking out onto a transparent balcony that they know to be extremely robust. Despite their reflective belief that they are safe, the person will feel and act (and perhaps think) as though they are in danger. They *alieve* that they are unsafe: they have a mental representation with the content *that I am unsafe*, which influences cognition, emotion, and behaviour despite their metacognitive verdict that it is inaccurate.

If my prediction above is borne out and mystical-type experience predicts clinical improvement more strongly than metaphysical belief change, this would spell trouble for the MBT. But it would be consistent with a *Metaphysical Alief Theory* the (MAT), which holds that patients' mental health is improved not by beliefs but by acquired or strengthened *aliefs* in a Joyous Cosmology. It is a familiar fact that fiction in various media can evoke strong emotions—inspiration, fear, sorrow, wonder—and perhaps even change lives. Something similar may be happening in psychedelic therapy. Perhaps patients who have mystical-type experiences acquire an extremely vivid mental representation of a transcendent universal consciousness, or of 'love as the fundamental and primary cosmic Fact', and vividly representing these things causes psychological benefits, regardless of whether the representation is metacognitively endorsed. This is similar to the idea that psychedelic therapy is a kind of 'inverse PTSD [post-traumatic stress disorder]' (Garcia-Romeu et al. 2014) in which a single, overwhelmingly intense, emotional episode has lasting *beneficial* effects on emotional processing.

In a related vein, Benny Shanon discusses the possibility of adopting the ayahuasca-inspired pantheist-idealist metaphysical vision in a poetic or pragmatic spirit, for its beauty and for the joy and wonder that it brings, regardless of its objective veracity or plausibility (Shanon 2010, p. 270). Perhaps this is exactly what successfully psychedelically treated but sceptically minded patients do, knowingly or otherwise: they *alieve* the psychedelically induced vision of a Joyous Cosmology, and are thereby uplifted. As we saw above, Harman explicitly rejects the MAT—but Flanagan and Graham seem to endorse something in its vicinity:

> ... it is best, probably, not to conceive of the hallucinatory state(s) as involving primarily belief, but something more like full-on imagination and a powerful desire to make something that is not yet real, real ... Metaphysical hallucinations involve having certain experiences, embracing how things seem while having those experiences, and then trying to imaginatively project oneself into a world in which

the relevant experiences or thoughts seem as real as real can be … and are thus spirit constituting and action guiding … The noetic confidence attaches perhaps not to believing that things are in fact such and so (although it might involve some of that), but wanting the world to be a certain way, a way one experiences as good, better, excellent.

(Flanagan and Graham 2017, p. 306).

Unlike the MBT, the MAT would be untouched by the confirmation of my prediction above—namely, a dissociation between rates of mystical-type experience and increased non-naturalistic metaphysical belief, with the former a stronger predictor of lasting benefits. If it is aliefs, not beliefs, that do the heavy lifting, then there is no reason to expect that metaphysical belief change will predict benefits more strongly than mystical-type experience.

However, the MAT still founders on the fact that many successfully treated patients do not emphasise non-naturalistic metaphysical contents in their retrospective descriptions. If a vivid metaphysical vision of a Joyous Cosmology were the primary factor reshaping a patient's psychology after a psychedelic session then, even if this vision were merely alieved, we would still expect it to figure prominently in their account of the experience—perhaps in the context of grappling with issues about how to regard its epistemic status, which permeate the reflections of Shanon (2002, 2010) on his ayahuasca experiences. But many patients instead emphasise experiences of broadened perspectives, psychological insight, emotional catharsis, connectedness, and acceptance, with no non-naturalistic metaphysics in sight (Gasser et al. 2015, Watts et al. 2017). This fact is difficult to account for on the MAT.

Once again, straightforward empirical tests can be devised. We are assuming, based on the arguments of section 4.2, that some aspect or consequence of the psychedelic experience is the main therapeutic mechanism. There are three possibilities under consideration: (1) it is sub-acute beliefs in a Joyous Cosmology that do the heavy lifting (the MBT); (2) it is acute experiences as of a Joyous Cosmology, and sub-acute recollections of them, irrespective of whether these are regarded as veridical (the MAT); (3) it is some other aspect of the experience, independent of non-naturalistic metaphysical contents (my conjecture). A dissociation between mystical-type experiences and metaphysical belief changes, with the former predicting benefits more strongly, would tell against (1) but would *not* discriminate between (2) and (3), being equally consistent with both hypotheses.

To my mind, the qualitative evidence surveyed in Chapter 3, and analysed in section 4.3 above, gives considerable prima facie reason to favour (3) over (2). This evidence is not logically inconsistent with (2), of course: it is a matter of abductive inference. Hypothesis (3) explains the qualitative evidence more simply than does hypothesis (2) (i.e., the MAT).

However, this argument could be bolstered further if we had a way of quantifying rates of *metaphysical hallucination*, as distinct from mystical-type experience or metaphysical belief change. In other words, we need a way of measuring the extent to which a given psychedelic *experience* represents the existence of a cosmic consciousness, or of non-physical or supernatural realms. (I am assuming that such a measure would correlate reasonably well with sub-acute aliefs). The MBQ introduced by Timmermann et al. is not adequate for this purpose, because an experience might contain non-naturalistic contents that are not subsequently endorsed or believed by the subject. And the various instruments for measuring mystical-type experience are not adequate because, as we have seen above, an experience can score highly on these questionnaires despite lacking non-naturalistic metaphysical contents.

One approach would be to adapt the MBQ into a Metaphysical Experience Questionnaire. The current MBQ contains such items as:

1. There exists another separate realm or dimension beyond this physical world that can be experienced and visited.

2. Visiting such immersive 'realms' or 'worlds' can sometimes depend on a supernatural / magical transition process or event.

3. There are two separate realms of existence, the physical (body, brain and external world) and the mind, the latter being non-physical/non-material.

4. There is just one primary reality: the mind and/or consciousness and all material things derive from it.

5. There is just one primary reality: the physical; the mind (and/or consciousness) is just physical/functional properties of the brain and has an entirely material explanation.

6. There are other realms of existence which are more important than everyday reality.

(Timmermann et al., in preparation)

Some of these items are intended to quantify subjects' changing credences in generic versions of standard philosophical positions, such as substance dualism (item 3), idealism (item 4)[6], and physicalism (item 5). Others, such as items 1, 2, and 6, refer instead to non-naturalistic or supernaturalistic beliefs that have sometimes been espoused by psychedelic users, or that are suggested by some psychedelic experience reports.

Here, then, is a simple method for quantifying the apparent metaphysical contents of the acute psychedelic experience: present subjects with these same items, but instruct them to rate the extent to which the statement *seemed* to be true during their experience, rather than the extent to which they now (post-experience) believe that the statement is true.

---

[6] A limitation, as Timmermann et al. acknowledge, is that item 4 in its current form does not discriminate between idealism and solipsism. I discuss possible relations between idealistic and solipsistic epiphanies induced by psychedelics in Chapter 7.

Suppose this were done. Suppose, that is, that in a rigorous double-blind random-ised controlled trial of psychedelic therapy for anxiety, depression, or addiction,[7] subjects were administered (a) the current MBQ; (b) the MBQ adapted, as just de-scribed, into a test of metaphysical-type *experiences* (metaphysical hallucinations); and (c) a standard measure of mystical-type experience such as the MEQ. My predic-tion is that: (1) results of all three measures would vary somewhat independently; and (2) of the three measures, mystical-type experience would prove to be the strongest predictor of lasting clinical benefits.[8]

No doubt increases in non-naturalistic metaphysical beliefs or aliefs contribute to therapeutic outcomes, when they do occur. However, my view is that there is a core mechanism of change in mystical-type experiences that is independent of non-naturalistic metaphysical beliefs and aliefs, and operative even when both of these are absent. Psychedelic therapy is not a pure pharmacotherapy: the experience matters. But mystical-type experience does not cause lasting psychological benefits primarily via non-naturalistic metaphysical ideations.

4.5 Conclusion

When psychedelic therapy is viewed as a pharmacotherapy, it is tempting to explain it in terms of low-level enhancements to the molecular mechanisms of neuroplasticity. However, I have argued that the pure Molecular Neuroplasticity Theory founders empirically on the dose-independent correlation between mystical-type experience and lasting psychological benefits. This correlation suggests that the core mechanism of psychedelic therapy is psychological, not an experience-independent pharmaco-logical process.

Thus, the Metaphysical Belief and Metaphysical Alief theories become appealing. Perhaps psychedelics cause lasting benefits by inducing transcendent visions of a Joyous Cosmology, whether it is subsequent beliefs in the veracity of the vision, or simply the vision itself (and imaginative recollection thereof) that does the work. However, both views struggle to explain the qualitative evidence of successfully treated patients, even in end-of-life contexts, who do not emphasise metaphys-ical themes in their retrospective reports. In my view, if these patients had under-gone metaphysical hallucinations, then they would be talking about them. Since they are not talking about them, we can conclude that they did not undergo them. This leads to an important point: not all experiences that satisfy psychometric criteria for a mystical-type experience are experiences as of non-naturalistic metaphysical real-ities. Or, in accordance with my new terminology, some mystical-type experiences are not metaphysical hallucinations.

---

[7] Or transformative administration in healthy subjects.
[8] A stronger predictor still might be ratings of psychological insight, which I discuss in Chapter 5.

My conjecture—which is subject to further empirical test, as described in section 4.4—is that the acute mystical-type experience is important for lasting benefits, but *not* because of the non-naturalistic metaphysical contents that sometimes feature in it. Rather, there is some other aspect of mystical-type experiences, independent of non-naturalistic ideations, that constitutes the core psychological mechanism of psychedelic therapy. Although we have seen several promising candidates, the nature of this factor remains unspecified. In Chapter 5, I will argue that the relevant factor is changes to the sense of self.

If the arguments of this chapter are sound, then a key assumption underlying the Comforting Delusion Objection is undermined. Psychedelic therapy does not, after all, work mainly by inducing or strengthening non-naturalistic metaphysical beliefs in a Joyous Cosmology. However, even if this is not the central therapeutic mechanism, there is no doubt that psychedelic experience sometimes promotes such beliefs. My ultimate contention that the Objection fails depends on the further claim that such epistemic risks are offset by significant epistemic *benefits*; and to assess this claim, we need a positive picture of how psychedelic therapy does work. Developing such a picture is the task of the next three chapters.

5
The role of self-representation

Still, if chemistry does not tell the whole story, what is that story? And what part do chemicals, replacing angels as divine intermediaries, play in it?
Huston Smith, *Cleansing the Doors of Perception.*

5.1 Introduction

According to the arguments of Chapter 4, psychedelic therapy is neither a low-level pharmacotherapy nor a matter of inducing mental representations of a Joyous Cosmology. What does the transformative work is some genuinely psychological factor, other than belief or alief in a cosmic consciousness or divine Reality, that correlates reasonably well with the construct of a mystical-type experience. What might this factor be?

The qualitative evidence surveyed in section 3.4 suggests several possibilities. Besides experiences as of non-naturalistic realities, successfully treated patients also report experiences as of psychological insight, emotional catharsis, connectedness, and acceptance. We want to know which, if any, of these factors is causally responsible for beneficial outcomes. But—but here, qualitative evidence has its limits. Are there other quantitative findings, besides the correlation between mystical-type experience and lasting benefits, that speak to this question?

There are, and they fall into three categories. The first is a small set of studies implicating experiences of *psychological insight* in lasting benefits. The second is a growing body of evidence that psychedelics durably elevate *mindfulness-related capacities* for taking an open, accepting, non-reactive attentional stance toward inner experience. The third is a set of findings concerning the neural correlates of psychedelics' lasting psychological benefits. While neuroimaging of the psychedelic experience in general has produced somewhat heterogeneous results, the picture becomes a little clearer when we focus on correlates of lasting therapeutic and transformative effects. Every relevant study that I know of has found changes to one or the other of two key neurocognitive systems: the *Default Mode and Salience networks*.

In this chapter, I review these three lines of evidence and argue that, collectively, they support the following simple hypothesis: the central mechanism of psychedelic therapy is the disruption and subsequent revision of mental representations of the self. The kinds of psychological insights captured by relevant psychometric instruments almost all concern the self in some way, especially the narrative self. The mindfulness-related capacities fostered by psychedelics involve a shift in the individual's sense of identity relative to her own thoughts and feelings. Specifically, they involve a kind of 'disidentification' and the creation of felt distance between the self and its mental states. And the Default Mode and Salience networks have both independently been identified as plausible neural substrates of self-representation. Changes to self-representation are the common factor that connects these three bodies of evidence, as well as the varieties of mystical-type experience—those that feature non-naturalistic metaphysical ideations and those that do not.

The task of the present chapter is to marshal evidence for the hypothesis that changes to self-representation are, in fact, the central causal factor in psyche-delic therapy. Speculating about how this might work mechanistically is the task of Chapters 6 and 7.

5.2 Psychological factors

If we think that psychedelics' therapeutic benefits are due to some aspect of the acute experience, and we want to know which aspect, then an obvious strategy is to look for correlations between (a) variables quantifying aspects of the experience and (b) variables quantifying lasting psychological benefits (cf. Letheby 2015). The most robust such correlation, as we have seen, is between ratings of acute mystical-type experience and measures of symptom reduction, personality change, and so forth. However, a few studies have also found a relationship between acute experiences of *psychological insight* and lasting benefits. Of course, we already saw in Chapter 3 that experiences of psychological insight are a common theme in qualitative studies. However, we are now going beyond this to examine *quantitative* evidence linking such experiences to lasting psychological benefits.

5.2.1 Psychological insight

In their open-label study of psilocybin for treatment-resistant depression, Carhart-Harris et al. (2018b) used the 11D-ASC scale (11 Dimensions of Altered States of Consciousness; Studerus et al. 2010) to quantify aspects of the acute psyche-delic experience. They combined three dimensions of this scale—'Unity', 'Spiritual Experience', and 'Blissful State'—into a single factor, 'USB', that serves as a reason-able proxy for the construct of a mystical-type experience. Unsurprisingly, they found a significant correlation between scores on the USB factor and lasting reductions in depressive symptoms. However, reductions in depressive symptoms correlated *more* strongly with scores on the 'Insightfulness' dimension of the 11D-ASC. This dimen-sion comprises the following three items:

'I felt very profound'
'I gained clarity into connections that puzzled me before'
'I had very original thoughts'

(Studerus et al. 2010, p. 9).

It seems that having this 'insightful' sort of experience under psilocybin correlates fairly strongly, but not perfectly, with having a mystical-type experience, and is a *better* predictor of antidepressant effects than the latter. Moreover, in the same cohort of patients, acute Insightfulness correlated with positive personality change (decreased Neuroticism and increased Extraversion) three months after the psilocybin treatment (Erritzoe et al. 2018).

This gives us some reason to suspect that experiences as of insightfulness are the real driver of change in psychedelic therapy. However, the three items comprising the Insightfulness sub-scale of the 11D-ASC do not tell us much about the content of these insights, nor about how they might transform personality and remediate pathology.

Intriguing clues on this score are provided by the findings of Davis et al. (2020), who administered a large-scale online survey to people who reported gaining *psychological* insight from a psychedelic experience. Davis et al. developed their own psychometric instrument, the Psychological Insight Questionnaire (PIQ), designed to assess 'the degree to which respondents experienced acute insight (e.g., gained an awareness [of their] emotions, behaviours, beliefs, memories, or relationships)'. The PIQ is considerably more detailed and fine-grained than the Insightfulness sub-scale of the 11D-ASC. Items from the PIQ are as follows:

Realized how current feelings or perceptions are related to events from my past
Awareness of uncomfortable or painful feelings I previously avoided
Realized ways my beliefs may be dysfunctional
Discovered how aspects of my life are affecting my well-being
Gained a deeper understanding of events/memories from my past
Experienced validation of my life, character, values, or beliefs
Realized the importance of my life
Awareness of dysfunctional patterns in my actions, thoughts, and/or feelings
Discovered specific techniques for coping with difficulties
Realized how critical or judgmental views I hold towards myself are dysfunctional
Discovered I could explore uncomfortable or painful feelings I previously avoided
Gained a deeper understanding of previously held beliefs and/or values
Discovered a vivid sense of the paradoxes in life
Realized I could experience memories previously too difficult to experience
Awareness of beneficial patterns in my actions, thoughts, and/or feelings
Discovered a clear pattern of avoidance in my life
Realized the nature and/or origins of my defenses or other coping strategies
Discovered new insights about my work or career

Gained resolution or clarity about past traumas or hurtful events

Discovered clear similarities between my past and present interpersonal relationships

Discovered new feelings or perspectives about significant relationships in my life

Realized certain actions I should take in regards to important relationships in my life

Discovered new actions that may help me achieve my goals

Realized the point of view or actions of others that had been difficult to understand previously

Discovered clarity or creative solutions about how to solve a problem in my life

Awareness of information that helped me understand my life

Discovered ways to see my problems with more clarity

Awareness of my life purpose, goals, and/or priorities

(Davis et al. 2020, p. 41).

Recall the distinction, introduced in section 3.3, between narrative and minimal forms of self-awareness. The narrative self is the rich and complex set of mental representations a person harbors of her identity over time, as a specific individual with an autobiographical history and a distinctive set of traits (Gallagher 2000). The minimal self, on the other hand, is a bare sense of being a subject of experience at a moment in time, prior to any specific character traits or diachronic continuity. On some accounts, the minimal self is a form of bodily awareness rooted in interoceptive processing (Seth 2013)—a hypothesis we will return to in Chapter 7.

The important point is this: virtually every item on the PIQ describes some kind of change to the narrative self. Almost all of these statements describe an epiphany, realisation, or change of perspective concerning *who one is* as a specific individual—one's beliefs, goals, values, memories, behaviours, problems, prospects, and relationships. This is especially clear when it comes to the items most commonly endorsed by participants in the survey. The four most common items, each endorsed by more than 95% of participants, were:

Discovered how aspects of my life are affecting my well-being

Gained a deeper understanding of previously held beliefs and/or values

Awareness of information that helped me understand my life

Discovered ways to see my problems with more clarity

(Davis et al. 2020, p. 41).

Clearly, the kind of psychedelic-induced 'psychological insight' being tracked by the PIQ has a lot to do with gaining, or seeming to gain, new information, understanding, or awareness pertaining to aspects of oneself and one's life. In other words, the psychological insight experience quantified by this measure centrally involves changes to the narrative self.

Most importantly for our purposes, the findings of Davis et al. mirrored those of Carhart-Harris et al. earlier: lasting psychological benefits—in this case, reductions in depression and anxiety—correlated with both acute mystical-type experiences and acute insightfulness experiences, but *more strongly* with the latter. We do not know for certain whether the PIQ is tracking the same phenomenon as the Insightfulness sub-scale of the 11D-ASC. However, given the similar findings from the two studies, it seems reasonable to assume that they are measuring broadly similar phenomena. This assumption receives further support from the findings of Watts et al. (2017), who conducted a qualitative study with the patients treated by Carhart-Harris et al., and reported that a 'sense of connecting to a new version of themselves was a very strong theme. Most patients reported having gained a fresh perspective on their lives' (p. 532). Here is an example that clearly would have been captured by the PIQ:

> I was thinking about relationships I had with other people and thinking I could see them clearly almost as if for the first time. I had fresh insight into things. It was almost as if suddenly the scales dropped from my eyes, I could see things as they really are.
>
> **(Watts et al. 2017, p. 532).**

Of 20 patients in this study, 14 reported 'visions of an autobiographical nature', with most being regarded as 'insightful and informative' (Carhart-Harris et al. 2018b, p. 403). Also interesting in this context is the finding of Kaelen et al. (2018) that increased responsiveness to music under psilocybin correlates with both mystical-type experience and insightfulness.

In a similar vein, Carhart-Harris et al. (2012a) found increases in self-reported well-being, two weeks after intravenous psilocybin, in healthy volunteers who were prompted to recall autobiographical memories while under the influence. Unsurprisingly, autobiographical memory recall was rated as more vivid, and featured more visual imagery, under psilocybin than placebo. Importantly for our purposes, increases in well-being at the two-week follow-up correlated with the vividness of memory recollection under psilocybin. This is more evidence that changes to narrative or autobiographical self-representations are causally relevant to psychedelics' lasting benefits.

A fourth finding connecting acute experiences of psychological insight to lasting benefits is reported by Garcia-Romeu et al. (2019). These researchers conducted an online survey study of people addicted to alcohol who had reduced their drinking after using psychedelics in a non-clinical setting. Participants filled out various measures quantifying the psychedelic experience and its after-effects. Most participants met the *Diagnostic and Statistical Manual of Mental Disorders* (DSM) criteria for severe alcohol use disorder prior to their psychedelic experience; most no longer met criteria for *any* alcohol use disorder after it. Most relevant to our concerns is the finding that reductions in drinking correlated with acute mystical-type experience and with acute psychological insight experience. The authors comment: 'Although this finding is preliminary, it suggests that psychological insight is also an important mechanism of behaviour change following a psychedelic experience.' (Garcia-Romeu et al. 2019, p. 1096).

In a fifth and final finding, Garcia-Romeu et al. (2020) reported a survey study of people who had experienced persisting reductions in the use of cannabis, opioids, or stimulants after a psychedelic experience. Reductions in use of these substances were associated with ratings of the psychedelic experience as mystical-type, insightful, and personally meaningful. The measure of psychological insight, used in both this study and the prior one assessing reductions in alcohol consumption, was as follows:

How **personally psychologically insightful** to you were the experiences?
(Circle the highest number that applies)
[Note: Personal psychological insight refers to realizations about personality, relationships, behavioral patterns, or emotions. Personal psychological insight can occur in complete absence of a spiritual/mystical insight, although spiritual mystical insight can sometimes prompt personal psychological insight.]

1. No more than routine, everyday psychologically insightful experiences
2. Similar to psychologically insightful experiences that occur on average once or more a week
3. Similar to psychologically insightful experiences that occur on average once a month
4. Similar to psychologically insightful experiences that occur on average once a year
5. Similar to psychologically insightful experiences that occur on average once every 5 years
6. Among the 10 most psychologically insightful experiences of my life
7. Among the 5 most psychologically insightful experiences of my life
8. The single most psychologically insightful experience of my life
(Roland Griffiths, personal communication, 17 July 2020).

It is clear that this description overlaps significantly with items from the PIQ.

Collectively, the studies we have just surveyed give some initial support to the conjecture that changes to the sense of self, especially the narrative self (Amada et al. 2020), are a central causal factor in psychedelic therapy. As we will see shortly, other quantitative findings support this conjecture too.

One possible objection relates to the findings of Roseman et al. (2019) that 'emotional breakthrough' under psychedelics predicts subsequent improvements in well-being. Roseman et al. conducted a prospective web-based survey study of people who were independently planning to undergo a psychedelic experience. They quantified the acute state using the commonly used Mystical Experience Questionnaire (MEQ), the Challenging Experiences Questionnaire (CEQ), which measures psychologically difficult or challenging experiences under psychedelics (Barrett et al. 2016), and their own new measure: the Emotional Breakthrough Inventory (EBI). They found that high MEQ and EBI scores, and low CEQ scores, predicted increases in well-being. Furthermore, they concluded that 'the EBI does not render either the CEQ or MEQ redundant but rather a multifactorial predictor model that combines all three measures performs better than any alternative that neglects any one of them' (Roseman et al. 2019, p. 1083). It might be thought, then, that this study provides evidence against my conjecture, pointing to emotional breakthrough rather than changes to self-representation as the central causal factor.

The first point to make is that, in my view, other psychological factors almost certainly play a causal role. I am not claiming that changes to self-representation are the *only* psychological mechanism of psychedelic therapy, just that they are the main one—the one that is doing most of the work and that is common to otherwise disparate cases.

The second point is that the putative distinction between emotional breakthrough and changes to self-representation may be spurious. Emotion and the sense of self are intimately bound up in the human mind. The autobiographical representations and simulations that constitute the narrative self need to be integrated with emotional feelings to drive behaviour (Damasio 1994, Gerrans 2014). Moreover, it has been argued that the pre-reflective minimal self is generated by the same neural mechanisms that underlie emotional feelings: in other words, that affect and the sense of self are intertwined all the way down (Damasio 1999, Seth 2013). We will return to these ideas in Chapter 7. For now, a brief inspection of EBI items reveals considerable overlap with the types of experiences measured by the PIQ:

> I faced emotionally difficult feelings that I usually push aside.
> I experienced a resolution of a personal conflict/trauma.
> I felt able to explore challenging emotions and memories.
> I had an emotional breakthrough.
> I was able to get a sense of closure on an emotional problem.
> I achieved an emotional release followed by a sense of relief
>
> **(Roseman et al. 2019, p. 1082).**

Although they emphasise the affective rather than noetic aspects, several of these items describe processes of autobiographical reappraisal and perspective-shifting that might well be captured by PIQ items. In my view, the finding that EBI scores predict changes in well-being does not undermine, but underscores, the importance of changes to self-representation.

We already know that the sense of self is disrupted dramatically in the mystical-type experience: the sense of unity is the cardinal feature of such experiences, whether or not any non-naturalistic ideations are involved. Perhaps such experiences are therapeutically valuable because this transient but dramatic disruption to self-representations affords an opportunity for the beneficial revision of such representations. Perhaps mystical-type experiences alleviate pathology and transform personality because they allow us to change *how we see ourselves*—how we relate to and understand our own minds and lives—at a deep and fundamental level.

5.2.2 Mindfulness-related capacities

The case for this view is bolstered by the further findings of Davis et al. (2020). Not only did they find that insightfulness experience outperformed mystical-type experience as a predictor of anxiolytic and antidepressant effects: they also found that the relationship between insightfulness and symptom reductions was fully mediated by increases in the construct of *psychological flexibility*. This construct is central to contextual behavioural therapies such as Acceptance and Commitment Therapy (ACT) and Dialectical Behavioural Therapy (DBT) and is closely related to the kinds of attentional skills cultivated in mindfulness meditation.

At first, it may be unclear how psychological flexibility relates to the sense of self. However, this becomes clearer when we examine the construct more closely. The measure of increased psychological flexibility used by Davis et al. was *decreased* scores on the Acceptance and Action Questionnaire II (AAQ-II), an instrument designed to quantify psychological inflexibility and 'experiential avoidance'—known transdiagnostic predictors of psychiatric distress (Bond et al. 2011). The AAQ-II is based on the core idea at the heart of contextual behavioural therapies that 'mental health and behavioural effectiveness are influenced more by how people relate to their thoughts and feelings than by their form (e.g., how negative they are)' (Bond et al. 2011, p. 677). As such, these therapies aim primarily at changing, not the kinds of thoughts and feelings that patients have, but how they relate to those thoughts and feelings.

The AAQ-II includes such items as 'My painful experiences and memories make it difficult for me to live a life that I would value'; 'I'm afraid of my feelings'; and 'My painful memories prevent me from having a fulfilling life'. High scores reflect psychological inflexibility and experiential avoidance; low scores reflect psychological flexibility and experiential acceptance. Each item probes some aspect of how a person conceives of herself, relates to her own mental states, and experiences the relationship between her inner and outer worlds.

Contextual behavioural therapies such as ACT and DBT are predicated on the existence of a psychological capacity known as the 'perspective-taking self': the ability to 'step back' from one's specific first-order thoughts and feelings, to disidentify with the contents of these, and to identify instead with the bare quality of consciousness or subjectivity—the context in which all thoughts and feelings come and go (Hayes et al. 2020). The perspective-taking self refers to a sense of identifying with the subject who experiences thoughts and feelings, rather than with any of the thoughts and feelings themselves. Psychological flexibility and experiential acceptance are theorised to result from increased identification with this perspective-taking self—a bare subject of experience, reminiscent of the minimal self—and a correspondingly detached and flexible relationship with the contents of the narrative self.

This is similar to the construct of *decentring*, developed to quantify the effects of mindfulness meditation, which measures the ability to take an 'objective, distanced, and open approach toward one's internal experiences' (Naragon-Gainey and DeMarree 2017, p. 935). It is interesting to note that increases in decentring, as well as greater acceptance, enhanced emotion regulation, and changes to the sense of self, have been postulated as mechanisms underlying the psychological bene-fits of mindfulness-based interventions (Creswell 2017). The phenomenology of (i) identification with the minimal perspective-taking self, and (ii) corresponding disidentification with the contents of the narrative self is described by some of the psychedelic experience reports that we saw in Chapter 3. These reports also highlight the potential of such a shift to foster psychological flexibility:

> Two related feelings were present. One was a tremendous freedom to experience, to be I. It became very important to distinguish between 'I' and 'Me', the latter being an object defined by patterns and structures and responsibilities—all of which had vanished—and the former being the subject experiencing and feeling. My normal life seemed to be all Me, all demands and responsibilities, a rushing burden which destroyed the pleasure and freedom of being 'I'. Later in the evening the question of how to fit back into my normal life without becoming a slave of its patterns and demands became paramount.
>
> **(Durr 1970, p. 79).**

> For a few seconds, it was just like 'I'm me, and there are no defining characteristics!' ... that made me realise that I'm not a 'smoker'.
>
> **(Noorani et al. 2018, p. 759).**

Thus, the finding that anxiolytic and antidepressant effects are mediated by increased psychological flexibility suggests that these effects might be caused by an increase in felt identification with the minimal, perspective-taking self, and a concomitant de-crease in felt identification with specific contents of the narrative self (the 'patterns and structures and responsibilities', such as being a 'smoker')—making the latter less rigid and more malleable (cf. Watts and Luoma 2020). This is how findings of increased psychological flexibility implicate changes to the sense of self (Hayes et al. 2020).

In a prospective online survey study, Close et al. (2020) replicated some of the cen-tral findings of Davis et al. Volunteers with a prior intention to have a psychedelic experience (self-guided or in a psychedelic retreat) filled out various psychometric questionnaires before and after their experiences. Psychological flexibility increased after the psychedelic experience, and this increase correlated with reductions in de-pressive symptoms, as well as with acute mystical-type and emotional breakthrough experiences (albeit weakly). No measures of psychological insight were administered to this cohort. However, these findings provide further support for the idea that the lasting benefits of psychedelics importantly involve decreased subjective identifica-tion with specific mental contents (i.e., increased psychological flexibility).

This idea receives convergent support from studies implicating increased *mindfulness-related capacities* in the therapeutic process. Mindfulness medita-tion, also known as *Vipassana* or 'insight' meditation, is a practice drawn from the

Buddhist tradition. It consists of a body of techniques for systematically cultivating the ability to bring a steady, open, non-reactive attention to whatever contents arise in the phenomenal field—thoughts, feelings, sensations, and so on—without becoming 'caught up' or unduly invested in any of them. The practice typically begins with the stabilisation of attention and the development of concentration by focused attention to bodily sensations, including the breath. On the basis of meditative concentration, the practitioner then engages in 'open monitoring'—giving a bare, even attention to all mental contents without attempting to restrict or direct them in any way. Ideally, the successful practitioner will ultimately be able to retain her equanimity and tranquilly observe or witness the passing flux of experience, without identifying with or getting 'caught up in' any of its transient contents (Brewer et al. 2013; cf. Fasching 2008).

The purpose of mindfulness in the traditional Buddhist path is to foster direct experiential insight into the putatively liberating truths of impermanence (*anicca*) and non-self (*anatta*)—the transience and insubstantiality of all phenomena, including the meditator herself (Goleman 1972). However, mindfulness techniques have been adapted for secular purposes, notably in the form of the Mindfulness Based Stress Reduction (MBSR) programme developed by Jon Kabat-Zinn (2013), and a large body of evidence suggests that secular mindfulness practices have beneficial effects in stress, chronic pain, and many other conditions—including anxiety, depression, and addiction (Wielgosz et al. 2019).

Based on this brief description, we can see clear similarities between the attentional skills cultivated in mindfulness practice and the notion of the 'perspective-taking self' invoked in contextual behavioural therapies. Indeed, the theoretical basis of these therapies was derived, in part, from an attempt to render the psychological benefits of spiritual practices naturalistically comprehensible and scientifically tractable (Hayes 1984). Moreover, therapies such as ACT often incorporate mindfulness-based interventions for the purpose of promoting psychological flexibility (Levin et al. 2012).

Psychometric instruments have been developed for quantifying the psychological capacities cultivated in mindfulness practice. For example, the Five Facet Mindfulness Questionnaire (FFMQ) measures mindfulness capacities in terms of five distinct subskills: 'observing, describing, acting with awareness, nonjudging of inner experience, and nonreactivity to inner experience' (Baer et al. 2008, p. 329). Intriguingly, several recent studies have found evidence that a single psychedelic experience can durably increase some of these capacities.

In a survey study, Mian et al. (2020) used the FFMQ and the Experiences Questionnaire (EQ; Fresco et al. 2007), the latter of which measures the construct of 'decentring', to track changes in mindfulness capacities in the month following an ayahuasca ceremony. They found that depressive symptoms were significantly reduced after the ceremony and that these reductions correlated strongly with increases in mindfulness capacities. Similarly, Murphy-Beiner and Soar (2020) found that FFMQ and EQ scores, as well as cognitive flexibility (a construct distinct from psychological flexibility) were increased in the 24 hours following an ayahuasca session.

These studies build on earlier findings that ayahuasca can increase mindfulness capacities: Soler et al. (2016) found that capacities for decentring, non-judging, and non-reactivity were significantly elevated 24 hours after a single ayahuasca session. Uthaug et al. (2018) reported increases in mindfulness and life satisfaction the day after a single ayahuasca session, and reductions in stress and depression lasting four weeks. All changes correlated with the degree of ego dissolution during the acute effects. Later, Soler et al. (2018) reported that four weekly ayahuasca sessions led to increases in non-judging comparable to those observed in a control group who undertook a standardised 8-week MBSR course.

To my knowledge, medium- or long-term follow-ups with these cohorts have not been reported. However, in another study, Sampedro et al. (2017) found that a single ayahuasca session led to significant increases in non-reactivity and non-judging the following day, with the increases in non-judging maintained at two month follow-up. (These increases in non-judging also correlated with distinctive brain changes, discussed in section 5.4 below.)

Over the course of a year, González et al. (2020) administered psychometric measures to a sample of bereaved volunteers who participated in traditional ayahuasca ceremonies during that year. They found a correlation between reductions in grief and (a) increases in decentring, as well as (b) decreases in experiential avoidance, lasting up to a year post-ayahuasca. They relate this to earlier qualitative findings reporting 'experiences of emotional release, biographical memories, and experiences of contact with the deceased' (González et al. 2019, p. 260) among bereaved participants who consumed ayahuasca.

Similar results have been found concerning the intense, short-acting psychedelic 5-MeO-DMT. Uthaug et al. (2019) reported that a single inhaled dose of 5-MeO-DMT led to immediate increases in satisfaction with life that remained significant four weeks after the session. Scores on the non-judging and 'awareness' sub-scales of the FFMQ also increased, with these increases *reaching* significance at the four-week follow-up point. Finally, in a separate sample, Uthaug et al. (2020) found that a single inhaled dose of 5-MeO-DMT led to increases in non-judging and reductions in depressive symptoms seven days after the experience, and that both changes correlated with ratings of ego dissolution during the psychedelic session.

As well as ayahuasca and 5-MeO-DMT, psilocybin has shown the potential to durably enhance mindfulness capacities. Madsen et al. (2020) used the Mindful Attention Awareness Scale (MAAS; Brown and Ryan 2003) to measure the effects of a single psilocybin session on psychedelic-naïve participants. They found that both MAAS scores and Openness to Experience were significantly elevated three months after the psilocybin experience. The authors note the potential implications: 'Considering MBSR effects on clinical symptoms, it is possible that increases in mindfulness constitutes [*sic*] a key element of psilocybin therapy' (Madsen et al. 2020, p. 6; cf. Heuschkel and Kuypers 2020).

Finally, in a fascinating study we encountered in Chapter 2, Smigielski et al. (2019a) investigated the interactions between psilocybin and intensive meditation training.

Experienced practitioners of Zen meditation (*zazen*), a form of mindfulness practice, undertook a standard five-day group retreat (*sesshin*) involving several hours per day of silent meditation. On day four, volunteers received either psilocybin or placebo in a randomised, double-blind fashion and continued their meditation routine. Psilocybin induced positively valenced experiences of ego dissolution and oceanic boundlessness, with low levels of anxiety.

Immediately before and after the retreat, subjects completed a mindfulness questionnaire. Unsurprisingly, all subjects showed an increase in trait mindfulness from pre- to post-retreat. However, as the researchers had hypothesised, the increase was larger in the psilocybin than the placebo group. Thus, not only can psychedelic administration alone increase mindfulness capacities—it seems that psychedelics, under suitable conditions, can enhance the efficacy of traditional mindfulness practice.

To recap: several studies show that psychedelics can durably increase mindfulness capacities, and related constructs such as psychological flexibility. In some cases, these increases correlate with therapeutic benefits, such as reductions in depressive symptoms. As Madsen et al. note, this raises the possibility that changes in mindfulness constitute a key element of psychedelic therapy. Given that mindfulness capacities centrally involve changes in the sense of self—changes that are a traditional goal of mindfulness practice—this bolsters the case that such changes are of paramount importance.

There is a third and final line of evidence implicating changes to self-representation in psychedelic therapy. This comes from studies investigating the neural correlates of psychedelics' lasting psychological benefits. Evidence to date suggests that therapeutic and transformative effects of psychedelic experiences are consistently accompanied by changes to neural networks that have independently been implicated in generating the sense of self.

5.3 Neural correlates

Today's psychedelic researchers possess sophisticated tools and techniques unavailable to their forebears—notably, advanced neuroimaging technologies such as positron emission tomography (PET) and functional magnetic resonance imaging (fMRI). Neuroimaging studies of the psychedelic state have yielded fascinating but tantalising results. Not all findings have been replicated, which may be due partly to the variability of the psychedelic state itself, and partly to the variability of other relevant factors. Perfect consistency would be surprising across studies using different imaging methods to assess the effects of different substances, with different time courses, given in different doses via different routes of administration to different populations of volunteers in different laboratory settings.[1] In particular, the question

---

[1] It is also important to appreciate that the psychedelic state unfolds in time—within a single six-hour psilocybin session, the same subject will undergo radically different conscious experiences at different points in time (Preller and Vollenweider 2016, Fox et al. 2018).

whether psychedelics cause an overall increase or decrease in neural activity remains unresolved (Vollenweider et al. 1997, Carhart-Harris et al. 2012b, Lewis et al. 2017; see Müller et al. 2018a for discussion).

However, when we narrow our focus, matters become somewhat clearer.[2] Every neuroimaging study that has investigated neural correlates of *lasting therapeutic and transformative effects* has found changes to one or both of two important neural systems: the Default Mode and Salience networks. This bolsters the case that I am making in this chapter because a considerable body of non-psychedelic evidence links these two networks to different aspects of self-representation—to the narrative self and the minimal self, respectively (Lou et al. 2017). Moreover, every study examining neural correlates of acute *insightfulness* or *ego dissolution* experiences under psychedelics has found changes to one or both of these systems.

This is not to deny that other regions are involved in these extraordinarily complex effects: clearly, they are. For instance, changes to thalamus activity seem to be a common feature of the psychedelic state, highlighted by several studies (Müller et al. 2018a). Furthermore, I am not proposing any simplistic one-to-one relation between self-representation and the relevant neural networks—other systems participate in self-representation, and these systems participate in multiple functions. However, modulation of the Default Mode and Salience networks seems to be an especially consistent correlate of (i) *insightfulness experiences*, (ii) *ego dissolution*, and (iii) *lasting psychological benefits* induced by psychedelics.

5.3.1 The Default Mode Network

A key discovery of twenty-first century cognitive neuroscience is that the healthy adult human brain is organised into large-scale *intrinsic connectivity networks*—coalitions of regions that exhibit high levels of mutual 'functional connectivity'[3] at rest, prompting the inference that they comprise a functionally unified system (Fox et al. 2005). Most famous is the Default Mode Network (DMN), centred on cortical midline structures such as the medial prefrontal cortex (mPFC) and the posterior cingulate cortex (PCC). The DMN displays high levels of activity during conditions of wakeful, task-free rest, as well as during self-referential, metacognitive, and socially oriented tasks. During impersonal and externally oriented tasks, its hubs tend to collectively quiet in favour of activity in anti-correlated 'task-positive networks' (TPNs) (Raichle et al. 2001, Fransson 2006). The discovery of the DMN was important because, among other things, it helped to undermine traditional conceptions of the

---

[2] Which is not to say *entirely* clear.

[3] The functional connectivity between two regions is defined as the temporal correlation between their activity levels: the stronger the correlation between increases and decreases in activity in two distinct regions, the higher their functional connectivity. Such correlation is standardly interpreted as indicating functionally significant interaction, hence the name.

brain as an essentially reactive, stimulus-driven organ, raising the question of what exactly all this 'spontaneous' or 'intrinsic' neural activity was for (Bechtel 2013).

The DMN has repeatedly been linked to the narrative self for both direct and indirect reasons. Activity in its nodes is reliably increased by high-level self-referential tasks, such as making conceptual judgements about one's character or personality. Moreover, the other functions with which DMN activity is associated are precisely those that might contribute to a diachronic or narrative self-concept: rumination or mind-wandering during the task-free 'resting state', which often concerns self-referential themes; the attribution of mental states ('theory of mind'); and the autobiographical simulation of past and future events ('mental time travel'; Gusnard et al. 2001, Davey et al. 2016, Davey and Harrison 2018).

Further anatomical and physiological facts suggest that the DMN plays a pivotal role in our mental economy. Its main nodes are pivotal 'hub' regions with unusually high levels of metabolic activity and anatomical connectivity. Evidence suggests that these hubs are involved in regulating or 'tuning' the activity and connectivity profiles of multiple far-flung neurocognitive systems throughout the brain (Leech et al. 2012, Braga et al. 2013, Leech and Sharp 2014). Relevantly to our concerns, abnormal activity and connectivity of DMN hubs have been documented in multiple psychiatric pathologies (Broyd et al. 2009, Whitfield-Gabrieli and Ford 2012). The activity and connectivity of these regions is also altered by meditation practices (Fox et al. 2016). Notably, these regions are unusually rich in the 5-HT2A receptors that are psychedelics' main molecular target (Carhart-Harris et al. 2014).

The hypothesis that coherent functioning in the DMN is a neural substrate of the narrative self receives convergent support from psychedelic neuroimaging results. In a magnetoencephalography (MEG) study of healthy volunteers, Muthukumaraswamy et al. (2013) found that psilocybin reduced the power of synchronised neuronal oscillations across a wide range of frequency bands, in multiple brain regions. Notably, they reported strong decreases in the power of alpha (8–13 Hz.) oscillations in the PCC—a highly active and densely connected region that has been called the 'core node' of the DMN (Davey and Harrison 2016, p. 390; cf. Fransson and Marrelec 2008)—and found that these decreases correlated with subjective ratings of ego dissolution under psilocybin.[4] Based on these and other findings, Carhart-Harris et al. proposed that:

within-default-mode network (DMN) resting-state functional connectivity (RSFC) and spontaneous, synchronous oscillatory activity in the posterior cingulate cortex (PCC), particularly in the alpha (8–13 Hz) frequency band, [could] be treated as *neural correlates of 'ego integrity'.*

(2014, p. 2; my emphasis).

---

[4] Interestingly, decreased alpha power in the PCC also correlated with participants' level of agreement that the experience had 'a supernatural quality' (Muthukumaraswamy et al. 2013, p. 15178).

This idea is broadly consistent with findings linking PCC down-regulation to meditatively induced disruptions of self-awareness (e.g., Brewer and Garrison 2014, Winter et al. 2020).

Further evidence comes from the findings of Speth et al. (2016) that disintegration of the DMN (i.e., decreased functional connectivity between its constituent regions, as measured by fMRI) correlated with a decrease in mental time travel to the past under LSD. Healthy volunteers were administered LSD or placebo and then underwent a neuroimaging scan. They subsequently described their experiences and thought processes during the scan. Descriptions of LSD sessions featured significantly fewer references to past autobiographical events than did descriptions of placebo sessions,[5] correlating with reductions in DMN integrity. While reduced mental time travel to the past may not explicitly be described as 'ego dissolution', it is a disruption to one aspect of the narrative self (cf. Millière et al. 2018). This is a crucial point: not all psychedelic-induced changes to self-representation amount to a 'dissolution' or 'disintegration' of the ego, so the hypothesis that changes to self-representation are the central factor is *not* equivalent to the hypothesis that ego dissolution is the central factor.

Finally, Mason et al. (2020) found that changes to regional neurotransmitter levels correlated with distinct types of ego dissolution experience induced by psilocybin. In healthy patients, negatively valenced states of ego dissolution were associated with higher levels of glutamate in the mPFC—a major node of the DMN. Positively valenced states of ego dissolution, however, were associated with lower levels of glutamate in the hippocampus, a memory-related structure that is also an important component of the DMN (Greicius et al. 2004).

As well as acute changes to the sense of self, modulation of the DMN has been linked to acute experiences of *insightfulness*. In the only neuroimaging study that I am aware of to probe the correlates of this specific psychedelic-induced experience, Kometer et al. (2015) conducted electroencephalography (EEG) studies of healthy volunteers who received psilocybin or placebo, and quantified their subjective experiences using the 11D-ASC. Scores on the Insightfulness and Spiritual Experience sub-scales correlated strongly with lagged phase synchronisation of neuronal oscillations in the delta frequency band (1.5–4 Hz.) within a network comprising the parahippocampal cortex (PHC), the retrosplenial cortex (RSC), and the lateral orbitofrontal cortex. The RSC and the adjacent PCC are sometimes jointly described as the 'posterior DMN' (Kaboodvand et al. 2018, p. 2020). Moreover, the RSC and the PHC have both been hypothesised to facilitate information flow between cortical DMN nodes and memory-related structures in the medial temporal lobes, such as the hippocampus (Ward et al. 2014, Kaboodvand et al. 2018). As Kometer et al. put it:

---

[5] This is consistent with the idea that autobiographical insights are important parts of the therapeutic mechanism. Presumably, psychedelics decrease the overall frequency of mundane, everyday mind-wandering to the past by disintegrating the DMN, which also creates the conditions for qualitatively unusual and intense autobiographical insights to occur.

Because phase synchronization of parahippocampal oscillations in this frequency range has previously been linked to autobiographical memory retrieval ... and to the attribution of valence in memory ... our finding suggests that psilocybin-induced insightfulness may be associated with increased retrieval and reattribution of autobiographic memories... The RSC has previously been implicated in coding the location of oneself within a global spatial context ... and therefore, our finding may suggest that with increasing intensity of spiritual experiences, the self is reorganized within the global spatial context through phase synchronization of delta oscillations.

(2015, p. 3672).

Of course, the idea that psilocybin-induced insightfulness is associated with 'increased retrieval and reattribution of autobiographic memories' fits well with many of the items on the PIQ developed by Davis et al. (2020) and discussed in section 5.2.1 above.

Finally, changes to the structure and function of the DMN have been found to correlate with lasting psychological benefits of psychedelics. I will discuss therapeutic benefits first, and then transformative effects in healthy subjects.

In their study of psilocybin for treatment-resistant depression, Carhart-Harris et al. (2017) conducted fMRI scans of patients' brains pre- and post-treatment. They found *increased* functional connectivity within the DMN post-treatment—a surprising result given that heightened DMN activity and connectivity have previously been linked to depressive symptoms (e.g., Hamilton et al. 2015). Specifically, Carhart-Harris et al. found that antidepressant effects at five-week follow-up were predicted by (i) increased functional connectivity between the ventromedial prefrontal cortex (vmPFC) and the inferior lateral parietal cortex, and (ii) decreased functional connectivity between parahippocampal and prefrontal cortical regions, the day after psilocybin. They explain these surprising findings by positing that distinct *patterns* of activity and connectivity within the DMN are associated with distinct mental health profiles. Thus, by acutely disintegrating this network, psychedelics in effect 'shake the snow globe', allowing the system to be subsequently reset into a healthier configuration. We will discuss this *Reset Theory* of psychedelic therapy further in Chapter 6.

Separate analyses of data from the same cohort also highlight the involvement of DMN changes in antidepressant effects. Roseman et al. (2018b) reported that patients showed increased amygdala reactivity when viewing emotional face expressions the day after psilocybin, and this increase predicted antidepressant effects a week later. (The amygdala is a node of the Salience Network (SN), not the DMN—but we will see momentarily that DMN changes were involved too). Once again, this is a surprising finding, because prior research has shown that selective serotonin reuptake inhibitors (SSRIs) *decrease* amygdala reactivity to emotional stimuli. Roseman et al. suggest that SSRIs and psilocybin may alleviate depressive symptoms via fundamentally different mechanisms, with SSRIs reducing emotional responsiveness across the board, thereby masking symptoms (but sometimes inducing undesirable 'affective blunting'), while psilocybin increases emotional responsiveness and facilitates a cathartic confrontation with psychological problems underlying symptoms. This hypothesis is based partly on the spontaneous comments of patients, many of whom contrasted the psilocybin treatment with other antidepressant treatments in just these terms. These patients reported that psilocybin helped them to discover and deal with the psychological causes of their depression, confronting and accepting difficult emotions and memories, whereas previous treatments had tended to 'reinforce [the] sense of disconnection and [emotional] avoidance' (Watts et al. 2017, p. 520) that characterised their depression.

Most importantly for present purposes, a subsequent analysis by Mertens et al. (2020) found that not only was amygdala activity during emotional face processing increased post-psilocybin, but functional connectivity between the right amygdala and the vmPFC—a core DMN node—was *decreased*. The authors speculate that this might reflect decreased top-down inhibitory influence of the vmPFC over the amygdala, in line with their hypothesis of restored emotional responsiveness following psilocybin treatment. Interestingly, the *reduction* in right amygdala-vmPFC functional connectivity was not significantly correlated with any psychological variables, but *absolute* levels of functional connectivity between these regions post-treatment correlated negatively with levels of rumination, a known predictor of depressive symptoms (Nolen-Hoeksema 2000).

We turn now to transformative effects and positive personality change in healthy subjects. Bouso et al. (2015) conducted fMRI scans of long-term, religious ayahuasca users and matched controls in the sober state. Relative to controls, ayahuasca users showed cortical thinning in the PCC, and thickening in the anterior cingulate cortex (ACC; a key node of the SN, discussed further in section 5.3.2). The PCC thinning was not associated with any cognitive impairment or psychiatric distress: users' mental health and neuropsychological function were comparable to those of controls. However, the degree of PCC thinning was correlated with both (a) the duration of prior ayahuasca use and (b) elevated psychometric scores for the personality trait of 'Self-Transcendence'—a construct that measures both religious and spiritual beliefs and feelings of identity or unity with a reality larger than the individual self.

As we saw in section 5.2.2, Sampedro et al. (2017) found that mindfulness-related capacities for non-judging were increased in healthy volunteers two months after a single dose of ayahuasca. They also conducted neuroimaging scans of their subjects before and after the psychedelic experience. They found reduced levels of multiple neurotransmitters in the PCC, as well as increased functional connectivity at rest between (a) the PCC and the ACC, and (b) the ACC and medial temporal lobe structures involved in memory and emotion (including the hippocampus, a subcortical DMN node, and the amygdala, a subcortical SN node). These reductions in neurotransmitter levels and increases in functional connectivity correlated with the sustained increases in non-judging.

Finally, in their study of a psilocybin-assisted meditation retreat, Smigielski et al. (2019b) conducted neuroimaging scans of their subjects before and after the retreat.

Each scanning session contained periods of task-free rest, focused attention (concentration) meditation, and open awareness (mindfulness) meditation. From pre- to post-retreat, meditators who received psilocybin, but not those who received placebo, showed changes in DMN connectivity during open awareness meditation—specifically, a reduction in functional connectivity between the PCC and the mPFC, the main posterior and anterior cortical nodes of the DMN. Moreover, the degree of this reduction correlated with the degree of 'oceanic boundlessness' experienced during the psilocybin-enhanced meditation session.

Post-retreat, meditators in the psilocybin group showed *increased* connectivity between the PCC and the mPFC in the task-free resting state—reminiscent of the findings of Carhart-Harris et al. in their depressed patients—and decreased connectivity between the mPFC and the angular gyrus during focused attention meditation. Both these changes correlated significantly with sustained increases in well-being four months after the retreat. The authors comment:

> These dissociable effects of psilocybin on task-versus-rest and acute-versus-intermediate network dynamics point to a complex, yet behaviorally relevant modulation of DMN function. The psilocybin experience of [oceanic boundlessness] might increase the meditators' capability of down-regulating DMN integration during OA [open awareness] practice, representing a neural mechanism frequently found during states of self-transcendence. In contrast, higher DMN integration at rest was predictive of lasting behavioral outcomes at the 4-month follow-up. This is consistent with the idea that psychedelics increase context-dependent DMN flexibility, enabling more adaptive allocation of brain resources. Although higher DMN integration in the psilocybin group predicts the long-term transformative impact of the retreat on core life attitudes and behaviors, experienced meditators were still able to down-regulate DMN connectivity during OA to reach states of self-transcendence. Hence, the dynamic repertoire of DMN function may be increased following psychedelic drug administration, which aligns with recently proposed therapeutic mechanisms of 'brain resetting' that mediate psilocybin's antidepressant properties . . .
>
> **(Smigielski et al. 2019b, p. 213).**

In sum, a considerable body of evidence suggests that complex modulations of DMN activity and connectivity are involved in (a) acute experiences of insightfulness and ego dissolution, and (b) lasting psychological benefits—including increased mindfulness capacities, positive personality change, and reduced psychiatric symptoms—resulting from psychedelic use.

5.3.2 The Salience Network

The other network that seems to be involved in these effects is the SN, which incorporates the ACC, the anterior insular cortex (AIC), and subcortical structures including the amygdala (Seeley et al. 2007). As its name suggests, this network is involved in the detection of salient (i.e., behaviourally relevant) events and the coordination of adaptive responses. The insula has been implicated in many different functions, including interoception—sensing the internal physiological condition of the body—as well as empathy and conscious emotional feelings.[6] Menon and Uddin (2010) attempted to unify these findings by proposing that the essential function of the AIC is to (i) detect salient stimuli across cognitive and perceptual modalities, and (ii) work in concert with other structures such as the ACC to coordinate an effective response. This involves, inter alia, regulating switching between the DMN and anti-correlated TPNs, allocating processing resources in accordance with the nature and location of the salient stimulus:

> [We view] the anterior insula as an integral hub in mediating dynamic interactions between other large-scale brain networks involved in externally oriented attention and internally oriented or self-related cognition [i.e., the DMN]. The model we present postulates that the insula is sensitive to salient events, and that *its core function is to mark such events for additional processing and initiate appropriate control signals*. The anterior insula and the anterior cingulate cortex form a 'salience network' that functions to segregate the most relevant among internal and extrapersonal stimuli in order to guide behavior ... with the insula as its integral hub, the salience network assists target brain regions in the generation of appropriate behavioral responses to salient stimuli.
>
> **(Menon and Uddin 2010, p. 655; my emphasis).**

However, this hypothesis does not address an important question: why should the SN be associated with the minimal self? One reason is the known involvement of the AIC in both interoception and the 'experience of body ownership': the sense of inhabiting or owning a specific physical body (Craig 2009, Seth 2013). Another reason comes from studies of pathologies of selfhood, such as depersonalisation disorder (DPD), in which patients report feeling as though they have died or no longer exist. Some such studies have shown hypoactivity of SN nodes, particularly the AIC, in patients relative to controls (Phillips et al. 2001, Medford 2012). At a first pass, we could describe the link as follows: the SN attributes salience to stimuli as a function of their hypothesised relevance to the goals and interests of the self; thus, to attribute salience, it needs a representation of the self and its goals and interests.

We will examine the nature of this link more closely in Chapter 7. At present, we are concerned with converging evidence for the *existence* of such a link, which can be found in psychedelic neuroimaging studies. Lebedev et al. (2015) conducted fMRI scans of healthy volunteers who received intravenous psilocybin or placebo. In contrast with the earlier findings of Muthukumaraswamy et al. (2013), they found that

---

[6] There is also evidence that multiple forms of meditation practice affect the structure and function of SN nodes, especially the insula (Fox et al. 2014, 2016).

subjective ratings of ego dissolution correlated, not with changes in the DMN, but with disintegration of the SN—as well as with decoupling of medial temporal structures from various cortical regions, and decreased communication between cerebral hemispheres. Referring to the apparent conflict with earlier findings, Lebedev et al. appeal to the distinction between narrative and minimal/embodied forms of self-awareness, noting that the DMN is often associated with the former and the SN with the latter. Their implicit suggestion seems to be that psychedelics disrupt different forms or aspects of self-awareness in different subjects at different times—depending, perhaps, on such factors as set, setting, dosage, and route of administration.

Two subsequent studies have also implicated the SN in altered self-experience under psilocybin. First, Lewis et al. (2020) conducted morphological scans of the brains of healthy volunteers prior to a psilocybin experience. As hypothesised, they found that thickness of the rostral ACC predicted ratings for the four sub-scales of the 11D-ASC that have significant emotional content: Feeling of Unity, Bliss, Spiritual Experience, and Insightfulness. At least two of these four (Unity and Spiritual Experience) clearly involve changes to the sense of self; I argued above that Insightfulness does too. Second, Smigielski et al. (2020) administered psilocybin or placebo to healthy volunteers who then engaged in a 'source monitoring' task, which involved discriminating between one's own and others' voices, while being scanned by EEG. Psilocybin decreased the difference between neural responses to own-voice versus others' voices. This neural change was 'driven by current source density changes within the supragenual anterior cingulate and right insular cortex' and correlated with 'the intensity of psilocybin-induced feelings of unity and changed meaning of percepts' (Smigielski et al. 2020, p. 1).

Meanwhile, a fMRI study of LSD in healthy volunteers found that ego dissolution under this drug was associated with changes to the connectivity profiles of *both* the DMN and the SN. Tagliazucchi et al. (2016) found that LSD increased functional connectivity between multiple regions throughout the brain, disrupting its normally stable network architecture. When they searched for correlations between neural changes and phenomenological effects, they found that subjective ratings of ego dissolution correlated with increased functional connectivity in both the temporoparietal junction (TPJ), a key DMN node, and the bilateral insula, a key SN node[7]. These correlations were specific to ego dissolution: no correlations between functional connectivity changes and other phenomenological features survived rigorous statistical testing. The increases in functional connectivity in the TPJ and insula were heavily weighted toward sensory areas, suggesting that systems involved in emotion and self-awareness engage in increased cross-talk with 'exteroceptive'[8] perceptual systems under LSD. It is intriguing, to say the least, that a blurring of the experiential subject/object boundary should correlate with increased communication between systems that represent the internal and external worlds.

---

[7] Its anterior sub-division, at least.

[8] Pertaining to the sensing and perception of the extra-organismic world; opposite to 'interoceptive'.

Changes in SN function have been linked, not just to acute alterations in self-awareness, but also to therapeutic effects of psychedelics and transformative effects in healthy subjects. Beginning with therapeutic effects: as we saw above, Roseman et al. (2018b) reported increased amygdala reactivity to emotional faces the day after psilocybin, correlating with reductions in depressive symptoms a week later. In a separate analysis of data from the same cohort, Mertens et al. (2020) reported decreased functional connectivity between the amygdala and the vmPFC the day after psilocybin; *absolute* levels of functional connectivity between these regions correlated negatively with levels of rumination.

Turning now to transformative effects: as we saw in section 5.2.2, the findings of Sampedro et al. (2017) linked both DMN and SN modulation to elevated mindfulness capacities following an ayahuasca session. Sustained elevations in non-judging two months post-ayahuasca were predicted by decreased neurotransmitter levels in the PCC immediately post-ayahuasca, but also by increased functional connectivity of the ACC—a key SN node—both to the PCC and to medial temporal regions, including the amygdala. Increased functional connectivity between the ACC and medial temporal regions correlated with elevated scores for self-compassion, a construct adapted from Buddhist psychology (Neff 2003, Garcia-Campayo et al. 2014). However, these increases in self-compassion were not sustained at two-month follow-up.

Finally, Lebedev et al. (2016) found that Openness to Experience was increased in healthy volunteers a fortnight after a single LSD session. These personality changes were predicted by acute increases in the *entropy*—roughly, the disorderliness or unpredictability—of brain activity during the psychedelic session. These increases in entropy were observed in multiple networks, including the DMN and the SN. But, of these two networks, only increases in SN entropy were significantly correlated with personality change at two-week follow-up.

In sum, while more evidence points to the DMN, there is also evidence that alterations to the SN are involved in (a) acute experiences of insightfulness and ego dissolution, and (b) lasting psychological benefits—including increased mindfulness capacities, positive personality change, and reduced psychiatric symptoms—resulting from psychedelic use.

5.4 Neurocognitive explanation

We have seen both psychological and neuroscientific evidence that (I argue) implicates changes to self-representation as a central causal mechanism of psychedelic therapy. The psychological evidence consists in:

(i) correlations between acute insightfulness experiences and lasting benefits, and
(ii) durable increases in mindfulness-related capacities and psychological flexibility, sometimes correlating with therapeutic effects.

(i) implicates changes to self-representation because the relevant kinds of insights seem mainly to concern autobiographical themes, and (ii) implicates changes to self-representation because psychological flexibility, and mindfulness-related capacities such as decentring, involve a shift in the felt sense of identity—away from specific contents of the narrative self, and towards a bare, minimal, 'witnessing' self, leading to a more flexible sense of identity.

The neuroscientific evidence consists in correlations between

(i) relevant psychological variables—namely, acute ego dissolution experiences, acute insightfulness experiences, and lasting psychological benefits—and

(ii) acute and lasting modulation of the DMN and SN.

These findings implicate changes to self-representation because the DMN and SN are independently plausible neural substrates of narrative and minimal forms of self-representation, respectively.

However, all of this leaves an important question unanswered: What exactly is the relationship between these two distinct bodies of evidence? Is it possible to theoretically integrate psychological and neuroscientific perspectives—to turn these mere *correlations* between psychological and neural variables into explanatory relations? If so, how? Psychedelic therapy is a profoundly multilevel phenomenon, involving complex interactions between phenomena at multiple spatiotemporal scales, studied by different disciplines, and described in different proprietary vocabularies (Carhart-Harris et al. 2014, p. 4). As such, it is impossible to pursue a convincing integrative understanding of this novel treatment without considering how different levels of description and explanation are related in the sciences of mind and brain.

My position, in brief, is that it is possible to explain psychological phenomena in neuroscientific terms, by means of *neurocognitive theory* that specifies the computational or information-processing functions of neural structures (Gerrans 2014, Boone and Piccinini 2016). This epistemological approach is rooted in an influential metaphysical doctrine: the *computational theory of mind* (CTM), which holds that the mind is a computational system implemented in the 'wetware' of the biological brain. The idea is simple and intuitive enough at heart, but requires some unpacking.

CTM has served as the conceptual foundation for cognitive science and cognitive neuroscience for several decades. Both enterprises are interdisciplinary attempts to explain psychological phenomena in terms of computational operations performed by neural structures.[9] The computational framework is arguably the most empirically successful general theory of human mentality ever devised, but is often misinterpreted (Piccinini 2009). One example is popular talk of the 'computer metaphor' of mind, which belies the fact that, on standard formulations, CTM is a straightforwardly literal

---

[9] This characterisation has become more controversial since the advent of non-computational and anti-representational approaches to the study of cognition (e.g., Hutto and Myin 2012) but it is certainly historically sound, and arguably still accurate with respect to the majority of cognitive (neuro-)scientific research programmes today (Boone and Piccinini 2016, Thomson and Piccinini 2018).

assertion: mental (or cognitive) processes just *are* computational processes (Rescorla 2020). Of course, to appreciate why a literal reading of this claim might be thought plausible, one needs a basic grasp of the central concept of computation, and of the crucial fact that there are many possible kinds of computational systems—most of which bear little obvious resemblance to those that populate our laptops and desktops.

This is not the place for a detailed treatment of these issues. For classic introductions to these themes, see Haugeland (1985) and Copeland (1993); for more recent developments, see O'Brien and Opie (2006), Piccinini and Bahar (2013), and Rescorla (2020). Here I will simply outline the view that I favour, and its consequences for the matter at hand: the integration of psychological and neuroscientific evidence concerning psychedelic therapy.

To understand and assess any version of CTM, we need to know what conception of computation is at play in the assertion that mental or cognitive processes are computational. Here I assume, without argument, the *semantic conception* of computation, which holds that computation consists in the manipulation of *representations* in a manner systematically sensitive to their semantic properties (O'Brien 2011). What, then, is a representation? In the philosophy of mind and cognitive science, a representation is understood most generally as something which *stands in for* something (Bechtel 1998, pp. 297–298). The English word 'dog' stands in for a particular class of mammals. A portrait of a person stands in for that person. The arbitrary numerical symbols that we manipulate in arithmetic stand in for, and systematically correspond to, numbers or quantities—whatever in the world those might be. And so it goes.

Thus, on this conception of computation, CTM amounts to the view (i) that there are states of the brain, such as patterns of synaptic strength, patterns of neural firing rates, or both—that stand in for aspects or features of the world (including the organism itself)—i.e., there are neurally implemented *mental representations*—and (ii) that cognitive processes consist in the manipulation of these representations in ways that are sensitive to their semantic properties—i.e., their meanings or contents. Of course, this leaves many details unspecified, such as the format(s) of these representations, the type(s) of computational processes operating on them, and the nature of the relation(s) between *representing vehicle* (the physical structure in the head) and *represented object* (that which it represents in the world). But the basic idea is intuitive and eminently plausible. A perceptual (auditory) representation of a knock at the door causes the generation of a representation with semantically related content along the lines of *I wonder who is at the door.* An interoceptive representation of the sensation of hunger causes the generation of a representation with content along the lines of *Is it nearly lunchtime yet?* A representation with content along the lines of *Where did I leave my keys?* causes the generation of a representation with content along the lines of *Well, when I came in last night, I went straight to the kitchen*—accompanied, perhaps, by an 'offline' visual representation of the scene in question—and so it goes. Across cognitive and sensory modalities, states with certain contents cause the activation of states with systematically related contents, in a manner so ubiquitous as to go unnoticed, but crucial to the coordination of adaptive behaviour (Clark 2001, pp. 2–3).

Not only is this framework independently plausible, but it offers an attractively simple picture of how to integrate psychological and neuroscientific evidence in the explanation of cognitive and behavioural phenomena. On the version of CTM that I have sketched, the brain is in the business of constructing and manipulating neurally implemented representations of entities, properties, and states of affairs, and using the results to guide behaviour. Note that many of these representations exist, and are processed, outside of conscious awareness. A classic example is the sophisticated mental representations of the grammar of one's native language, which are deployed in unconscious parsing processes that yield, as their outputs, virtually instantaneous comprehension and judgements of grammaticality whose grounds typically elude articulation (Chomsky 1959; cf. O'Brien and Jureidini 2002a). However, the contents of some of our mental representations *do* enter conscious awareness. For example, as I look out my window and see a tree gently swaying in the breeze, part of the explanation of the occurrence of this experience is that there are, in my visual system, representations of the relevant shapes, colours, locations, movements, and so forth, and that these representations possess some 'consciousness-making' property that other, unconscious, mental representations lack.

Just as I have remained neutral on the details of representational format, etc., here I remain neutral on the specific property that demarcates conscious from non-conscious mental representations. Perhaps it is being a local maximum of integrated information (Gallimore 2015); perhaps being broadcast into the 'global workspace' (Grinde and Stewart 2020); perhaps being a stable activation pattern in a 'neurally realised PDP Network' (O'Brien and Opie 2015). Irrespective of which property is at issue, we have a simple and attractive way of conceptualising what in the (natural) world conscious experiences *are*: they are nothing other than complexes of neurally implemented mental representations, all of which bear some consciousness-making property in addition to semantic properties (i.e., representational contents) that determine the qualitative properties of the experience.[10] And this, in turn, offers a straightforward methodological prescription for integrating psychology and neuroscience: to explain psychological (including experiential) phenomena in neuroscientific terms, identify (i) the neural structures involved and (ii) the computational functions performed by those structures, such that (iii) the organised interaction of those structures performing those functions gives rise to the psychological phenomenon to be explained (Machamer et al. 2000, Craver 2007, Bechtel 2008, Piccinini and Craver 2011).

Within this framework, we can explain psychedelics' psychological effects in terms of their neurobiological effects by constructing *neurocognitive theories* that (i) attribute specific computational or information-processing functions to specific neural structures, and (ii) specify how the performance of those functions by those

---

[10] Philosophers, please note: My view is that phenomenal properties supervene on narrow, not wide, content. In other words, the qualitative character of experience is fixed by intrinsic properties of the organism, not by any organism–environment relations. This point will come up, in different terms, in Chapter 6.

structures is altered by pharmacological perturbation. This is essentially the approach laid out by Philip Gerrans (2014) in his neurophilosophical treatment of clinical delusions. As he puts it:

> I advocate *neurocognitive psychiatry*, that is, the use of neurocognitive theory to explain psychiatric disorder ... the mechanisms involved in psychiatric disorder necessarily include cognitive—that is, information-processing—ones. This is a general truth about human psychology. Genes build proteins, which build neurons, which build neural circuits, which process information in representational formats that allow organisms to control their behavior. Tracing the psychological effects of a genetic deletion, a neurotransmitter imbalance, a head injury, a childhood trauma, a private school education, or a conversation requires us to treat the mind as an integrated set of computational mechanisms implemented in neural wetware.
>
> **(Gerrans 2014, p. 28; emphasis original).**

Here I am proposing to extend the project of neurocognitive psychiatry to the explanation of psychiatric *treatment* (cf. Gerrans and Scherer 2013): in this case, psychedelic treatment. Of course, this project does not constitute a solution to the Hard Problem of Consciousness: that remains unsolved. However, it does give us the resources to pursue 'a type of contrastive explanation aimed, not at consciousness itself, but at why specific aspects of conscious contents are the way they are, rather than another way' (Hohwy 2007a, p. 16). Why, for example, should lesion to cortical area V5 lead to akinetopsia, or visual motion blindness? (Zeki 1991). Why should heightened activity in Brodmann Area 17 correlate with increased vividness of mental imagery rather than, say, feelings of anger or olfactory hallucinations? (de Araujo et al. 2012). Such correlations are mysterious unless we postulate that the relevant neural structures are specialised for the processing of various kinds of visual information (cf. Hohwy 2007b, p. 317). This hypothesis gives us the resources to explain the links between such neurophysiological and phenomenological changes.

The framework of neurocognitive psychiatry constitutes a distinctive metatheoretical stance in psychedelic science.[11] It allows us to see, for example, what is right and what is wrong about Benny Shanon's contention that 'biological accounts—detailed as they might be—[cannot] offer viable psychological explanations' (2002, p. 35). In his seminal cognitive psychological study of the ayahuasca experience, Shanon embraces the classic thesis of the *Autonomy of Psychology* from neuroscience (cf. Bechtel 2006). He acknowledges the obvious causal relation between ingestion of psychoactive molecules and psychedelic experiences, but contends that theoretical frameworks drawn from neurobiology are pitched at the wrong level of description

---

[11] Others have suggested that a multilevel explanatory framework of this general kind might be useful in the multidisciplinary study of psychoactive substances (e.g., Móró 2010, Díaz 2013); here I am simply putting a little flesh on the bones of this suggestion.

to explain the properly psychological features of the ayahuasca state. On this view, the biological action of DMT and other alkaloids may *cause* a psychedelic experience, but their effects on the brain, described in solely biological terms, cannot adequately *explain* that experience. Trying to explain ayahuasca-induced visionary experiences in biological terms would be like trying to understand Macbeth via a chemical analysis of the ink on the page, or a 'rigid geometric analysis of the script' (Shanon 2002, p. 363). This is reminiscent of a remark by Alan Watts (1960) that a 'chemical description of spiritual experience has somewhat the same use and the same limits as the chemical description of a great painting.'

As far as it goes, this is correct. Explanations confined to the vocabularies of action potentials and ion channels, receptor conformations and functional connectivity, are separated by a vast conceptual gap from the type of phenomenological psychology that Shanon practices. It is true that neuroanatomical and neurophysiological accounts cannot *in themselves* 'serve as explanations in psychology' (Shanon 2002, p. 363). But neuroscience is not limited to pure neuroanatomy and neurophysiology (Gold and Stoljar 1999). In particular, as we have seen, *cognitive* neuroscience is founded on the premise that neurocognitive theory provides the necessary conceptual and explanatory tools to bridge the gap between biological and psychological descriptions of the human brain/mind (Boone and Piccinini 2016). Adopting a neurocognitive approach allows us to avoid the implausible conclusion that recent findings from psychedelic neuroscience have nothing to tell us about why psychedelic experiences feel the way they do. At the same time, it allows us to avoid the equally implausible conclusions that (a) the psychedelic state can be characterised in wholly biological terms, or that (b) neuroscientific knowledge makes psychological investigations obsolete (cf. Bechtel 2006). All levels of the mechanistic hierarchy are real and important. Molecular neuroscience can no more replace psychology than chemistry can replace sociology.

The approach I propose is also distinct from the suggestion of Robin Carhart-Harris (2018) that the construct of *entropy* constitutes a unique conceptual bridge between neurobiological and phenomenological accounts of the psychedelic state. Carhart-Harris suggests that elevated neural entropy under psychedelics can directly explain phenomenal feelings of uncertainty and informational richness experienced by subjects. Since entropy is formally defined in terms of uncertainty and information content, it offers 'a unique bridge across the physical and experiential divide that demands no special extrapolation' (2019, p. 18). In the seminal paper that introduced the entropic brain theory, Carhart-Harris et al. write:

> Entropy is a powerful explanatory tool for cognitive neuroscience since it provides a quantitative index of a dynamic system's randomness or disorder while simultaneously describing *its informational character, i.e., our uncertainty* about the system's state if we were to sample it at any given time-point. When applied in the context of the brain, this allows us to make a translation between mechanistic and qualitative properties. Thus, according to this principle, increased subjective uncertainty or 'puzzlement' accompanies states of increased system entropy.
>
> **(2014, pp. 1–2; my emphasis).**

However, an increase in *our* uncertainty about a system's state (because its behaviour has become more random or disorderly) need not lead to an increase in the *system's* subjective or phenomenal feelings of uncertainty. Indeed, empirical evidence suggests that it sometimes does not: at certain points during high-dose, presumably highly entropic, psychedelic states, subjects experience the noetic quality—the vivid phenomenal feeling of *certainty* that is criterial of the mystical-type experience. Also, there is some evidence that high-dose, presumably highly entropic, psychedelic states can feature episodes of 'pure consciousness', devoid of all ordinary perceptual and cognitive content, which have been described as having a maximally sparse phenomenology (Millière et al. 2018, p. 16). Both observations would seem to undermine any direct link between (i) high levels of neural entropy and (ii) phenomenal feelings of uncertainty and informational richness. The sense in which entropy is defined, mathematically, in terms of uncertainty and information content offers no a priori answer to the question of how such phenomenal feelings are implemented mechanistically in actual cognitive systems. As such, it is not clear that entropy describes the 'informational character' of a system in the sense relevant to explaining that system's phenomenal properties.

I do not mean to deny that there is any theoretically interesting link between entropic brain activity and psychedelic phenomenology. However, my view is that specific phenomenal qualities do not, in the philosophical jargon, *supervene* directly on quantitative properties of brain dynamics. If this is correct, then the concept of entropy—important though it may be—is not the conceptual bridge needed to link psychedelic neurobiology and phenomenology. Entropy is a quantitative property of brain dynamics that abstracts away from specific neurocomputational states and processes, but it is those states and processes that determine the contents of phenomenal consciousness. Phenomenal qualities supervene on, and are explained by, the semantic contents of mental representations within neural networks; the concepts of representation and computation provide the necessary conceptual bridge.

What, then, is the nature of the link between entropy and phenomenal properties, such as feelings of uncertainty? In my view, it is simply this: highly entropic brain states often, but not always, feature specific sorts of representational contents, and it is the latter that explain the phenomenal properties. Increased neural entropy correlates, imperfectly, with increased conscious mental representations of uncertainty. For instance, according to a neurocognitive theory proposed by Carhart-Harris and Friston (2019) and discussed more in Chapter 6, psychedelics alter consciousness by perturbing neural processes that encode the *precision* (or 'confidence') that the brain assigns to its own high-level beliefs. Since these high-level beliefs play a central role in the cognitive economy, one flow-on effect is to induce an unconstrained mode of cognition, sending the system on a whirlwind tour (or 'trip') through an expanded state space. When phenomenal feelings of uncertainty or puzzlement occur, they result from specific representational activity: from the brain representing its own beliefs as highly imprecise or uncertain. As such, phenomenal feelings of uncertainty and increases in neural entropy are distinct effects of a common cause: decreasing the brain's confidence in its high-level beliefs. This is consistent with the idea that, during its entropic trip, the brain may visit states in which it represents its own informational state as highly precise or reliable. Indeed, it is hard to see how else we might explain the occurrence of the noetic quality during a period of elevated neural entropy. So, in my view, facts about neural entropy do have explanatory relevance to facts about conscious experience, but this relevance is indirect: some extrapolation *is* required. Entropy levels underdetermine representational contents, and therefore phenomenal character.

In closing, it is worth reiterating that the approach I am proposing is not to sideline psychedelic consciousness itself in favour of a focus on its neural and cognitive underpinnings. Rather, I propose to try to *understand* the remarkable properties of the former, as described by subjects and patients, by explaining them in terms of the latter. Explanation in this context amounts neither to elimination nor to reduction (except in a weak and innocent sense of the latter; Bechtel 2006). Once again, Gerrans puts the point well:

> the type of cognitive explanation I propose does not involve ignoring personal experience and thought or explaining it away by redescribing it as something else. My aim is to show that personhood is a cognitive phenomenon constituted by the fact that personal-level phenomena such as feelings, beliefs, emotions, and desires arise at the highest levels of a cognitive processing hierarchy whose nature can be described and explained. Delusions, like many psychiatric disorders, emphasize the dependence of personal-level phenomena on the complex layers of processing that support personhood.
>
> (Gerrans 2014, pp. 3–4).

The same could be said of the remarkable states of consciousness involved in certain novel psychiatric treatments. My conviction is that attempting to explain the distinctive phenomenology of psychedelic experience in terms of underlying neurocognitive mechanisms will enhance, not replace, our understanding of the former in its own right.

5.5 Conclusion

The conclusion of Chapter 4 was that psychedelic states cause lasting benefits via some genuinely psychological aspect of the ASC that correlates with the construct of a mystical-type experience, but is somewhat independent of non-naturalistic metaphysical ideations. Alteration of self-representation is an independently plausible candidate. For one thing, the dissolution of the ego and the concomitant sense of unity are regarded by some as the cardinal, defining features of the mystical experience (Stace 1960). Moreover, altered self-awareness has repeatedly been nominated as one of the most distinctive, consistent, and theoretically significant effects of psychedelics (Watts 1964, Tagliazucchi et al. 2016). Finally, qualitative evidence of the kind we examined in Chapter 3 suggests a role for experiences of psychological insight, autobiographical reappraisal, and connectedness in the mechanisms of psychedelic therapy.

In this chapter, we turned to quantitative evidence and found further support for the conjecture that alteration of mental representations of the self is the central causal factor. Psychological evidence implicates acute insightfulness experiences and lasting elevations in mindfulness-related capacities; neuroscientific evidence implicates modulation of the DMN and SN. All of these factors have plausible links to changes in self-representation.

At this point, a question arose about how to understand the relations between these two bodies of evidence. I suggested that we can integrate neuroscientific and psychological findings about psychedelics by way of neurocognitive theory, which links neurobiology to phenomenology via the computational functions of neural structures. This means that, to understand how psychedelic therapy works, we need to know something about the cognitive properties of the neural networks that are involved: the DMN and the SN. This is the topic of Chapters 6 and 7.

6
Resetting the brain

The Brain—is wider than the Sky—
For—put them side by side—
The one the other will contain
With ease—and You—beside –

The Brain is deeper than the sea—
For—hold them—Blue to Blue—
The one the other will absorb—
As Sponges—Buckets—do—

The Brain is just the weight of God—
For—Heft them—Pound for Pound—
And they will differ—if they do—
As Syllable from Sound—

Emily Dickinson, 'The brain'.

6.1 Introduction

Psychedelic therapy involves changes to both neural and phenomenological markers of self-representation. Some have suggested that the therapeutic value of psychedelics lies in their ability to disintegrate rigid and dysfunctional patterns of connectivity in networks such as the Default Mode Network (DMN) and the Salience Network (SN). However, this *Reset Theory* of psychedelic therapy does not, on its own, illuminate the link between such neural changes and their characteristic phenomenological and behavioral correlates. In Chapter 5, I proposed that this link can be illuminated by neurocognitive theories that specify the information-processing functions of relevant neural systems. Therefore, in this chapter and the next, I will outline a neurocognitive theory of self-representation that connect these levels of explanation. This is the *predictive self-binding* account introduced by Letheby and Gerrans (2017), which promises to explain psychological facts about psychedelic therapy in terms of their neurocognitive underpinnings.

The predictive self-binding account invokes key principles from the predictive processing (PP) theory of cognition. According to PP, the brain is an inference engine that builds hierarchical models of the world and uses them to predict its future inputs. These models are updated on principles of error detection and correction.

Lower levels model more concrete perceptual features over smaller spatiotemporal scales, whereas higher levels model increasingly abstract features over larger scales. Each level attempts to predict the activity in the level below, and cognitive processing is driven by the imperative to minimise upward-flowing prediction error. On this view, conscious experience is a 'controlled hallucination'—an internal virtual reality or world-simulation created by this modelling process. However, the mental models that constitute the furniture of our experiential worlds are *transparent*, meaning that they cannot easily be recognised *as* models. Phenomenologically, it is as though self, body, and world are simply, immediately, and unquestionably present (Metzinger 2003, 2014).

Carhart-Harris and Friston (2019) have proposed a PP-based account of psychedelic action that they call the REBUS model ('RElaxed Beliefs Under pSychedelics'). According to the REBUS model, the most important and distinctive effects of psychedelics, especially at high doses, result from the weakening or relaxation of abstract, domain-general beliefs that reside toward the highest levels of the brain's hierarchical predictive models. These fundamental beliefs, or high-level *priors*, are implemented in multimodal association areas such as the cortical midline hubs of the DMN and SN. In sober waking cognition, they structure and constrain the process of probabilistic inference that generates our phenomenal models of reality. Pharmacological disruption to these networks decreases the brain's confidence in these foundational hypotheses, leading to an 'unconstrained' mode of cognition.

According to the REBUS model, the therapeutic effects of psychedelics stem from the fact that, by temporarily relaxing high-level beliefs, they afford an opportunity to revise deleterious beliefs that become rigidly entrenched in pathology. This raises the question: what specific beliefs are revised in the process of successful psychedelic therapy? The evidence surveyed in Chapter 5 suggests that beliefs about the self are the most plausible candidate. This is what the predictive self-binding account claims: that psychedelic therapy involves the temporary disintegration, and subsequent beneficial revision, of predictive models of the self. I begin the present chapter by sketching the Reset Theory, and then assemble ideas from PP and the REBUS model that can ground a neurocognitive interpretation thereof. In Chapter 7, I put these ideas to work in outlining the predictive self-binding account and showing how it can explain important facts about psychedelic therapy.

6.2 The Reset Theory

In order to understand how psychedelic therapy works, we need to know something about the cognitive (i.e., computational, or information processing) functions of the neural systems involved: the DMN and the SN. We saw in Chapter 5 that these networks have been linked to narrative and minimal/embodied forms of self-representation, respectively, and that abnormal activity and connectivity in them has been linked to symptoms of multiple psychiatric pathologies (Broyd et al. 2009, Peters et al. 2016, Sha et al. 2019).

This last point provides the impetus for a class of theories based on a simple, common idea. We can call this idea the *Reset Theory* of psychedelic therapy. It says that (i) large-scale neural networks such as the DMN and SN become stuck in rigid and dysfunctional configurations in pathology, and (ii) psychedelics are therapeutic because they disintegrate these networks, creating an opportunity to 'reset' them to a healthier configuration. We encountered a sketch of the Reset Theory in section 5.4.1: Carhart-Harris et al. (2017) explained their findings of *increased* DMN integrity after psilocybin for treatment-resistant depression by suggesting something along these lines. This echoes the earlier suggestion by this research group, in the context of the Entropic Brain Hypothesis, that inducing a transient state of neural entropy or disorder can be therapeutic because it provides an opportunity to disengage from inflexible cognitive configurations characteristic of anxiety, depression, addiction, and obsessive-compulsive disorder (Carhart-Harris et al. 2014).

A version of the Reset Theory is formulated by Nichols et al. in terms of *hub dismantling*. As we have seen, the core nodes of the networks affected by psychedelics are densely connected 'hub' regions that facilitate communication and functional integration between multiple far-flung systems throughout the brain. Nichols et al. (2017) cite evidence of changes in the activity and connectivity profiles of these hub regions across various pathologies (pp. 214–215), and echo the suggestion of Stam (2014) that *hub failure* might be a unifying, transdiagnostic marker of psychiatric pathology. This could explain the remarkable apparent transdiagnostic efficacy of psychedelics, given that their network-level target seems to be precisely the connectivity profiles of these pivotal hub regions (Müller et al. 2018b, Carhart-Harris 2019). Perhaps by dismantling pathological patterns of hub connectivity, psychedelics provide an opportunity to reset these networks into a healthier state. Nichols et al. even suggest that the mystical-type experience might be a mere 'behavioural marker' for the real, underlying therapeutic mechanism of hub dismantling:

[There has been] debate among researchers studying psychedelic-assisted therapy as to whether the therapeutic improvements seen are due to some receptor-based change in neurochemistry, or whether the transcendent/mystical/religious experience is itself the change agent. Both of these points of view may miss the mark, however, as we will argue here that the mystical or transcendent experience may actually be a behavioral marker for the underlying therapeutic mechanism of psychedelics ... following psychedelic-induced disintegration within local networks, as well as increased global interconnectivity, connections responsible for psychiatric-disorder-associated hub failures are disrupted ... as the effect of the drug wears off, networks can reconnect in 'healthy' ways, in the absence of the pathological driving force(s) that originally led to hub failure and disease.

(Nichols et al. 2017, p. 215).

The suggestion that the mystical-type experience may be a therapeutically epiphenomenal 'behavioural marker' is ambiguous. It could mean that the non-naturalistic metaphysical ideations—the 'mystical' aspects of the experience, in an intuitive sense—are therapeutically unnecessary. I defended this view in Chapter 4. Or it could mean that the experience *in toto* is therapeutically epiphenomenal, because all the *real* causal action takes place at the level of hub dismantling and network rewiring. This second interpretation merits caution. Even if we grant that psychedelic therapy is, in some sense, a matter of 'resetting the brain' and rewiring dysfunctional neural networks, it does not follow that the experience is causally irrelevant. On a naturalist view of the type that I favour, conscious experiences are real, physical events that occur within the brain and participate in causal relations, just as much as action potentials and alpha oscillations. Neuroscience is a multilevel field, and there is no principled basis on which to single out one level of scale or description as the site of all the 'real' causal action (Craver 2007).

Indeed, if the ideas that I outlined in section 5.4 are on the right track, then we must go beyond *mere* talk of hub failure and network disintegration to arrive at a satisfactory integrative account of psychedelic therapy. On their own, correlations between hub failure and pathology, between hub dismantling and mystical experience, between network rewiring and symptom reduction, are mysterious. However, a neurocognitive theory that specified the computational or information-processing functions of these systems would allow us to understand why specific changes to their activity and connectivity profiles should have distinctive phenomenological and behavioural manifestations. Correlations between such neural and psychological variables can become explanatory if we can determine which cognitive functions are ordinarily performed by the regions and networks in question, and how the performance of these functions is affected by the relevant changes to these structures.

We cannot yet answer these questions definitively. However, enough evidence exists to make some informed conjectures. In collaborative work, Philip Gerrans and I have developed a neurocognitive account of self-representation in the DMN and SN, and its alteration by psychedelics (Letheby and Gerrans 2017). This account, while speculative, is consistent with the available neural and phenomenological evidence about psychedelic experience, and promises to shed light on its lasting psychological benefits. The account invokes key tenets of the PP theory of cognition; as such, a little background is in order.

6.3 Predictive processing

PP depicts the brain as an inference engine that builds hierarchical models of the world in order to predict its future inputs. Any discrepancy between predicted and actual input generates an error signal that must be cancelled, either by updating the model or by acting in the world to alter the source of the discrepant input. The overarching imperative of the brain, on this view, is to minimise error signals by optimising its predictions of sensory inputs (Hohwy 2013, Clark 2016).

In pursuit of this aim, over a lifetime, the brain builds highly sophisticated internal models that replicate the causal structure of the extracranial world. Specifically, the predictive brain develops a *generative model*: a model[1] that recreates, or generates, a pattern of observed effects by representing the hidden causes that give rise to them (Clark 2016). In this case, the 'observed' effects are the brain's sensory (including interoceptive) inputs: the hidden causes, which the brain must model, are simply the objects, properties, and events that populate the extracranial world, including the organism's own body.

The generative model created by the brain is hierarchical, as mandated by the hierarchical causal structure of the actual world (Hohwy 2013). Lower levels model more concrete regularities at narrower spatiotemporal scales, such as basic perceptual features and objects. These are subsumed by more general or abstract regularities encoded at higher processing levels—from concrete events and situations, through (auto-) biographical narratives and social information, to unchanging fundaments such as space, time, and self. If all goes well, the result will be a detailed and relatively accurate intracranial facsimile, encoded in patterns of synaptic connectivity, of the actual structure of the world (Gładziejewski 2016)—or, at least, of the relatively narrow portion of it that is ecologically relevant to human beings.

PP inverts traditional views of perception as a process of bottom-up, feedforward feature detection. On the received view, the process of perception begins with inputs to primary sensory areas specialised for the detection of elementary features. Feature representations generated in these areas are fed forward to areas specialised for the detection of increasingly complex and abstract patterns. As information propagates up the processing hierarchy, feature representations are integrated into percepts, which are multimodally integrated into object representations, situation models, and so on, in a linear accumulation of representational complexity (Clark 2016, p. 12).

In contrast, PP holds that perception begins from the top down, with the derivation of predictions from an existing generative model. Each level in the hierarchy generates predictions of activity in the layer below. As such, the entire model conspires to generate predictions of expected sensory inputs. (Like a Quinean web of belief, the hierarchical generative model makes direct contact with the empirical world only at the periphery.) Any successfully predicted signals are 'cancelled out' and travel no further up the hierarchy. Andy Clark (2016) likens the arrangement to a hierarchical corporation in which busy superiors instruct their juniors: 'Only tell me the news!' Only the unexpected commands valuable bandwidth. The brain endeavors to stay one step ahead of the world and stem the tide of prediction error so thoroughly that sensory surprises are almost eliminated. It is important to note that the process of error-driven

---

[1] For present purposes, the term 'model', in the context of PP, can be treated as synonymous with the term 'mental representation' as I defined it in section 5.4.

model updating happens rapidly and largely outside conscious awareness. In general, our experience is populated by the outputs of this modelling process, not by the process itself.

With its top-down, internalist vision of perception, PP has the startling consequence that conscious experience is little more than a 'controlled hallucination'. The contents of our phenomenal awareness are simply a subset of the contents of the generative model assigned the highest probability by the brain based on its total inputs to date. Conscious experience is sometimes described as 'transparent', meaning that it does not wear its representational or simulatory nature on its sleeve. In ordinary waking life, it does not seem to us as though our experience is comprised of generative models, virtual simulations, or intracranial mental constructions. Rather, it seems that the world itself in all its glory, with our own bodies and minds at the centre of everything, is simply, immediately, and unquestionably present. To say that consciousness is transparent, in this sense, is to say that we do not experience our mental models of the world *as* models: it is as though we look 'through' them and see only the world itself. This property of *phenomenal transparency* has been defined in many different ways; here, I adopt the following simple definition given by Thomas Metzinger:[2]

> 'Transparency' refers to a property of conscious representations, namely, that *they are not experienced as representations*. Therefore, the subject of experience feels as if [they are] in direct and immediate contact with [the] content [of the representations]. Transparent conscious representations create the phenomenology of naïve realism. An opaque phenomenal representation is one that is experienced as a representation, for example, in ... lucid dreams.
>
> **(Metzinger 2014, p. 123).**

According to PP and related views, this transparency is profoundly misleading (Metzinger 2003, Revonsuo 2006). All the furniture of our waking experience—the people, animals, plants, tables, chairs, and our own bodies and selves—is as thoroughly virtual, internally constructed, and simulatory as the fantastic creations of nocturnal dreams and psychotic hallucinations. The main difference is that, in normal waking consciousness, the contents of the models that populate consciousness are strongly constrained (hence '*controlled* hallucination') by complex streams of multimodal sensory inputs from the actual extracranial world. (PP as a theory of cognition only makes sense on the assumption that there *is* an external world whose structure the brain must track in order to guide adaptive behaviour.)

---

[2] Here I remain neutral on other, related claims, such as Metzinger's contention that the phenomenal feature of transparency results from the attentional or introspective unavailability of the earlier processing stages in which conscious representations are constructed. Such claims are, strictly speaking, distinct from the mere definition of transparent phenomenal representations as *phenomenal representations not experienced* as *representations*.

Thus, in the usual course of things, our models approximate the structure of this world well enough for practical purposes. The point, however, is that the experiential contents of veridical waking perception and the experiential contents of dreams and hallucinations are ontologically equivalent, and result from the same basic mechanism: the intracranial, inferential construction of a virtual, phenomenal model of reality. The core difference consists in modulations to the processing that determines the contents of those models—but in either case, an internal model is an internal model is an internal model. As Metzinger puts it:

> Phenomenal experience during the waking state is an online hallucination ... Phenomenal experience during the dream state, however, is just a complex offline hallucination ... the human brain [can be viewed] as a system that constantly simulates possible realities ... a fruitful way of looking at the human brain, therefore, is as a system which, even in ordinary waking states, constantly hallucinates at the world, as a system that constantly lets its internal autonomous simulational dynamics collide with the ongoing flow of sensory input, vigorously dreaming at the world and thereby generating the content of phenomenal experience.
>
> (Metzinger 2003, pp. 51–52).

The transparency noted above arises partly from the fact that our conscious reality-models or world-simulations inherit a high degree of structure, coherence, and volition-independence from the actual world that they seek to emulate. As Antti Revonsuo (2006) puts it, our brains give us a thoroughly realistic and convincing 'out-of-brain experience': an experience as of simply being immediately present in a real, objective, extracranial world. The simulatory nature of our conscious reality is difficult to take seriously, other than as a merely intellectual proposition. Most of the time we cannot easily regard the constituents of our experiential worlds as virtual entities, or as products of a modelling process. Phenomenologically speaking, they simply appear as reality, and we automatically regard them as such: transparency in action.

Occasionally, however, this transparency is undermined by glitches in the neurocognitive Matrix: stubborn and startling perceptual illusions that expose the constructed and probabilistic nature of experience. One example is the Hollow Mask Illusion, in which a mask of a human face, presented in the concave orientation, is nonetheless perceived as convex (Hill and Bruce 1993). The assumption that human faces are always convex is assigned such a high probability by the brain that it simply overrides any apparent sensory evidence to the contrary. Conflicting inputs are dismissed as unreliable noise, and the perceptual model settled on by the brain represents the object in a manner that we know, intellectually, to be inaccurate. In such cases, it becomes obvious that the contents of experience are determined by a fallible sub-personal process of probabilistic inference. Our phenomenal representations become somewhat opaque: we can, unusually, experience them *as* representations—at least to an extent. (Perceptually, of course, the illusion persists, despite our metacognitive awareness of its true nature.)

The example of the Hollow Mask Illusion illustrates another central aspect of the PP scheme: the process of error-driven model updating requires the brain to estimate the relative *reliability* of both its prior expectations and its various input channels.[3] In the Hollow Mask case, the prior assumption that faces are convex is assigned such a high probability that it outweighs sensory evidence to the contrary. Such evidence, no matter how persistent, is never deemed sufficiently trustworthy by the brain to over-ride such a well-confirmed prior belief. Indeed, the sensory evidence is deemed un-trustworthy precisely *because* it conflicts with such a deeply entrenched assumption. In such cases, sub-personal mechanisms in the predictive brain engage in something analogous to David Hume's refusal to countenance reports of miracles *qua* violations of natural law, on the grounds that our evidence for the inviolability of natural laws is sufficiently strong to outweigh any possible testimonial evidence for their violation.

The same principle can be seen at work in the phenomenon of binocular rivalry. When a different stimulus is presented to each half of a subject's visual field—say, a face to the left half, and a house to the right—we might expect the subject to perceive a mish-mash of a face and a house, reflecting the actual pattern of retinal stimula-tion. Instead, subjects alternate between seeing only a face and only a house, with brief periods of 'mixed percept' in between. The PP explanation is that the generative model maintained by the typical human brain harbors a deep-seated assumption that distinct objects never occupy the same spatial position. As such, a perceptual model positing only a house, or only a face, will always be deemed more probable than one positing a co-located house-face. But, whichever model is settled on, the conflicting input will generate high volumes of prediction error, forcing a revision. In other words, while the brain has 'decided' that there is only a house, the face-related input will generate an error signal, and vice versa: hence the alternation (Hohwy et al. 2008).

According to PP, then, evidence inconsistent with a sufficiently well-confirmed or deeply entrenched model will simply be filtered out by the brain, dismissed as noise. This leads to a crucial aspect of the PP story: as Andy Clark puts it, prior knowledge in the predictive brain is 'always both constraining and enabling' (2016, p. 288). Prior knowledge is enabling because, without predictive models, we could not perceive anything at all. Models are needed to extract the signal from the noise of our sparse and ambiguous sensory inputs, to impose coherence and structure on what would otherwise be a buzzing, blooming confusion. It is a familiar but remarkable fact that we can effortlessly recognise most instances of the letter 'A' as instances of the same category, or tokens of the same type, despite large variations in handwriting, lighting conditions, and so forth. Likewise, we can recognise the same person from multiple perspectives, in multiple modalities, across extensive changes in appearance and be-haviour. All this is possible thanks to predictive models that carve away inessential detail to extract the essential, latching onto the higher-order invariant patterns that unify instances of a category.

---

[3] Technically, these estimates of reliability are known as 'precision expectations', and are central to the PP account of attention (Hohwy 2013).

Nonetheless, extracting the essential requires dismissing and ignoring the (deemed-to-be) inessential, and this is where predictive models can carry epistemic costs as well as benefits. In the examples given above, unconscious prior beliefs that play vital roles in generating accurate reality-models can be seen, under ecologically anomalous conditions, to impede veridical perception. In these specific cases, the consequences are not too dire: the relevant situations are low-stakes, and we are able to deploy theoretical knowledge to generate accurate propositional judgements about the true states of affairs—albeit the process of perceptual inference itself remains unaffected. In other situations, however, the constraining influence of prior knowledge can cause more serious harms—psychological, social, and even epistemic. As such, weakening its constraining influence can have corresponding benefits.

6.4 Relaxed beliefs under psychedelics

The hierarchical structure of the generative model posited by PP mirrors known facts about the functional anatomy of the cortex. Lower-level regions nearer the periphery are specialised for more concrete and modality-specific processing, while higher-level supramodal areas perform more abstract, domain-general, and integrative functions.

The networks modulated in psychedelic therapy, such as the DMN and SN, lie towards the top end of this hierarchy. The cortical midline hubs of these networks are high-level multimodal 'association' areas rich in the 5-HT2A receptors that are psychedelics' primary molecular target (Carhart-Harris et al. 2014). According to Carhart-Harris and Friston (2019), while disruption at lower levels may play a role, it is disruption to these high-level networks that explains the most distinctive and important effects of psychedelics.

In a recent review, Carhart-Harris (2019) outlines a multilevel account of how psychedelics work in the brain: they bind to 5-HT2A receptors, which are densely expressed in high-level cortical networks, especially on layer V pyramidal cells. By activating these receptors, they induce an irregular or asynchronous mode of glutamate release in the relevant cells, causing them to 'spike' (generate action potentials) more erratically. The net, macroscopic effect of this is to weaken the power of synchronous neuronal oscillations across multiple frequency bands, but especially in low frequencies such as the alpha rhythm. This broadband decrease in oscillatory power (Muthukumaraswamy et al. 2013) leads to three neural signatures of psychedelics. The first two are *disintegration* and *desegregation* of resting-state networks: reductions in functional connectivity within networks, and increases in functional connectivity between networks, blurring the boundaries between usually distinct systems. The third is *entropic brain activity*—an increase in the randomness, disorderliness, or unpredictability of brain activity[4] (Carhart-Harris et al. 2014).

---

[4] Interestingly, a recent study found that various meditation practices, but especially Buddhist Vipassana, also increase entropic brain activity (Vivot et al. 2020).

The obvious question is: why should this 'cascade of neurobiological changes' (Carhart-Harris et al. 2014, p. 16) manifest phenomenologically as experiences of ego dissolution, strange visions, intense emotions, and insights? According to the view outlined in section 5.4, it is because some of these neurobiological changes also constitute specific neuro*cognitive* changes—i.e., changes to neurally implemented computational processes that generate and transform phenomenally conscious mental representations. So, the question becomes: which physiological processes are at issue, and what cognitive functions do they implement?

On the PP scheme, the networks targeted by psychedelics implement the highest levels of the brain's generative model. This is to say that, among other things, they encode our most abstract, fundamental beliefs about self and world—our bedrock, largely unconscious, domain-general assumptions concerning space, time, and causality, the laws of logic, and the existence of the self. Philosophers have repeatedly noted the existence and significance of these foundational beliefs. Riding roughshod over important subtleties, we might liken them to Kantian categories, to Wittgensteinian 'hinge' or 'framework' propositions, to the constituents of a Kuhnian paradigm, or to the central nodes of a Quinean web of belief. In ordinary cognition, these 'hyperpriors' play a crucial role in constraining the brain's hypothesis space, drastically limiting the kinds of world-models that it can generate, and thereby making the process of probabilistic inference computationally tractable (Swanson 2016).

According to the REBUS model ('RElaxed Beliefs Under pSychedelics') proposed by Carhart-Harris and Friston (2019), low-frequency neuronal oscillations in high-level cortical networks have the cognitive function of encoding high-level *priors* (i.e., prior beliefs) of this kind. As such, the basic cognitive effect of psychedelic-induced neuronal desynchronisation and network disintegration is to reduce the brain's confidence in these fundamental beliefs—to 'relax' the beliefs by decreasing their *precision weighting*, in the jargon. Carhart-Harris and Friston suggest that 'this straightforward model can account for the full breadth of subjective phenomena associated with the psychedelic experience' (2019, p. 319). Given the picture of conscious experience outlined in section 6.3—that it is a controlled hallucination or virtual reality whose content is fixed by the brain's probabilistic models—relaxation of high-level beliefs certainly offers compelling explanations of many psychedelic phenomena.

Nowhere is this clearer than when it comes to the mystical-type experience. The standard criteria for a 'complete' mystical-type experience read like a checklist of negated framework propositions. The *transcendence of time and space* is self-explanatory. *Paradoxicality* might result from weakening something functionally akin to the law of non-contradiction. The senses of *internal and external unity* plausibly result from a weakening of the assumption that the self exists as an entity distinct from the rest of the world (much more on this shortly).

Interestingly, the *noetic quality*—the feeling of certainty or direct knowledge—might also result from a weakening of the sense of separate selfhood. The idea here is that the sense of being an entity distinct from the object of knowledge is a prerequisite for conceiving of the possibility of error: with no sense of a distinct knowing subject, there is no sense of a fallible epistemic connection between that subject and a distinct object of potential knowledge. Hence, doubt is inconceivable. This principle is illustrated clearly by Michael Pollan's report of his 5-MeO-DMT experience, which we encountered in Chapter 3:

> I felt a tremendous rush of energy fill my head ... and then ... 'I' was no more, blasted to a confetti cloud by an explosive force. I could no longer locate [myself] in my head, because it had exploded that too, expanding to become all that there was. Whatever this was, *it was not a hallucination. A hallucination implies a reality and a point of reference and an entity to have it. None of those things remained.*
> **(Pollan 2018, pp. 276–277; my emphasis).**[5]

From the standpoint of the REBUS model and the controlled hallucination view of phenomenal consciousness, the significance of this report is as follows: to experience a mental state *as* a hallucination requires the experience as of being an entity standing in (fallible) representational and epistemic relations of truth and error, accuracy and inaccuracy, to a world external to itself. This corresponds to what Metzinger (2003) calls the 'Phenomenal model of the intentionality relation' (PMIR). Pollan's inability to conceive of his experience as hallucinatory, and the noetic quality, can both be explained by the absence of the phenomenal self-model (PSM) and concomitant PMIR. It is because such experiences lack the seemingly ubiquitous, transparent sense of being an experiencing, knowing entity—a 'point of reference' on reality—that those who undergo them cannot readily conceptualise them as hallucinatory.

Alleged *ineffability* might not result directly from the relaxation of high-level priors, but simply from the fact that human languages have evolved to communicate representational content generated in the ordinary waking state, content consistent with the beliefs that psychedelics undermine. As such, no language has the words, or perhaps even the structure, for the sorts of mental contents inconsistent with those beliefs that emerge when their influence is diminished.[6] The *sense of sacredness* and *deeply felt positive mood* are a little less straightforward, but it seems likely that a relevantly similar story could be told.

Thus, there is a noteworthy correspondence between defining phenomenological features of the mystical-type experience and (the negations of) the sorts of abstract beliefs that have been proposed independently as the bedrock of the standard-issue human reality-model. Moreover, increasing evidence suggests that psychedelics disrupt precisely the neural networks that encode those beliefs, according to the PP scheme. In light of these facts, the case for a naturalistic view of the psychedelic

---

[5] Incidentally, when Pollan filled out the MEQ, he found that this experience scored above the threshold for a 'complete' mystical-type experience. However, this led him to conclude that the MEQ was a 'poor net' for capturing the experience (Pollan 2018, pp. 283–284).

[6] This might also form part of the explanation of paradoxicality: Perhaps the inapplicability of ordinary language to the relevant kinds of representational contents results in an unavoidable sense of ambiguity regarding whether certain terms apply correctly or not.

experience looks quite persuasive. If key tenets of PP, such as the hierarchical structure of the brain's generative model and the controlled hallucination view of consciousness, were true, mystical-type phenomenology is *exactly the sort of thing* one should expect to result from the disintegration of high-level cortical networks. This can be construed as a naturalistic error theory of psychedelic mysticism: it explains why we should expect psychedelics to induce vivid experiences as of a cosmic consciousness, even if no such thing existed. In light of this, positing an actual cosmic consciousness to explain such experiences seems superfluous, and a naturalistic explanation more parsimonious. (We might wonder why such experiences so often seem to involve a cosmic *consciousness*, specifically, rather than simply a cosmic unity. I will return to this question in Chapter 7).

Meanwhile, when we shift our focus to the other varieties of psychedelic experience, we can see why high-level priors should constrain cognition, and relaxing them unconstrain it. The abstract beliefs disrupted by psychedelics constrain cognition in several ways. Most basically, as we have seen, they limit the brain's hypothesis space. While these foundational assumptions are deeply entrenched, the sub-personal process of probabilistic inference will never settle on a model of a spaceless, timeless, selfless, unitive world. It will never settle on a model of a world in which distinct objects stably occupy the same spatial position, or human faces are concave. And it will never settle on a model of a world in which walls 'breathe' or undulate, fractal patterns overlay the surfaces of objects, plant spirits communicate telepathically, humans shrink to the size of a thumbnail, or writhing multicoloured snakes emerge from the carpet. Hyperpriors constrain cognition by deeming many logically possible (and, indeed, logically impossible) worlds so improbable that they become cognitively and phenomenologically impossible. By diminishing the brain's confidence in its foundational axioms, psychedelics expand the phenomenological possibility space (cf. Metzinger 2003, 2011).

6.5 Resetting beliefs under psychedelics

According to the REBUS model, psychedelics alter consciousness by disintegrating high-level cortical networks, thereby decreasing the precision-weighting of domain-general high-level priors. This weakens the constraining influence of those priors on the process of probabilistic inference, thereby expanding the space of phenomenologically possible worlds. We have seen, in brief outline, how this model might explain some key phenomenological features of the psychedelic state. But what does it have to tell us about the therapeutic mechanisms of psychedelics?

A simple answer would be that the pathologies for which psychedelics show therapeutic promise are characterised by *deleterious high-level beliefs*, and undermining the brain's confidence in those beliefs, by pharmacologically disrupting their neural substrates, creates an opportunity to revise them for the better. This would amount to a neurocognitive version of the Reset Theory, which identifies the cognitive process implemented by the relevant networks as the encoding of high-level beliefs, and the cognitive process implemented by the disintegration and 'resetting' of those networks as the relaxation and revision of those beliefs. This is precisely what Carhart-Harris and Friston propose:

> With regard to their potential therapeutic use, we propose that psychedelics work to relax the precision weighting of pathologically overweighted priors underpinning various expressions of mental illness. We propose that this process entails an increased sensitization of high-level priors to bottom-up signaling ... and that this heightened sensitivity enables the potential revision and deweighting of overweighted priors.

> **(2019, pp. 316–317).**

This raises the question: which specific priors are revised in the process of successful psychedelic therapy? It cannot be metaphysical beliefs about the ultimate nature of reality, or about the existence or non-existence of a divinity: as we saw in Chapter 4, successful psychedelic therapy can occur without any change in such beliefs. Moreover, several other classes of high-level beliefs disrupted by psychedelics seem like poor candidates. It is hardly plausible, for instance, that patients' mental health is improved by adopting new beliefs about the nature of space and time, or by rejecting the law of non-contradiction.[7]

However, there is one class of beliefs that constitutes an eminently plausible candidate: beliefs about the self. The weakening or dissolution of ego boundaries is a central aspect of the psychedelic state that has repeatedly been singled out as distinctive and theoretically significant, and that unifies non-naturalistic cosmic consciousness experiences with more naturalistic 'mystical-type' experiences of connectedness, wonder, and awe. Moreover, as we saw in Chapter 5, both neuroscientific and psychological evidence implicates changes to self-representation in the mechanisms of psychedelic therapy.

Letheby and Gerrans (2017) propose a neurocognitive account of self-representation in the predictive brain, its disruption by psychedelics, and the potential therapeutic effects thereof. This *predictive self-binding* theory can be viewed as a special case of the REBUS model. Like the REBUS model, it holds that signature phenomenological effects of psychedelics result from the relaxation of high-level priors via the disintegration of high-level cortical networks that implement those priors. Moreover, it holds that psychedelic therapy works because this transient belief relaxation provides an opportunity to revise those beliefs for the better.

The further, distinctive emphases of the predictive self-binding account include:

(i) the idea that the DMN and the SN encode distinct layers of a hierarchical predictive self-model;

---

[7] I know of no evidence that dialetheists are, on average, more mentally healthy than monoletheists.

(ii) the idea that this model plays a cognitive *binding* function, integrating information across modalities and levels of processing, by positing the existence of a simple, indivisible, and enduring entity; and

(iii) the idea that this model functions as a *centre of representational gravity*, governing and constraining the construction of our world-models by allocating salience, attention, and processing resources in accordance with the hypothesised goals and interests of the self.

Equipped with conceptual tools from our discussion of PP and the REBUS model, in Chapter 7, I will outline the predictive self-binding theory and its picture of how psychedelic therapy works.

7
Unbinding the self

An eminent philosopher among my friends, who can dignify even your ugly furniture by lifting it into the serene light of science, has shown me this pregnant little fact. Your pierglass or extensive surface of polished steel made to be rubbed by a housemaid, will be minutely and multitudinously scratched in all directions; but place now against it a lighted candle as a centre of illumination, and lo! the scratches will seem to arrange themselves in a fine series of concentric circles round that little sun. It is demonstrable that the scratches are going everywhere impartially, and it is only your candle which produces the flattering illusion of a concentric arrangement, its light falling with an exclusive optical selection. These things are a parable. The scratches are events, and the candle is the egoism of any person . . .

George Eliot, *Middlemarch* .

7.1 Introduction

Many psychiatric disorders feature deleterious changes to self-related beliefs, and many treatments aim at 'resetting' these beliefs—at changing them for the better (Zhao et al. 2013, Moutoussis et al. 2014, Sui and Gu 2017). This is very difficult to do, however, when the beliefs themselves are heavily weighted, or assigned high prior probabilities, by the brain, and thus recalcitrant in the face of counter-evidence. The difficulty is exacerbated by the fact that high-level self-related beliefs typically exhibit the feature of phenomenal transparency introduced in Chapter 6: they do not manifest in the patient's experience *as* beliefs, models, or representations, but simply as reality itself. Phenomenologically speaking, the interpersonal world simply *is* threatening, or the self simply *is* powerless: they are not (merely) *believed* to be so. Even when this transparency breaks to an extent, and these beliefs are recognised as such intellectually, they typically continue to exert representational dominance, filtering incoming information and determining what permeates our conscious reality-models.

By disrupting the neurocognitive substrates of the brain's high-level beliefs, psychedelics can change this situation transiently but dramatically. They diminish the brain's confidence in its deepest assumptions about reality, including about the self, and thereby weaken the influence of those beliefs on the contents of the phenomenal world. This has two important effects. First, subjects experience new phenomenal worlds inconsistent with, and previously precluded by, those beliefs. Second, as a corollary, the beliefs themselves become phenomenally *opaque* as their representational nature becomes vividly apparent. Through radically altered forms of self-experience, subjects discover the contingency, mutability, and simulatory nature of their own sense of identity and habitual modes of attention. They learn directly that there are other ways of being, and other ways of seeing, because their ordinary ways of being and seeing result from a malleable modelling process.

In this chapter, I sketch a speculative account of psychedelic therapy along these lines. On a neural level, psychedelic therapy involves transient network disintegration and subsequent 're-wiring'. On a cognitive level, it involves decreasing the precision-weighting of high-level priors, especially concerning the self, facilitating revision of those priors. According to Letheby and Gerrans (2017), predictive self-models—priors concerning the self—perform a cognitive *binding* function: they integrate information across multiple modalities and levels of processing into a representation of a unified subject of experience. Hubs of the Salience Network (SN) integrate bodily and affective information into a model of a momentary subject of experience (i.e., the minimal self), while hubs of the Default Mode Network (DMN) situate this information in an autobiographical context, creating a story of a persisting protagonist (i.e., the narrative self). The 'self-binding' function of these systems parses the world into 'me' and 'not-me' and filters incoming information for self-relevance, attributing salience and allocating attention in accordance with the goals and interests of the hypothesised self. Hence, disruption to this function permits re-evaluation of basic assumptions concerning the properties and relations of the self. On a phenomenological level, this leads to changes in 'existential feelings' (Ratcliffe 2005): the pervasive but elusive background sense, rooted in bodily awareness, of one's orientation to the world and the possibilities it affords. Many candidate psychological mechanisms of psychedelic therapy—including connectedness, acceptance, awe, emotional breakthrough, psychological insight, and enhanced meaning—can be subsumed by this general account of (i) disrupted self-binding leading to (ii) altered existential feelings. The common denominator is unbinding and revising predictive models of the experiencing subject and its relations to various aspects of the internal and external worlds.

The upshot is a two-factor theory of psychedelic therapy. The induction of neural, cognitive, and phenomenological plasticity, via multiple pathways, may be necessary but is not sufficient for long-term benefit. In line with Thomas Kuhn's (1970) account of scientific paradigm shifts, it is not enough merely to undermine a dysfunctional self-model for a spell: for durable change to result, new forms of self-modelling must be discovered during the acute experience and consolidated during the subsequent period of integration.

I conclude the chapter with some brief remarks on philosophical questions about self and self-consciousness. The self-binding account might seem to license two controversial claims: that there can be states of phenomenal consciousness totally lacking self-consciousness, and that the self does not exist. I have defended both claims elsewhere (Letheby 2020, Letheby and Gerrans 2017), but neither follows straightforwardly from the evidence, and the very real difficulties must be acknowledged. For present purposes, we can content ourselves with two weaker, but still extremely interesting, claims: (i) There can be states of consciousness lacking anything like the *ordinary* sense of self, and (ii) the *kind* of self that we ordinarily seem to be does not exist. Theoretically and existentially, this is plenty to be getting on with.

The structure of the chapter is as follows. The first three sections are devoted to outlining the predictive self-binding account of self-representation (sections 7.2, 7.3, and 7.4). The next three sections are devoted to showing how this account can explain important facts about psychedelic therapy: its beneficial effects on symptomatology and personality (sections 7.5 and 7.7), and some of the non-naturalistic metaphysical ideations that it can promote (section 7.6). One section is devoted to philosophical issues concerning self and self-consciousness (section 7.8), and a final section to summarising the discussion (section 7.9).

7.2 Predictive self-binding

In its quest to minimise prediction error, the brain builds complex hierarchical models of the world. These models must account for regularities at multiple scales and levels of abstraction. Like scientific theories, they need to latch onto the genuine, projectible patterns in past observations in order to generate accurate future predictions. And like successful scientific theories, they achieve this predictive feat by *going beyond the evidence*: by positing unobservable hidden causes whose existence would account for the relevant regularities (Yon et al. 2019).

One crucial inferential leap that the predictive brain makes is to the existence of a world of substantial objects. This leap is underdetermined by the evidence, as intractable philosophical disputes attest: our total sensory evidence is consistent with any number of metaphysical schemes, including bundle theories, varieties of nominalism, and processual and structuralist ontologies. But, whatever our reflective convictions, the sub-personal mechanisms that conjure our phenomenal worlds are congenital substantialists. Watching a gull glide over the ocean, we do not experience a free-floating mishmash of properties and parts—whiteness, wings, location, motion, and so forth—but a coherent, unified object that bears these properties and persists through time. This is remarkable given that these different properties are processed in distinct cortical regions. The question of how the brain integrates them into coherent object representations is known as the 'binding problem' and is a major unresolved issue in the philosophy and science of consciousness (Revonsuo 1999). The existence of binding mechanisms is demonstrated by their failure in pathological and experimental conditions—for example, a subject presented briefly with a blue circle and a red square might report perceiving a red circle and a blue square (Burwick 2014).

The predictive processing (PP) framework offers an elegant solution to the binding problem via its top-down inversion of the process of perception. PP holds that the process begins with the issuing of predictions by a pre-existing generative model. When inputs are accurately predicted, the feedforward signal is 'cancelled out' and propagates no further up the hierarchy. The predictively successful model is reinforced. Only error signals resulting from unpredicted inputs demand a response.

The relevance to the binding problem is this: on PP, the brain does not start with separate property representations and face the problem of subsequently recombining them correctly (e.g., binding the whiteness to the gull and the blueness to the ocean, rather than vice versa). Rather, the process of perception begins with a rich and complex set of top-down expectations issuing from models that *already* populate the world with objects bearing properties, standing in relations, and persisting through changes. Such models are assigned high prior probabilities because of their past predictive success. Assuming such an ontology is an efficient strategy for prediction error minimisation. Regardless of the actual metaphysics of the world, postulating particulars is a parsimonious way to track regularities in complex and noisy streams of sensory input. In effect, a substantialist ontology is a data compression strategy. As Hohwy puts it:

> The binding problem is … dealt with by default: the system assumes bound attributes and then predicts them down through the cortical hierarchy … This as it were turns the binding problem inside out because bound percepts are predicted and evidence sought in the input that will confirm the prediction.
>
> **(Hohwy 2013, p. 103).**

To the extent that evidence from the input confirms the prediction—that the relevant properties do systematically co-occur—the model is reinforced. On this view, 'binding is inference' (Hohwy 2013, p. 103)—specifically, *abductive* inference, or inference to the best explanation. The analogy with scientific theorising is illustrative: just as the theoretician populates the unobservable world with entities bearing properties, and derives observational predictions from this ontology, so too does the predictive brain populate the 'hidden' extracranial world with substantial objects and thereby derive expectations of future sensory inputs.

A key difference, of course, is that the brain's error-minimising posits become the very stuff of our phenomenal worlds—the tables, chairs, people, birds, and trees that we encounter in everyday experience. No wonder the Ship of Theseus still evokes puzzlement, after millennia: the substantialist ontology simulated by the predictive brain gives us the irresistible feeling that there is some underlying object that is *the* original ship, and a corresponding fact of the matter as to whether *that very object* remains after gradual, piecemeal, wholesale change (cf. Metzinger 2011). Of course, as Derek Parfit (1984) pointed out, this intuition is even more compelling, but every bit as questionable, when it comes to that axiologically central but ontologically elusive entity that we call 'I'.

According to Letheby and Gerrans (2017), this symmetry is no accident, but stems from a deep symmetry between self-representation and object-representation in the predictive brain. Just as sub-personal mechanisms minimise prediction error by modelling the existence of substantial entities in the extra-organismic world, so too do they minimise prediction error by modelling the existence of a substantial entity in the intra-organismic world: the self. As Hohwy and Michael (2017) point out, one of the major sources of inputs to the brain is the organism itself. Innumerable streams of interoceptive and proprioceptive input require prediction and regulation, and, at higher levels, abstract correspondences between internal and external variables demand explanation—as when thirst causes muscle contractions resulting in distinctive patterns of visual, proprioceptive, and gustatory feedback, or when the auditory perception of a threatening yell modulates levels of cortisol, adrenaline, and blood pressure. An efficient way to track these complex regularities is to attribute them to the actions and fluctuating fortunes of a single underlying entity—a simple and unitary particular that persists across changes in its properties.

On this view, predictive self-modelling is just another instance of a ubiquitous cognitive binding strategy. The brain needs to track stably co-instantiated collections of properties by integrating representations of those properties into unified object representations. On PP, this integration is achieved via the top-down postulation of particulars: substantial objects that bear properties and persist through time. Likewise, self-representation is a matter of integrating information across modalities, time-scales, and levels of processing into a unified representation of a simple and persisting entity—in this case, the subject of experience, the author of actions, the one to whom it all happens. Binding is a matter not just of integration, but of *segregation*: it is a process of parsing or segmenting the world into distinct objects and distinguishing them from each other by the attribution of properties. Binding makes boundaries. Likewise, *self-binding* (Sui and Humphreys 2015, Letheby and Gerrans 2017) is a matter of parsing and segmentation along the lines of a primordial division: subject and object, self and world, I and it. Metzinger speaks of the 'phenomenal unit of identification' (2013b, p. 5): the sub-section of the total phenomenal field that the brain represents or tags as being 'me', and which we therefore experience ourselves, quite simply, as *being*. In our terms, this is the sub-section of the phenomenal field whose contents are determined by representations bound to the self-model.

The basic idea of Letheby and Gerrans (2017) is that we can explain key features of self-awareness and its psychedelic disruption by integrating (i) the work of Sui and Humphreys (2015) on self-binding with (ii) the PP account of binding as top-down abductive inference. Sui and Humphreys review evidence that cognitive binding processes are enhanced at all levels, from basic perceptual processing through to higher cognition, for information deemed self-relevant. They suggest that this integrative advantage for self-relevant information is best explained by the existence of a 'core self-representation' implemented in cortical midline structures, including nodes of the DMN and SN, that is accessed rapidly in most cognitive tasks and unifies the otherwise disparate varieties of self-representation. Stimuli deemed as relevant to, belonging to, or constituting 'me' are integrated or bound into a model of a unified and persisting entity—a model that must represent not only the entity itself but also its various properties and relations. PP provides a cognitive account of how this self-binding process is performed: the core self-representation posited by Sui and Humphreys is a hierarchical model of a unified entity underlying the flow of experience, and the top-down attribution of properties and relations to this entity binds self-relevant information across domains and levels of processing.

At the end of Chapter 6, I said that the predictive self-binding account has three distinct emphases, over and above the general principles embodied in the REBUS model (RElaxed Beliefs Under pSychedelics) of Carhart-Harris and Friston (2019):

(i)   the idea that the DMN and the SN encode distinct layers of a hierarchical predictive self-model;

(ii) the idea that this model plays a cognitive *binding* function, integrating information across modalities and levels of processing, by positing the existence of a simple, indivisible and enduring entity; and

(iii) the idea that this model functions as a *centre of representational gravity*, governing and constraining the construction of our world-models by allocating salience, attention, and processing resources in accordance with the hypothesised goals and interests of the self.

In the present section, we have examined the second of these three features: the cognitive binding function of the self-model. We turn now to the first, which concerns the hierarchical structure of the self-model and its neural implementation.

7.3 Selfhood embodied and (temporally) extended

The view I have just outlined can readily explain the respective association of the SN and the DMN with minimal and narrative forms of self-awareness. As I have emphasised, the predictive brain needs to track the internal world, like the external world, at multiple spatiotemporal scales and levels of abstraction. One fundamental aspect of phenomenal selfhood is 'spatiotemporal self-location': the sense of occupying a particular point in space at a particular point in time. In ordinary waking consciousness, the relevant point in space is usually within the physical boundaries of the organism (Blanke and Metzinger 2009).

However, we do not merely experience ourselves as located *within* our bodies. We also have the *experience of body ownership* (EBO): the pre-reflective, unquestioned sense that 'this is *my* body'. Like many aspects of self-awareness, the EBO can be introspectively elusive, but its existence is revealed by conditions in which it is absent or altered, such as pathologies or ingenious experimental manipulations. In depersonalisation disorder (DPD), patients sometimes report a global loss of the EBO (Sierra and David 2011). Meanwhile, in the rubber hand illusion (Costantini and Haggard 2007), a carefully calibrated combination of visual and tactile feedback tricks the predictive brain into inferring that a visually perceived rubber hand is part of the subject's own body, resulting in a striking local alteration to this experience.

Anil Seth (2013) has argued from a PP standpoint that aspects of the minimal self, notably the EBO, depend on computational processes implemented in the anterior insular cortex (AIC), a core node of the SN. As we saw in Chapter 5, the AIC has been implicated in many different functions, including interoception, empathy, nociception (i.e., pain perception), and conscious emotional feelings. The idea of a link between interoception and emotion was given influential articulation in the nineteenth century by James and Lange, and has been revitalised in the context of modern cognitive neuroscience by the work of Antonio Damasio (1994, 1999). In philosophy, one recent exponent of an interoceptive theory of emotion is Jesse Prinz. Prinz (2004) argues that specific bodily states—'somatic markers', in Damasio's parlance—have the evolved function of signalling the presence of *core relational themes* (Lazarus 1991). In other words, specific internal bodily states have been 'set up [by evolution] to be set off by' the perceived occurrence of adaptively relevant situation-types, such as the presence of danger, the suffering of an irrevocable loss, or the attainment of progress towards a valued goal.

One challenge for bodily theories of emotion is the lack of a simple one-to-one mapping between bodily states and emotions (or emotional feelings). For instance, increased arousal might be experienced as anxiety or elation, depending on the context (Schachter and Singer 1962). Therefore, some computational process beyond the mere representation of bodily state is required to generate the emotions we experience. Seth identifies this process with top-down probabilistic modelling in the AIC that explains interoceptive changes in terms of core relational themes. Evidence suggests that the posterior insular cortex (PIC) generates a 'primary interoceptive image of homeostatic afferents' (Craig 2002, p. 660)—in other words, a purely descriptive read-out of changes to the internal physiological milieu (Gerrans 2019). What transforms such interoceptive representations into the feelings that populate our emotional lives? Interpreting existing theoretical ideas in PP terms, Seth proposes that what does the trick is top-down abductive inference that models the hidden causes of these changing bodily states: namely, core relational themes. Mere elevated arousal, registered by the PIC, is transformed into anxiety or elation when it is represented by the AIC (in communication with multiple other systems) as caused by possible danger or present reward, respectively.

The phenomenology of DPD suggests a deep link between affect and the sense of self (cf. Damasio 1999) and this, too, is explicable on Seth's hypothesis. If the AIC interprets interoceptive changes as signals of core *relational* themes, then the conclusion seems inescapable: relations require relata. If danger is present, it must be danger to someone; an opportunity must be an opportunity for someone; and so forth. DPD patients, who often display hypoactivity in the AIC, have not lost the ability to interpret bodily states as signals of importance or relevance simpliciter, but as signals of importance or relevance *to someone* (Gerrans 2015). This is why the EBO goes hand-in-hand with the minimal self—the bare feeling of being a subject or experiencing entity at a point in time. This also explains why such DPD patients may report feeling as though they have become unreal or ceased to exist.

As Klee put it in relation to ego dissolution under lysergic acid diethylamide (LSD): 'Lacking a reliable inflow (or integration) of stimuli, particularly from his body, the subject has lost much of the basis for his self-percept' (1963, p. 465). What DPD patients lack, on this view, is an integration of stimuli from their bodies with contextual information that reveals the significance of those stimuli for the fortunes of the organism. In healthy waking cognition, these representations are transformed into affects by top-down inferences that bind them to a representation of an entity to whom things matter (Gerrans 2015) This binding is evident phenomenologically: we do not experience a bodily feeling and a distinct thought that, for example, danger is present, but rather the feeling is simply (transparently) experienced as the very fact of danger's being present.

On Seth's view, then, emotional experience and the minimal self both depend importantly on top-down interoceptive inference in the AIC. He summarises the view as follows:

> emotion and embodied [i.e., minimal] selfhood are grounded in active inference of those signals most likely to be 'me' across interoceptive and exteroceptive domains. In humans, self-related predictive [processing] simultaneously engages multiple levels of self-representation, including physiological homeostasis, physical bodily integrity, morphology and position, and—more speculatively—the metacognitive and narrative 'I'.
>
> **(2013, p. 570).**

This is essentially the view taken by Letheby and Gerrans (2017), with a couple of additional emphases. One of these is on the content of the model generated by such inferential processes, which we explored in section 7.2: it represents the self as a simple indivisible entity, or Cartesian substance. Another is on the hierarchical relations between embodied and superordinate, narrative or autobiographical levels of self-modelling, to which we now turn.

Seth's mention of the 'metacognitive and narrative "I"' brings us to the role of the DMN in self-modelling. The need for this role stems from the fact that human life is not just a series of discrete, isolated, emotion-evoking encounters with the world. Such encounters form complex patterns and occur in spatiotemporally extended contexts. In many cases, especially when it comes to more abstract, evolutionarily recent (e.g., social), or long-term goals, the personal relevance of worldly encounters depends ineliminably on autobiographical information. Suppose that you end up in the elevator with someone who has your job application on her desk for review. This encounter will evoke all kinds of somatic, affective, cognitive, and attentional responses, due to the significance of this person to your long-term goals and interests, while another's encounter with the same person may go completely unnoticed. It is only in your specific autobiographical context that this encounter takes on its distinctive and salient character, with myriad potential psychological and behavioural consequences.

On the PP scheme, higher levels of the brain's generative model track regularities at greater spatiotemporal scales, and self-modelling is no exception. As we have seen, a large body of evidence links activity and connectivity of DMN regions to self-referential tasks of a high-level, conceptual, or autobiographical nature (such as 'mental time travel'—the simulation of past and future events—and making explicit judgements about one's own personality), as well as to theory of mind (the attribution of mental states) and to mind-wandering in the task-free resting state (which often concerns self-referential, social, or autobiographical themes). This body of evidence can be explained parsimoniously by the hypothesis that a core function of the DMN is to encode the highest layers of a hierarchical predictive self-model, representing the fortunes, goals, and interests of the postulated self at greater levels of abstraction and larger spatiotemporal scales than those tracked by SN nodes.

This is the proposal of Letheby and Gerrans (2017): a hierarchical predictive model of the self is implemented in the cortical midline nodes of the SN and DMN, which represent synchronic/minimal/embodied and diachronic/narrative/autobiographical aspects of selfhood, respectively, and these distinct layers of self-modelling are integrated 'vertically' by attributing these diverse properties and relations to a single underlying entity. It is the coherent functioning and interplay of these networks in healthy, sober, waking cognition that underlie the ubiquitous but introspectively elusive sense of being a coherent persisting subject, distinct from all of its mental and physical states, but standing to them in relations of ownership, authorship, and so forth; the one who thinks the thoughts, feels the feelings, owns and inhabits the body; the one to whom it all happens, and to whom events in the world matter.

As we saw in Chapter 5, psychological insights induced by psychedelics often involve changes to the narrative self (cf. Amada et al. 2020). Aspects of narrative selfhood also illustrate the epistemic and psychological costs that predictive models can have. Deeply entrenched 'core beliefs' about the self, such as 'I am unworthy', are characteristic of depression and other pathologies, and have been theorised to play a role in their genesis and maintenance (Waller et al. 2001). Such beliefs have obvious emotional costs. PP theory illuminates their potential *epistemic* costs: if such beliefs are sufficiently highly weighted by the brain (like the assumption that human faces are convex), then conflicting evidence will be dismissed as noise.

Thus, a profoundly depressed person may simply fail to notice evidence of her worthiness. If her belief that she is unworthy is sufficiently highly weighted, then conflicting evidence will be deemed unreliable—which, on PP, means that it will go unattended. As such, it will be unable to force an update of the model. Even if the evidence is brought directly to the patient's attention, she may simply attempt to reinterpret it or explain it away as an anomaly, rather than revising her deep-seated belief that she is unworthy. Similarly, an addicted person may be unable vividly to imagine, or simulate, a non-addicted future for herself, because her identity as a (currently using) addict is bound so tightly to the self-model that it is effectively posited as an essential property of the self (Philip Gerrans, personal communication). Thus, it becomes neurocognitively impossible to represent that very entity without those properties.

As I have emphasised, predictive models have both costs and benefits. They are the only means we have for picking up on the real higher-order patterns that characterise the complex thinking, feeling, and behaviour of creatures such as ourselves. But, in their quest for computational efficiency, our predictive brains are not just substantialists but also essentialists: they reify mere patterns and tendencies into intrinsic properties. Oversimplifying the situation and failing to appreciate that multiple, seemingly dissonant patterns can co-exist, they condense us representationally to a fraction of our actual complexity, and thereby create the corresponding reality. Epistemologically, predictive models can function as echo chambers: cognitively, emotionally, and behaviourally, as self-fulfilling prophecies. Of course, transiently disrupting these models can make their very real benefits temporarily unavailable. People on heroic doses of psilocybin should not be driving cars, teaching schoolchildren, or conducting business meetings. But such disruption can also afford an opportunity to improve these models, minimising their psychosocial and epistemic costs by rendering them temporarily more flexible, plastic, and permeable by new information (Carhart-Harris and Friston 2019).

7.4 A centre of representational gravity

The first two emphases of the predictive self-binding account are (i) that the DMN and the SN encode distinct layers of a hierarchical self-model, and (ii) that this model binds or integrates multimodal stimuli by relating them to a postulated substantial entity. We have just examined those two emphases in reverse order: section 7.2 was devoted to the idea of self-binding, and section 7.3 to the hierarchical structure of the self-model.

The ideas I have just discussed concerning attention bring us to the third emphasis of the account. Dennett (1992) famously described the self as a 'centre of narrative gravity.' Letheby and Gerrans (2017) describe the predictive self-model as a centre of *representational* gravity, positing that it serves as an organising principle for cognitive processing: it regulates and constrains the allocation of attention, the attribution of salience, and the construction of mental representations at all levels—not just that of explicit narrative reflection.

The self-centred structure of our default phenomenal worlds is most obvious at the concrete sensorimotor level. The physical world is represented in perception as being apprehended from a specific spatiotemporal vantage point (Blanke and Metzinger 2009). The ordinary perceptual space that we inhabit from day to day is an egocentric space, in the sense of being organised relative to a centre where the self or 'I' is experienced as residing (Revonsuo 2006). However, our phenomenal worlds are also self-centred in more abstract senses, determined at higher levels of processing.

In particular, as I suggested in section 7.3, our sense that events in the world matter depends on inferences, computed in the AIC, which model interoceptive changes as signals of core relational themes. The AIC and the anterior cingulate cortex (ACC), another major hub of the SN, then cooperate to initiate control signals appropriate to the content of the core relational theme—signals that allocate attention and processing resources to stimuli deemed relevant to the postulated goals and interests of the self (Menon and Uddin 2010). This underpins the phenomenal experience as of a world rich with meaning and significance, in which certain stimuli capture attention immediately and automatically, while others go unnoticed or ignored.

This process of salience attribution and attention allocation is informed by the hierarchical interactions between the SN and the DMN. The latter represents the properties, goals, and interests of the self at longer timescales and higher levels of abstraction than the former. One core function of the SN is regulating the contextually mandated switching between the DMN and anti-correlated 'task positive' networks (TPNs) in accordance with task demands (Sridharan et al. 2008). However, DMN nodes themselves have also been linked to attention regulation. The posterior cingulate cortex (PCC) has been called the 'core node' of the DMN (Davey et al. 2016) and has repeatedly been implicated in the psychedelic state (Carhart-Harris et al. 2012b, 2016c, Bouso et al. 2015, Smigielski et al. 2019b). According to one recent model, subregions of the PCC are involved in monitoring the balance (internal vs. external) and breadth (narrow vs. broad) of attention, by tuning the activity and connectivity profiles of multiple neurocognitive networks throughout the brain (Leech and Sharp 2014).

At lower levels of the processing hierarchy, the function of the amygdala deserves mention too. Findings from one cohort of patients have linked the therapeutic effects of psychedelics to changes in this region (Roseman et al. 2018b, Mertens et al. 2020), which is considered a subcortical node of the SN (Menon and Uddin 2010, Sui and Gu 2017) and was identified by Sui and Humphreys (2015) as part of the 'core self' network involved in self-binding. Multiple studies have found changes to amygdala activity and connectivity during the acute effects of psychedelics (e.g., Kraehenmann et al. 2015, Mueller et al. 2017, Grimm et al. 2018). Contrary to earlier descriptions as a 'fear centre', the amygdala has been described by one influential model as an evolved system for *relevance detection* (Sander et al. 2003) that plays a crucial role in orienting toward salient stimuli at the level of basic perceptual processing.

In a recent paper, Wanja Wiese (2019) has described the predictive self-model as a 'hierarchical salience model': a complex representation of the many classes, or dimensions, of stimuli that putatively matter to the organism, at multiple levels of abstraction. For Wiese, the phenomenal sense that the self is *substantial* arises from the fact that this hierarchical model unifies the many dimensions and levels of salience by attributing them all to an 'abstract salience object'—an object that, while not concrete, is represented as strictly numerically identical over time.

It seems that there is a bidirectional, mutually reinforcing relationship between the contents of the self-model and the patterns of attention and salience that characterise default waking consciousness. Representing the self as a specific entity with a specific set of goals and interests supports characteristic patterns of attention allocation and salience attribution—and these patterns, in turn, provide evidence confirming the hypothesis: that 'I' am a specific entity with specific properties, including a distinctive set of traits, goals, and interests. This illustrates the circular dynamic that can lead to the rigid entrenchment of dysfunctional self-models: the more heavily weighted are our beliefs about who we are, the less likely it is that we will think, feel, attend, or act in ways inconsistent with those beliefs, that generate high volumes of prediction error.

Thus, in ordinary waking life, our phenomenal worlds are not only organised around a central point at a basic sensorimotor level. Our attention is also captured selectively by stimuli that are represented as personally relevant and thus evoke feelings (whether subtle or intense) of salience or importance. When no stimulus in the immediate environment captures attention in this way, we often revert to the default mode of mind-wandering, whose topics typically concern self-referential themes (Smallwood and Schooler 2015). We travel mentally to the past and the future, spinning autobiographical narratives about where we have come from, where we are going, how we might seek or avoid desirable or undesirable stimuli (broadly construed), and how we might communicate these plans and motivations to conspecifics.

As Letheby and Gerrans put it:

Perceptual representations are organized in an egocentric space; interoceptive representations are interpreted as signals of adaptively relevant events or 'core relational themes' ... and [autobiographical] narratives are structured around the fortunes and prospects of a protagonist. At all levels, salience is attributed, attention directed, and information integrated in accordance with the [hypothesized] relevance of information to the organism's goals.

(2017, p. 9).

If this is correct, then disruption to the coherent functioning of the relevant systems should lead to an 'unconstrained' mode of cognition (Carhart-Harris et al. 2012b, Swanson 2018) in which 'consciousness itself, the basic sensation of being an 'I,' undergoes a remarkable change,' and 'the spotlight of consciousness [becomes] a floodlight which ... brings to light unsuspected details—details normally ignored because of their lack of significance' (Watts 1964).[1] And on moderate-to-high doses of psychedelics, this is exactly what we find.

---

[1] What explains the difference between the beneficial disruptions to self-representation that often result from controlled psychedelic ingestion, and the detrimental disruptions that characterise pathologies such as DPD and schizophrenia? (I am indebted to Miri Albahari for pressing this question.) A complete answer is not yet available, but there are a few points to make (see also Dambrun and Ricard 2011). First, subjects in controlled settings receive psychedelics voluntarily, with preparation and foreknowledge. This decreases the probability of dysphoric responses. When psychedelics are given to unprepared or unwitting subjects, the results often *are* detrimental (Masters and Houston 1966). Second, Albahari herself has speculated that differences in attentional capacity might constitute an important difference between beneficial and pathological disruptions to self-consciousness (Albahari 2006, pp. 208–209). In this light, it is interesting to note that the psychedelic state is often described in terms of expanded or heightened attention. While *voluntary* attention regulation may be impaired, subjects describe a greater attentional capacity than in normal waking consciousness. Third, and finally, it may be important that some minimal form of self-consciousness seems to be preserved in most psychedelic experiences. Even if all forms of self-consciousness are sometimes lost, it is likely that this happens relatively briefly, with the important therapeutic processes occurring either side. The typical retention of the minimal self in beneficial psychedelic

7.5 The self unbound

The most obvious application of the predictive self-binding framework is in explaining the experience of ego dissolution. We have already seen, in Chapter 6, how the REBUS model might explain defining phenomenological features of the mystical-type experience, such as the transcendence of space and time and the noetic quality. However, when it comes to the cardinal feature of the felt loss of individual identity, and the concomitant experience of unity and interconnectedness, the predictive self-binding framework offers further, specific insight: if the DMN and SN perform their integrative functions by modelling the existence of a simple, indivisible entity, sharply bounded and distinct from the external world, then this would explain why disruption to these systems should lead to the feeling that the individual is disintegrating, dying, or merging with the cosmos (cf. Nencini and Grant 2010). This also amply explains why significant anxiety, disorientation, and confusion can result from high-dose psychedelic administration—especially when subjects are not adequately prepared or supported, but sometimes even when they are (Griffiths et al. 2008).

More specifically, the hierarchical structure of the self-model explains why the supposedly unitary phenomenon of 'ego dissolution' should actually have distinct phenomenological profiles (Millière et al. 2018) and neural correlates (Muthukumaraswamy et al. 2013, Carhart-Harris et al. 2014, Lebedev et al. 2015). The idea is that psychedelics disrupt different neurocognitive networks, to different extents, under different conditions—depending, no doubt, on such factors as substance, dose, set, and setting—and this leads to distinct types of ego dissolution experiences (cf. Millière 2020). Specifically, disruption to the DMN should be associated selectively with disruptions to the narrative self, while disruption to the SN should be associated with disruptions to the minimal self. This fits well with early clinical accounts that distinguished between the losses of 'mental ego feeling' and 'bodily ego feeling' under LSD (Savage 1955). As we have seen, some such accounts explained these losses in terms of disrupted mechanisms of expectation and integration (cf. prediction and binding): 'Lacking a reliable inflow (or integration) of stimuli, particularly from his body, the subject has lost much of the basis for his self-percept' (Klee 1963, p. 465). This is a testable prediction of the self-binding account: that narrative and minimal self-dissolution should be associated with DMN and SN disintegration, respectively (Letheby and Gerrans 2017; cf. Lebedev et al. 2015).

However, the experience of ego dissolution per se—the phenomenal feeling as of disintegrating or losing one's identity—is not the most important factor in psychedelic therapy. What is more important is that the weakening of self-related beliefs creates an opportunity to revise these beliefs for the better. In successful psychedelic therapy, the

states may mark an important difference between these states and at least some pathological disruptions to self-awareness (Albahari, personal communication).

patient learns to see herself differently, which can encompass changes to many facets and dimensions of self-awareness. And this process can be facilitated by disruption to self-binding processes, even when they do not result in an experience that is naturally described as 'ego dissolution'. As we saw in Chapter 5, recent quantitative research into therapeutic mechanisms highlights two psychological factors: (i) experiences of psychological insight, and (ii) increases in mindfulness-related capacities and psychological flexibility. I now consider these in turn to see what light the self-binding account can shed. (Please note that, in this chapter, I am pursuing a purely descriptive account of the mechanisms of psychedelic therapy. A normative epistemological evaluation of these mechanisms and their products will be the task of Chapter 8).

On the first count, regarding psychological insight, the story is fairly straightforward: by weakening the brain's confidence in its fundamental hypotheses about who 'I' am—by relaxing the precision-weighting of self-related priors and unbinding the self-model—psychedelics induce different forms of self-modelling. Under the influence, patients can gain new perspectives on their lives, see things differently, and access information previously filtered out or ignored. They can thereby discover new and often healthier forms of self-modelling. This sort of process is described clearly by patients in clinical trials, as we saw in Chapter 3. Consider the example of a patient who received psilocybin-assisted therapy for alcoholism:

Lisa was a Latin-American female in her 50s with a family history of alcoholism, physical and emotional abuse, abandonment, and neglect. Her problematic drinking began around the age of 30 and resulted in social isolation, hangovers, strong feelings of guilt and shame, and severe self-critical thoughts . . .

During the initial [psilocybin] session, Lisa . . . examined the negative feelings that she harbored for herself and feelings of alienation from God . . .

In the second session, Lisa received a higher dose of [psilocybin] and experienced an amplification of thought moving her into a confused and chaotic state. Underneath the chaotic thinking, she identified a deep well of overwhelming sadness. She was able to eventually surrender control over her thoughts and entered into a state of peacefulness, until her thoughts quieted completely. She heard her own inner voice rupturing the quiet, whispering into her ear: 'I'm going to tell you a secret. It's the worst-kept secret in the universe because everyone knows it but you. You are a perfect creation of the universe.' At that moment she felt that everything in existence was unified and was made of love, though a part of her remained reluctant to fully believe this to be true. The voice repeatedly presented her with this reality, asking 'do you believe this?' over and over until each one of her objections had been addressed and dismissed. She examined herself and found that she finally did accept this to be true, which propelled her into a state of profound self-acceptance and wellbeing. She later said, 'All there is is love, this is all that you are, this is all that matters.'

Following her [psilocybin] session, Lisa reported that her self-critical thoughts had dissolved and that alcohol had lost almost all of its appeal. She said that the [psilocybin] sessions had illuminated how she had been unkind to her body and had been harming herself with alcohol. She noted her ability to manage stress and found that she was making time to care for herself through socialization, relaxation, and a resumed meditation practice. She reported improved concentration, a lack of negative self-talk, decreased anxiety, and a spacious quality of mind . . . At 54 weeks, Lisa reported a persisting reduction in alcohol consumption and alleviated anxiety.

(Bogenschutz et al. 2018, p. 5).

Clearly a key part of the therapeutic process for Lisa involved revising her self-conception on a deep level, abandoning the core beliefs underpinning her 'severe self-critical thoughts' and coming to see herself instead as a 'perfect creation of the universe'. By her own account, this dissolution of self-critical thoughts led to reduced urges to drink and reduced actual drinking, as well as improved capacities for stress management and self-care—not to mention 'a lack of negative self-talk, decreased anxiety, and a spacious quality of mind'. Her experience as described above corresponds to several items on the Psychological Insight Questionnaire (PIQ) of Davis et al. (2020), which we encountered in Chapter 5:

Realized ways my beliefs may be dysfunctional
Discovered how aspects of my life are affecting my well-being
Experienced validation of my life, character, values, or beliefs
Realized the importance of my life
Awareness of dysfunctional patterns in my actions, thoughts, and/or feelings
Realized how critical or judgmental views I hold towards myself are dysfunctional

A different sort of experience is described by a patient who received psilocybin with psychological support for treatment-resistant depression:

[This patient] described how in adult life he 'had always found it difficult to be emotional, found it uncomfortable to be around other people if they were emotional' and saw 'emotions as weakness'. As a child, his parents had told him that 'boys don't cry', and as he matured he had learned to 'put his feelings in a box because you can't be upset, you're a man'.

(Watts et al. 2017, p. 536).

Under psilocybin, this patient described reliving a pivotal event from his childhood that led him to internalise such attitudes:

[This patient] reported:

[I] became myself at age 7, after my [grandparent] had died. I totally was back there, so vivid, so real, I had the emotions that I would have felt at the

> time: fearful, why did this happen, the naivety, the shock and confusion.
> I was getting overly upset and my parents were saying 'boys don't cry'.

This helped him realize how his unhealthy emotional habits as an adult developed.

> I saw that it's not [a] weakness to be emotional, that's an unhealthy attitude.
> (**Watts et al. 2017, p. 539**)

At first glance, it might not seem obvious what this report has to do with revising the self-model. However, from his descriptions, it seems clear that this patient's habits of emotional avoidance were intimately bound up with his conception of his own identity—first as a boy and later as a man. It seems plausible that his psychological tendency to avoid, ignore, or repress emotions, to put them 'in a box', stemmed in part from the deep-seated belief that 'you can't be upset, you're a man'—a belief precisely about his identity and what it entailed.

Of course, the experience also involved autobiographical reappraisal: the patient vividly relived an early life event and gained a new understanding of its role in his psychological development. After the psilocybin session, he could see himself, for the first time, as someone who had developed dysfunctional emotional habits by internalising unhealthy attitudes in his childhood. This new self-conception was empowering because it suggested the possibility of alternative, healthier ways of relating to his emotions—some of which were experienced during the psilocybin session itself. This patient's experience also corresponds to several PIQ items:

> Realized how current feelings or perceptions are related to events from my past
> Realized ways my beliefs may be dysfunctional
> Gained a deeper understanding of events/memories from my past
> Awareness of dysfunctional patterns in my actions, thoughts, and/or feelings
> Realized how critical or judgmental views I hold towards myself are dysfunctional
> Discovered I could explore uncomfortable or painful feelings I previously avoided
> Discovered a clear pattern of avoidance in my life
> Realized the nature and/or origins of my defenses or other coping strategies
> Gained resolution or clarity about past traumas or hurtful events
> Awareness of information that helped me understand my life

In considering these first two examples, I have focused largely on changes to the narrative self. The following report illustrates how changes to narrative, minimal, and bodily (Ho et al. 2020) aspects of self-representation can be intertwined in psychedelic therapy:

> Victor, [who was] a 17-year-old high school student [at the time] when he was first diagnosed with leukemia, saw his body as riddled with cancer, and his narrative

suggested anger, grief, and an abiding rejection of his body. He described that during his psilocybin session, he experienced himself as a disembodied form and came to a point where he had to choose a body:

> Until this point in the experience, I did not have a body. I was just this kind of soul, this entity ... I was shopping for a body, and the only body I could choose was my body. And this is meaningful because I had a lot of body issues associated with being sick with what chemo did to my body and how it changed. And so I was circling my body, and I saw everything that has happened to my body, all the food I have eaten, the drugs I have taken, the alcohol, the people I have had sex with, the chemo, the exercise, everything that has ever happened to my body. I took it in at once ... I kind of accepted my body for what it is, and I think up until that point I resisted that ... I saw this body for what it's worth. I picked it, it's mine ... It's more matter-of fact— this is what it is. I think that acceptance has been liberating.
>
> **(Swift et al. 2017, p. 501).**

In this experience, at least one aspect of the minimal self seems to be retained: the bare sense of being an experiencing subject, or 'I'. Nothing in Victor's report suggests total ego dissolution. However, other aspects of minimal selfhood, such as the EBO and spatiotemporal self-location, are disrupted in the experience of being a disembodied 'soul' or 'entity'. We can also see changes to bodily dimensions of the narrative self (dealing with 'bodily issues' and seeing 'everything that has happened to my body'), as well as the quintessential psychedelic shift from rejection or avoidance to acceptance— dramatised metaphorically through the vision of 'shopping for', and choosing, a body.

Victor's vision of shopping for a body highlights another important point: often, the process of finding new and healthier forms of self-modelling involves an explicit sense of disidentifying with one's existing self-conception. This brings us to the second psychological correlate of psychedelic therapy: the increase in mindfulness-related capacities and psychological flexibility. What does the predictive self-binding account have to say about this?

The answer, in brief, is that when mental contents are unbound from the self-model they can attain a degree of *phenomenal opacity* that is closely related to mindfulness-related capacities and psychological flexibility. As we have seen, predictive models in general exhibit the property of phenomenal transparency: they are not experienced as models, but simply appear, phenomenologically, as reality itself. This applies at least equally to the self-model. The all-important substantial entity posited by the predictive brain does not appear to us as a model or a story. Rather, we experience it as nothing more or less than our own immediate, unproblematic existence. In Metzinger's words:

> We do not experience the contents of our self-consciousness as the contents of a representational process ... but simply as *ourselves, living in the world right now* ...

the experiencing system, by necessity, becomes entangled in a naïve realism with regard to the contents of its own mental self-representation.

(Metzinger 2003, p. 331; emphasis original).

Indeed, Metzinger posits that transparency is a *defining* feature of a phenomenal self-model (PSM): to the extent that a cognitive system operates with an opaque model of its own functioning, it will not have the phenomenal experience of 'being someone', which can only result from the 'naïve-realistic self-misunderstanding' (Metzinger 2003, p. 333) involved in transparent self-modelling. This connects with an important observation from the phenomenology of mindfulness meditation: to see thoughts and feelings as *mere* thoughts and feelings is ipso facto to disidentify with them (Albahari 2006, pp. 63–64; cf. Wright 2017, p. 71, Sierra-Siegert and Jay 2020). To the extent that elements of the self-model become phenomenally opaque, they no longer form part of a self-model proper, because they are experienced as objects in awareness, rather than as the subject who is aware of those objects. The induction of phenomenal opacity into mental models, especially self-models, has been described as a central aim of traditional Buddhist meditation practices (Metzinger 2003, p. 566, Lutz et al. 2019).

My suggestion is that it can go both ways. On one hand, rendering thoughts and feelings phenomenally opaque by watching them calmly and non-reactively in meditation, seeing them as '*just* thoughts and feelings', can lead to disidentification with them. On the other hand, disidentification with such mental contents, induced by psychedelic unbinding of the self-model, can confer an ability to watch them non-reactively. By reducing the brain's confidence in its hypotheses about who, what, and where 'I' am, the phenomenal unit of identification can be expanded, contracted, shifted, or rendered ambiguous, such that it no longer determinately includes many of the thoughts, feelings, and perspectives with which we usually identify. These mental contents can then enter an open, spacious, non-goal-directed attention in the phenomenal guise of *mere* thoughts and feelings. No longer identified with so strongly, they evoke less defensiveness and reactivity. And if the control of attention is itself decoupled from self-representation, then the normal motivations for avoiding, suppressing, or rationalising uncomfortable thoughts and feelings may not wield their usual influence.

Through disidentification, we come to see these mental contents from the outside, as it were—as representations, rather than as the fixed essence of a substantial entity. By disidentifying with our self-representations, we see that they are mutable: they can change while we remain. The connections with psychological flexibility, the perspective-taking self, and decentring are obvious. As we have seen, some psychedelic subjects spontaneously distinguish between 'I' and 'me'—the minimal experiencing subject, and the structures and roles of the narrative self, respectively—and describe an exhilarating sense of radical freedom that comes from a shift of felt identity away from the latter and towards the former. The therapeutic relevance of this experience is made clear by a patient who received psilocybin in a recent clinical trial:

> In deep meditation … there is a state which is not dissimilar to some aspects of being under the influence of psilocybin. Spaciousness, a realisation that much of what we think is concrete and can't be escaped from are actually just ways we think.
>
> **(Watts and Luoma 2020, p. 95).**

Other patients describe similar experiences, both during and after a psilocybin experience:

> [During the dose] It was like a holiday away from the prison of my brain, I was a ball of energy bouncing around the planet, I felt free, carefree, re-energised. [Patient 8]

> [After the dose] It was like this great shroud had been lifted. [Patient 1]

> You're not immersed in thought patterns, the concrete coat had come off. [Patient 4]

> I felt spatial, not depressed. [Patient 6]

> A feeling of space and openness. [Patient 17]
>
> **(Watts et al. 2017, p. 528).**

In some cases, the entire narrative self seems to become opaque, causing the phenomenal unit of identification to contract to the minimal self—the bare feeling of subjectivity:

> It became very important to distinguish between 'I' and 'Me', the latter being an object defined by patterns and structures and responsibilities—*all of which had vanished*—and the former being the subject experiencing and feeling. My normal life seemed to be all Me, all demands and responsibilities, a rushing burden which destroyed the pleasure and freedom of being 'I'.
>
> **(Durr 1970, p. 79; my emphasis).**

> For a few seconds, it was just like 'I'm me, and *there are no defining characteristics!*' … that made me realise that I'm not a 'smoker'.
>
> **(Noorani et al. 2018, p. 759; my emphasis).**

I am suggesting that such experiences result from the same basic mechanism as the observed increases in mindfulness-related capacities and psychological flexibility: the unbinding of mental contents (such as 'defining characteristics') from the self-model, diminishing the sense of fixed identity with them. What seems to persist for at least some time after the experience is a flattening of the 'prior landscape': various hypotheses about what kind of person 'I' am are put on a more level playing field, as the relative probabilities assigned to some are decreased, and to others increased. This flattening of the prior landscape plausibly underlies the feelings of openness, spaciousness, and freedom—the sense of being unburdened—that characterises the short-to-medium-term afterglow (Carhart-Harris and Friston 2019).

One quite general effect of supervised psychedelic administration seems to be increased *plasticity*, or capacity for change (Carhart-Harris and Nutt 2017, Carhart-Harris 2019). The sense of freedom that comes from rendering the self-model opaque could be seen as a phenomenological manifestation of this effect. This effect manifests at other levels, too. As we have seen, psychedelics seem to stimulate the molecular mechanisms of neuroplasticity independently of their variable effects on cognition and consciousness (Ly et al. 2018). However, the flattening of the prior landscape I have just described amounts to the induction of a kind of cognitive plasticity: removing steep valleys or basins of attraction by decreasing the difference between the probabilities assigned to various hypotheses. Under these circumstances, the brain can slide more readily between world-models, trying a range of different predictive hypotheses on for size—a plausible cognitive interpretation of the fact that the psychedelic brain explores a wider range of global functional configurations than the sober waking brain (Tagliazucchi et al. 2014, Atasoy et al. 2017). Of course, the net result of this at the level of global neurodynamics is increased entropy (Carhart-Harris et al. 2014).

When it comes to the self-model specifically, by reducing the brain's confidence in its assumptions about who, what, and where 'I' am, the cognitive playing field is levelled with respect to one's own identity, allowing all sorts of hypotheses to be entertained that normally would be ruled out. This cognitive effect manifests phenomenologically, not just as ego dissolution but also as the experiences of disidentification, decentring, spaciousness, and freedom. We feel deeply and vividly that there are many ways we can be, many ways we can see ourselves, many ways we can relate to our lives and experience. Contrastively, we appreciate the extent to which we have been unknowingly identifying with a highly specific and rigid set of assumptions about who and what we are. Psychedelics induce neural, cognitive, and phenomenological forms of plasticity; the cognitive plasticity of the self-model and its phenomenological manifestations are of primary therapeutic importance.

7.6 Opacity and mystical epiphanies

Interestingly, the induction of opacity by psychedelics is not limited to the self-model. A widespread induction of phenomenal opacity might furnish a partial naturalistic explanation of an otherwise-mysterious fact: that psychedelic experiences often promote metaphysical views, such as idealism, which hold mind or consciousness to be ubiquitous or fundamental in the universe. Metzinger (2003, p. 250) has speculated that an experience of global opacity—the profound and existentially destabilising insight that one's entire *experienced* world is a purely mental construction—might be at the root of idealist philosophies. The central task of the present chapter is to explain psychedelics' therapeutic effects, not their tendency to promote non-naturalistic metaphysical ideations. However, explaining the latter is sufficiently important for a naturalistic understanding of the psychedelic state that it warrants a brief detour from our main current concerns.

Could it be that psychedelics cause idealistic (and related) ideations by inducing global phenomenal opacity? There is ample evidence that they can, indeed, induce global opacity in a manner that is phenomenologically neutral between various theoretical or metaphysical interpretations. Here is an example induced by the N,N-dimethyltryptamine (DMT)-containing smoking mixture *changa*:

> All became very bright, it seemed fake, as if I was in a plastic world. I could see psychedelic patterns rising in the walls up to the ceiling; it felt like I was in an elevator. It all went very fast, unexpected. All of a sudden I lost control of myself. I fell down onto the carpet, drawn by a mysterious force. I began to feel like I was going mad. The force wanted me to surrender. So I did. And then I saw all the elements of my life disappearing, as if they had never existed. I saw my life falling into pieces. *It seemed that my reality was just a hallucination, created by myself.* Everything I believed to be real was dissolving. How could I explain to my friends, my relatives, that I was their creator? Everyday life is just an illusion. Then I realized I was dying. Alone, in my studio. I wanted to reach for my phone to call someone to help me. But why? I am just dying. It is best to surrender, I thought. When I stopped resisting the sensation of death I felt something incredibly calm and peaceful: the cosmic void.
>
> **(Gaia 2016, pp. 50–51; my emphasis).**

On my view, this person has had an accurate psychedelic-facilitated insight into the nature of their conscious experience. It is true that their (*experienced*) reality is just a (*controlled*) hallucination, created by 'themselves' (by *sub-personal mechanisms* in their predictive brain). But, importantly, there is nothing in the experience itself to discriminate between two different metaphysical interpretations: (i) that the mental construction of one's conscious reality is performed entirely within, and by, a biological brain that actually exists within a fundamentally non-mental, objective, mind-independent world; and (ii) that there is, after all, no such mind-independent world. The experience reveals that *what one has always taken for such a world* was a purely mental construction all along. But there is more than one metaphysical position consistent with this revelation.

Interpretation (i) is, of course, the naturalistic view that I favour, whereas (ii) corresponds most closely to metaphysical views such as solipsism (shades of which are evident in the report above) or idealism. My position is that (i) is more plausible on independent grounds, which I outlined in Chapter 2. However, (ii) is likely to seem far more plausible if one simply takes the experience at face value: this interpretation requires no extra theoretical assumptions. The experience is *as of* discovering that all of reality is mentally constructed, so it is very naturally interpreted in those terms.

If this speculative explanation of psychedelic-induced idealistic epiphanies is roughly correct, then such epiphanies embody a peculiar combination of increased opacity and retained transparency. The virtual entities that populate one's experiential world—phenomenal tables, chairs, people, and so forth—are recognised accurately as nothing other than mental simulations or models: opacity in action. However, rather than being recognised as purely *intracranial* simulations or models, they are still mistaken for the extracranial, trans-individual world, in a retention of a certain sort of transparency that begets an inaccurate metaphysical conclusion: that the entire world is constituted or permeated by mentality or consciousness.

Reflecting on the theoretical and philosophical significance of psychedelic experience, Sidney Cohen draws the conclusion, quite congenial to PP and its view of consciousness, that:

> ... believing is as much a part of seeing as seeing is believing ... Our notions of what is 'out there' seem to be based upon an indistinct uncertainty. For all we know, the thing called reality may exist, but we shall never see it. What we call reality is a shadow upon an imperfect screen ...
>
> **(Cohen 1970, p. 48).**

However, one might easily slide from such an insight into the constructed nature of the *phenomenal* world to a more metaphysically extravagant conclusion about the ultimate nature of the entire world. This possibility is illustrated by some remarks from Alan Watts:

> ... any chemically induced alteration of the nervous system must draw the attention of that system to itself ... Ordinarily, we remain quite unaware of the fact that the whole field of vision with its vast multiplicity of colors and shapes is a state of affairs inside our heads ... Psychedelics induce subtle alterations of perception which make the nervous system aware of itself, and the individual suddenly and unaccustomedly *becomes conscious of the external world as a state of his own body.*
>
> **(Watts 1964; my emphasis).**

On my view, it is entirely correct that the 'field of vision', in a relevant sense, is a state of affairs inside our heads; that we ordinarily remain quite unaware of this fact; and that psychedelics can make us startlingly, shockingly aware of it.[2] It is also true that, in many such experiences, the individual 'suddenly and unaccustomedly' becomes

---

[2] Another simple naturalistic explanation of the apparent idealistic insight is as follows: In a full-blown mystical experience, consciousness is unquestionably still (vividly, intensely) present, but, because of the dissolution of the self-model, there is no longer any point, phenomenologically, at which 'I' (and my consciousness) stop and the rest of the world begins. An experience as of boundarylessness, induced by disruption to binding processes, in which consciousness clearly remains, would automatically be an experience as of boundaryless consciousness. This is related to, but distinct from, the speculative explanation of the noetic quality that I discussed in Chapter 6.

aware that *what she ordinarily takes for* the external world is a state of her own body. But, absent further substantive assumptions, this is not the same as becoming aware that the *actual* external world is a state of one's own body. The former formulation extracts the accurate insight from psychedelic-induced phenomenal opacity without drawing unwarranted metaphysical conclusions.

If these speculations are on the right track, then this is what underlies many idealist-type metaphysical epiphanies induced by psychedelics: the philosophically illicit slide from (i) the realisation that what one has habitually taken for the mind-independent world is no such thing to (ii) the conclusion that there is no such thing at all. This is analogous to what Susan Haack (1999, pp. 196–197) calls the 'Passes-For Fallacy'— the argument, roughly, that:

1. Many things that have often *passed for* objective truth or honest unbiased inquiry have turned out to be no such thing
2. Therefore, there is no such thing as objective truth or honest unbiased inquiry

We will revisit inferences of this kind shortly, when we discuss the metaphysics of the self. Of course, Watts may simply be speaking loosely. But the ambiguity of his formulation shows how easily one might slide from one interpretation of this insight to another.

7.7 Psychedelic therapy: a two-factor theory

After a brief detour, we return to our scheduled programming. What sort of theory of psychedelic therapy falls out of the discussion of this chapter? On the view that I have outlined, psychedelics alter consciousness by changing the activity and connectivity profiles of pivotal hub regions at the top end of the brain's processing hierarchy. The disruption to synchronous neural oscillations in these regions amounts, cognitively, to a decrease in the precision-weighting of high-level priors, including self-related priors that integrate multimodal stimuli by attributing them to a single underlying entity. In philosophical terms, this basic cognitive effect of psychedelics is akin to striking at the heart of a Quinean web of belief. This informal observation goes some way to explaining why its downstream effects can be so variable: undermining these cognitively foundational representations, implemented in densely connected and functionally pivotal brain regions, can have unpredictable and far-reaching effects depending on the prior state of the system (Carhart-Harris and Friston 2019, p. 319).[3] Under psychedelics, our self-conceptions and habits of attention are disrupted,

---

[3] It also goes some way to explaining psychedelics' tendency to provoke explicitly philosophical reflection (i.e., reflection on fundamental questions), even in the philosophically uninitiated (Shanon 2001, 2002; cf. Langlitz 2016). I will return to this point in Chapter 9.

allowing us to experience alternative self-conceptions—in part, by attending to what we usually ignore.

In my view, this account supports a *two-factor theory* of psychedelic therapy. The first factor is the induction of plasticity at multiple levels: neural, cognitive, and phenomenological. Psychedelics induce molecular-level plasticity independently of their effects on cognition and consciousness (Ly et al. 2018), but also induce entropic brain activity by disintegrating cortical networks such as the DMN and SN. Cognitively, this network disintegration amounts to a form of plasticity because it flattens the prior landscape. At the phenomenological level, the unbinding of the self-model manifests in the increased opacity of the phenomenal self, especially its narrative layers. This leads to the feelings of freedom, spaciousness, and possibility that come from disidentifying with the contents of the narrative self, realising that there are other ways one can be, other ways one can see, and other ways one can parse experience. The sub-personal mechanisms that conjure our phenomenal worlds are not just substantialists but essentialists. Psychedelics can undermine both of these tendencies, but the weakening of tacit essentialism regarding the self is therapeutically central.

These feelings of freedom and possibility are examples of what Matthew Ratcliffe (2005, 2009) has called 'existential feelings': experiences of the body that also represent fundamental relations between self and world, and the space of possibilities afforded thereby. Many characteristic psychedelic experiences, including the sense of connectedness, fall into Ratcliffe's category of existential feelings (Saarinen 2014). Indeed, dramatic change to existential feelings is probably one of the safest general characterisations of psychedelics' variable phenomenological effects, especially at moderate-to-high doses. Drawing on Ratcliffe's work, Juusi Saarinen notes that such dramatic changes can also cause existential feelings to move along the gradient from phenomenal transparency to opacity:

> Although existential feelings generally remain in the background of experience … they may become objects of attention and rational reflection … Usually this happens when a notable change or shift in the existential feeling occurs, and the orientation one previously took for granted becomes conspicuous by its absence. In this process, the contingency of one's earlier orientation is revealed … Importantly, once an existential feeling becomes the object of attention, one's reactions and attitudes toward it can reshape its structure.
>
> **(Saarinen 2014, p. 14).**

The correspondence with descriptions of psychedelic therapy is obvious.

This first factor alone—the induction of plasticity—may be sufficient for the short-term 'afterglow' of several weeks, in which subjects report feeling lighter, freer, more energised and unburdened. (Incidentally, the afterglow seems to consist almost entirely of changes to existential feelings.) However, a second factor is required for truly durable change: the discovery of new forms of self-modelling during the experience, and the consolidation of these during the subsequent period of integration. It's not just the plasticity—it's the way you use it.

On this view, patients and subjects do not merely discover, under psychedelics, that 'much of what we think is concrete and can't be escaped from are actually just ways we think'—although they certainly do discover this. They also discover *other ways of thinking* (and feeling, and attending, and so forth). They discover new, alternative forms of self-modelling, and the consolidation of these new forms is what the durable 'resetting' or 'rewiring' of high-level networks amounts to on a cognitive level. This is exemplified by the many varieties of psychological insight and emotional break-through that subjects report under psychedelics, all of which amount to variations on a central theme: reaching some new perspective on, belief about, or feeling toward some aspect of one's self and one's life. During the experience, subjects discover new ways of seeing, conceptualising, or relating to themselves and their lives. Subsequently, if all goes well, these new ways become consolidated as habitual modes of interpreting the world. The fact that LSD, psilocybin, and so forth act as *psychoplastogens*—agents that increase the plasticity of the mind—is part of what explains their therapeutic effects (Ly et al. 2018, Olson 2018). But the other part of the explanation is that they act as *psychedelics*—agents that reveal, or make manifest, various aspects of the mind, such as its potential for alternative self-conceptions and patterns of attention. Psychoplastogenic and (certain) psychedelic effects interact synergistically in psychedelic therapy.[4]

The fact that network resetting amounts, cognitively, to discovering and consolidating new forms of self-modelling is exemplified by reports of a kind that we have revisited repeatedly. These reports show how the phenomenal awareness of plasticity—the feeling of freedom, disidentification with the narrative self, and identification with a more minimal experiential self—can lead directly to the discovery and adoption of new, more beneficial self-conceptions:

> There was a part there where I felt gone ... it wasn't like [the last psilocybin session] where I always remembered I was Adam. There was a part there where I was gone ... I remember telling myself you took this [the psilocybin] to try and help. And it is helping ... There's the old Adam, then the new Adam without alcohol.
>
> (Nielson et al. 2018, p. 8).

---

[4] The distinction between psychoplastogenic and psychedelic effects is similar to the distinction drawn by Andrew Jones (2018) between 'mind-modifying' and 'mind-manifesting' effects. However, Jones defines 'mind-manifesting' effects specifically in terms of the traditional idea that psychedelics facilitate access to previously *unconscious* mental contents. Here I remain neutral on whether psychedelics facilitate access to content that is unconscious in the classical psychoanalytic sense. My definition of psychedelic effects is broader: It encompasses any effect in which psychedelics make manifest an otherwise latent potential of the mind, such as its potential for alternative forms of self-modelling or patterns of attention.

It felt like I'd died as a smoker and was resurrected as a nonsmoker. Because it's my perception of myself, and that's how I felt. So I jumped up and I said 'I'm not a smoker anymore, it's all done.'

(Noorani et al. 2018, p. 759).

A report from a different patient in this second cohort illustrates how the process of revising one's self-conception can include metaphorical or imagistic aspects:

I used to hide sitting on the air conditioning unit on the side of my house, when I used to smoke. And so the image was me sitting there, smoking, all hunched over, stupid, smoking. And the vine just rising up and this purply flower face thing looking down at me like, 'how ridiculous!' And then I'm not really that [person], I'm really this vine, that's really me, and the Goddess within me ... how silly to think that [smoking] ... was going to do anything or solve anything. So it was really just that rising up feeling, and that powerful feeling, and it just filled me with such beauty and strength and life.

(Noorani et al. 2018, p. 759).

It is important to note that revisions to the narrative self need not only target one's fundamental attributes or roles (e.g., being 'a smoker' or 'not a smoker'). They can also involve, inter alia, increasing the overall coherence of one's autobiographical narratives by finding patterns, connections, and meaning within these narratives, bringing a new sense of order, unity, or satisfaction to the sense one has of one's life as a whole:

[One cancer patient] described how the psilocybin led him through a kind of life review where 'everything that had occurred to me since the day I was born until that very moment made sense.' He further explained that the psilocybin was:

... rolling back all the experiences of my life. Whether it's a sprained ankle, or a delicious meal, or my marriage, or the children, or the clothes I've bought all my life ... revealed in a more profound way ... So that everything had its place. I didn't think a lot about cancer, and in many ways, cancer wasn't in the room.

(Swift et al. 2017, p. 505).

This report clearly resonates with other descriptions, including by cancer patients (Gasser et al. 2015), of 'zooming out' and gaining *broader perspectives*. In such experiences, patients come to see their own lives and problems, including their illnesses, in a much larger context, leading to a diminished attentional fixation on prior topics of rumination. We will return to experiences of this kind momentarily.

Interestingly, in the qualitative study of psilocybin therapy for tobacco addiction conducted by Noorani et al. (2018), many patients described the transformation of their self-identity not in terms of learning something new, but in terms of reconnecting with 'core values' that had been forgotten or neglected over the years. So perhaps, in some cases, subjects do not discover new forms of self-modelling so much as rediscover old, disused forms. This fits well with the contention of Nichols et al., in their presentation of the Reset Theory, that:

> as the effect of the drug wears off, networks can reconnect in 'healthy' ways, in the absence of the pathological driving force(s) that originally led to hub failure and disease ... the brain is able to restore its network connectivity *to a predisease state*.
> **(2017, p. 215; my emphasis).**

As we have seen, the self-model is not just a model of one's body, thoughts, and biography, but also a model of what matters to one. This is why a rediscovery of, or reconnection with, 'core values' amounts to a revision of the self-model. As a hierarchical salience model (Wiese 2019), it represents the relative importance of various classes of stimuli to one's postulated goals and interests, and uses this information to allocate attention and processing resources. This is why pharmacological disruption of the self-model can lead subjects to become aware of, or even fascinated by, stimuli that they would normally ignore—such as the pattern of veins on a leaf (Watts 1962), or the fabric of a pair of trousers (Huxley 1954).

This fact about self-modelling has an important corollary, foreshadowed above: that some of the ways in which self-models can become dysfunctional in pathology, and can be restored to a more beneficial form through psychedelic treatments, have to do with the *patterns of attention* that they underpin. Many reports from patients speak to this point. Patients who receive psychedelics often discover new ways of paying attention during the drug-induced experience—ways less filtered through the hypothesised cares and concerns of a solid, sharply bounded, isolated self:

> It was less about my [terminal] illness. I was able to put it into perspective.... Not to see oneself with one's sickness as centre. There are more important things in life ... The evolution of humankind for example ... Your Inner Ego gets diminished, I believe, and you are looking at the whole ... you are indeed starting to build relations with plants or with the entire living world around. You think less about yourself, you are thinking—across borders.
> **(Gasser et al. 2015, p. 26).**

Moreover, they often make clear that these new patterns of attention outlast the acute experience, and sometimes describe making a deliberate effort, whether formal or informal, to consolidate these attentional changes:

> I feel like a whole bunch of crap has been dumped off the surface. This stuff that made my world shut down so much and made me look at the ground and watch the clock numbers clicking by. There's life and so many things going on, just watching that tree over there blowing in the breeze, seeing people in the street, and all the

different people in vehicles rushing by! I just feel good about being alive ... It's always there; we just don't notice, and *I'm trying to notice and not forget that I can see it at any time, I can hear it any time*. It's like waking up in the most profound way, that this is really what life is.

(Swift et al. 2017, p. 507; my emphasis).

I've been exploring whether I can bring back other sensations from [the psilocybin experience] ... I have been able to, and I've been doing a lot of meditating. I got into meditating afterward because it was like, 'I just don't want to lose this', ... I really felt like there was a real connection with Buddhism and meditation and the psilocybin experience for me. And I've been doing that everyday.

(Malone et al. 2018, p. 5).

Indeed, the predictive self-binding account of psychedelic therapy can subsume many psychological factors that have been proposed as potential therapeutic mechanisms. Shifts from feelings of disconnection to connection (Carhart-Harris et al 2018a) involve a change in the experienced boundaries or relations of the self. Shifts from attitudes of rejection or avoidance to acceptance (Watts et al. 2017) involve a change in how one experiences the relationship between the self and its thoughts, feelings, body, and world. Psychological insight (Davis et al. 2020) and emotional breakthrough (Roseman et al. 2019) are often focused on autobiographical themes, and mindfulness-related capacities (Madsen et al. 2020) centrally involve changes to the sense of self. Even the feeling of awe (Hendricks 2018) involves the experience of the 'small self': a sense of being small or insignificant relative to some vaster reality (Piff et al. 2015). Finally, changed perceptions of meaning (Hartogsohn 2018) are linked to self-representation via the functions of the SN (cf. Smigielski et al. 2020).

If these speculations are on the mark, then psychedelic therapy has a two-factor structure. The induction of plasticity at multiple levels—neural, cognitive, and phenomenological—is necessary, and may suffice for the relatively short-term afterglow. It also lays the foundation for truly durable change, because it includes the vivid experiential insight into the availability of other forms of self-modelling—other ways of seeing and being; other ways of paying attention and relating to one's world. This, I have suggested, is closely related to the induction of phenomenal opacity. But for truly durable change to occur, the induction of plasticity alone does not suffice. New, healthier forms of self-modelling must be discovered during the acute experience, and consolidated during the subsequent period of integration.

Earlier I invoked the popular analogy between the 'hypothesis-testing' predictive brain and a scientist formulating theories, generating predictions, and testing them against the evidence. In light of this analogy, it is interesting to note that psychedelic therapy is structurally analogous to a scientific paradigm shift as described by Thomas Kuhn (1970). The acute psychedelic experience amounts to a kind of neurocognitive crisis, featuring high levels of intractable anomalies (i.e., increased prediction error signalling) precipitated by disrupting the core tenets of the dominant paradigm.

(These are psychoplastogenic effects.) However, as Kuhn emphasised, crisis alone does not beget revolution. A new neurocognitive paradigm must be found that constitutes a viable replacement for the old. (This necessarily involves *psychedelic* effects.) Otherwise, once the afterglow wears off, business as usual, in the form of well-worn neural pathways and the cognitive habits that they underpin, will inexorably resume.

7.8 Self and self-consciousness

If the broad picture of psychedelic therapy and self-representation outlined here is correct, the philosophical implications are considerable. With respect to our main concerns in this book, the implications are twofold. First, the predictive self-binding account bolsters the claim that the epistemic risks of psychedelic therapy, given naturalism, are relatively small. Second, it provides a basis for the claim that the epistemic benefits of psychedelic therapy, given naturalism, are relatively large. I will argue for this second claim explicitly in Chapter 8. First, however, I should briefly mention some of the other apparent philosophical implications—specifically, for questions about self-consciousness and the metaphysics of the self.

7.8.1 Selfless consciousness

A controversial question in the philosophy of mind is whether there can be phenomenally conscious mental states that lack all forms of self-consciousness. Following Millière (2020), I will call these 'totally selfless' phenomenal states. (At this point, we are remaining neutral on whether any such things as selves actually exist. The question is simply whether there can be conscious experiences without the phenomenal feeling *as of* being or having a self.)

The claim that totally selfless phenomenal states are impossible has a long history. Recent empirically oriented debates have focused on putative counterexamples from pathological conditions such as akinetic mutism and epileptic automatism (Damasio 1999), as well as schizophrenic thought insertion and DPD (Graham and Stephens 1994, Billon and Kriegel 2015, Billon 2016). Other authors have examined mystical and meditative states (Forman 1998, Albahari 2006, Millière et al. 2018), and states of deep dreamless sleep in which phenomenal consciousness is allegedly retained (Thompson 2015, Windt et al. 2016). Of course, the induction of totally selfless phenomenal states has long been portrayed as an attainable goal by mystical traditions such as Buddhism and Advaita Vedanta (Albahari 2006, 2014, Metzinger 2003), and putative instances of such induction are now objects of empirical research (e.g., Winter et al. 2020). But the interpretation of relevant evidence is highly contentious.

Recently, several philosophers have turned to psychedelic research, in the hope that it might furnish clearer cases. Relatively few psychedelic experience reports describe, unambiguously, a *total* loss of self-consciousness, but some seem to. One of the clearest examples, to my mind, is Michael Pollan's description of his 5-methoxy-N,N-dimethyltryptamine (5-MeO-DMT) trip, which we encountered in Chapter 3, section 3.3:

> I felt a tremendous rush of energy fill my head ... and then ... 'I' was no more, blasted to a confetti cloud by an explosive force. I could no longer locate [myself] in my head, because it had exploded that too, expanding to become all that there was. Whatever this was, it was not a hallucination. A hallucination implies a reality and a point of reference and an entity to have it. None of those things remained.
>
> **(Pollan 2018, pp. 276–277).**

There are other reports that also seem to clearly and explicitly describe a total abolition of all forms of phenomenal selfhood. I quoted another, from a research subject administered intravenous DMT, in Chapter 3, section 3.3:

> I immediately saw a bright yellow-white light directly in front of me ... I was consumed by it and became part of it. There were no distinctions—no figures or lines, shadows or outlines. There was no body or anything inside or outside. I was devoid of self, of thought, of time, of space, of a sense of separateness or ego, or of anything but the white light. There are no symbols in my language that can begin to describe that sense of pure being, oneness, and ecstasy. There was a great sense of stillness and ecstasy.
>
> **(Strassman 2001, pp. 244–245.)**

According to the predictive self-binding account, the sense of self is ultimately just one more conscious experience among many. It is part of an intracranial virtual reality conjured by neurocomputational mechanisms that are susceptible to pharmacological disruption. This view suggests that the sense of self might be unnecessary for conscious experience, despite its ubiquity in the default waking state. Here, then, is a simple psychedelic argument for the existence of totally selfless phenomenal states:

> 1. If someone reports undergoing a phenomenal state of some kind, and there is no good reason to mistrust their report, then we should conclude that they did undergo a phenomenal state of that kind.
> 2. Some psychedelic users, such as those quoted above, report undergoing totally selfless phenomenal states during psychedelic experience.
> 3. There is no good reason to mistrust their reports.
> 4. Therefore, we should conclude that these psychedelic users have experienced totally selfless phenomenal states.
> 5. Therefore, no form of self-consciousness is necessary for phenomenal consciousness.
>
> **(Adapted from Billon and Kriegel 2015, p. 36).**

Personally, I find this argument quite persuasive, and I have defended something like it elsewhere (Letheby 2020). Premise 1 is a relatively uncontroversial methodological principle of consciousness science,[5] which I will take for granted here. But even with this premise granted, several difficulties arise.

Take premise 2, for instance. Do reports of this kind really describe conscious experiences without any sense of self? At first glance, it might seem that nothing could be clearer. Consider Pollan's insistence that neither 'a reality [nor] a point of reference [nor] an entity' remained, and the DMT subject's description of an experience devoid 'of self, of thought, of time, of space, of a sense of separateness or ego, or of anything but the white light'. What possible phenomenological report could describe a total loss of self-consciousness more explicitly or less ambiguously?

This interpretation has been contested, however. There are at least two other possibilities. The first is that reports such as these describe not ego dissolution but ego *expansion*: profoundly unitive experiences in which the phenomenal unit of identification, far from contracting to nothing, expands to coincide with the entire conscious field. In this case, such experiences would not be ones in which the phenomenal ego disappears, but simply ones in which phenomenal ego-*boundaries* disappear. They might nonetheless be described by subjects in terms of a loss of self or ego because, in ordinary waking consciousness, a sense of self is always accompanied by a sense of a self-other boundary. However, as Sebastián (2020) points out, it cannot be a *conceptual* truth that the existence of a self requires a self/other boundary, otherwise solipsism would be an incoherent (rather than a merely implausible) position. Sebastián contends that extant reports of psychedelic ego dissolution are ambiguous between these two interpretations—that they describe a conscious state lacking phenomenal selfhood, and that they describe a conscious state merely lacking a phenomenal self/other *boundary*—and, as such, that we lack sufficient justification for premise 2 of the argument above.

A second challenge to premise 2 appeals to the notion of 'for-me-ness', drawn from the phenomenological tradition in philosophy and championed most notably by Dan Zahavi (2011, 2014). For-me-ness is sometimes described as the most minimal form of self-consciousness possible. Its proponents hold that it is not one more content of consciousness among many, but an ineliminable structural feature of consciousness as such:

> ... the 'me' of for-me-ness is not in the first instance an aspect of *what* is experienced but of *how* it is experienced; not an object of experience, but a constitutive manner of experiencing. To deny that such a feature is present in our experiential life, to deny the for-me-ness or mineness [sic] of experience, is to fail to recognize the very subjectivity of experience [...] once *anything* occurs consciously, it must be given to the subject and thus exhibit for-me-ness. In other words, the 'me' of

---

[5] However, it is denied, at least according to some interpretations, by the methodological stance that Dennett (1991, 2003) dubs 'heterophenomenology'.

for-me-ness is not a separate and distinct item but rather a pervasive feature of experiential life as such.

(Zahavi and Kriegel, 2015, p. 38; emphasis original).

Some have argued that phenomenological reports of the kind above may unambiguously describe a total absence of narrative, bodily, and affective self-consciousness,
but do not unambiguously describe the absence of for-me-ness (Henriksen and
Parnas 2019). Furthermore, it has been suggested that for-me-ness, or something
like it, must have been present in these experiences; otherwise subjects could not
unhesitatingly ascribe the past experiences to *themselves*. On this line of reasoning,
these subjects have no doubt whatsoever that the remarkable states of consciousness
happened to them, rather than to somebody else, and this fact is only explicable on
the supposition that these experiences were 'given to [that] subject and thus [exhib-
ited] for-me-ness' (cf. Sebastián 2020). This is reminiscent of, although not identical
to, an argument from Metzinger against trusting phenomenological reports of this
kind. Metzinger (2003, p. 566) contends that giving a retrospective report of a totally
selfless state of consciousness creates a 'performative self-contradiction', because the
act of giving a retrospective autobiographical report presupposes that the self was
present in the earlier experience, but this presupposition is contradicted by the content of the report (i.e., that the experience was selfless; see Fink 2020 and Millière
2020 for discussion).

Metzinger's performative self-contradiction argument is probably best construed
as a challenge to premise 3: the claim that there is no positive reason to mistrust reports of this kind. Sebastián has also challenged this premise, arguing that there is
reason to suspect that subjects' retrospective conceptualisation of their experiences
is subject to cognitive bias arising from the cultural influence of neo-Buddhist frameworks in interpreting the psychedelic experience. He points out that, in some cultures,
traditional psychedelic use is viewed more as a means 'for meeting spirits and getting power and knowledge from them' than as a means to attaining 'ego-dissolution
or mystical union with the universe' (2020, p. 21). It is questionable how much explanatory work cognitive bias can do here. Investigators were describing the effects
of mescaline in terms of depersonalisation, derealisation, and the dissolution of
ego boundaries well before psychedelics were linked to Eastern spiritual disciplines
by the now-canonical writings of Huxley, Watts, and Leary (e.g., Guttmann 1936).
However, it is certainly interesting to compare the above description of DMT-induced
ecstasy by Strassman's subject with the passage, quoted by Sebastián, in which Leary
et al. describe psychedelic-induced, putatively Buddhist illumination as 'complete transcendence—beyond words, beyond space—time, beyond self. There are
no visions, no sense of self, no thoughts. There are only pure awareness and ecstatic
freedom' (Leary et al. 1964, quoted in Sebastián 2020, p. 20). Of course, there is more
than one way of explaining such commonalities—but cognitive bias and cultural
framing cannot be discounted.

In sum, inferring the existence of totally selfless consciousness from the extant psychedelic evidence is less straightforward than it initially appears. Of course, there are responses that can be made to the worries that I have just raised: see, for example, Fink (2020), Letheby (2020), and Millière (2020) for discussion. However, delving deeply into these issues would take us too far afield from our primary concerns in this book. As such, I will simply note two things. First, reports of the kind we have seen may not demonstrate that there can be states of consciousness totally lacking any sense of self. However, they do demonstrate quite clearly that there can be states of consciousness lacking anything like the ordinary sense of self—indeed, lacking anything that subjects recognise, or are willing to describe, as a sense of self. In the debate over whether there can be *totally* selfless experiences, it is easy to forget how remarkable a discovery this 'weaker' conclusion really is.

The second point is that, even if it does not prove the existence of totally selfless consciousness, psychedelic evidence inverts traditional wisdom about the relationship between self-consciousness and phenomenal consciousness. Often we are apt to think of the former as somehow a constitutive or enabling condition of the latter. It may yet turn out to be a necessary condition. But, if so, it is remarkable that, as its salience and influence diminish, the breadth, variety, vividness, and intensity of conscious experience in general seem to increase (Carhart-Harris et al. 2014). Even if there are no states of consciousness that lack self-consciousness altogether, it is still startling to note that a primary effect of self-consciousness seems to be to constrain, regulate, and limit the contents of phenomenal consciousness itself.

7.8.2 Does the self exist?

Perhaps psychedelic evidence more straightforwardly supports a second controversial but venerable philosophical thesis: that the self does not exist. This view is most often associated with Buddhism, but has also been defended in contemporary neurophilosophy and philosophy of mind, by philosophers such as Metzinger (2003), Albahari (2006), and Bayne (2010). According to Letheby and Gerrans (2017), the evidence concerning psychedelic ego dissolution supports eliminativism about selves. Their psychedelic argument for the no-self view can be summarised as follows:

1. We represent the self as having a particular set of properties.
2. No real entity has that set of properties.
3. Therefore, the self is not real.

(McClelland 2019, p. 25).[6]

---

[6] The argument as McClelland presents it has two further steps, and purports to establish a variant of the no-self view that he calls the 'virtual self theory'. However, this more limited argument for anti-realism about the self will suffice for present purposes.

The role of the psychedelic evidence is to provide support for premise 1. Part of the evidence for the predictive self-binding account is subjects' reports of dying, disintegrating, or merging with the cosmos, which can readily be explained if the brain normally models the self as a Cartesian substance: a simple, indivisible, persisting entity, sharply distinct from all of its properties. Premise 2 is supported by the fact that scientific investigations have never discovered such an entity anywhere in the brain or body. Moreover, it remains as mysterious as ever how such an entity would interact with the neurophysiological processes known to implement perception, cognition, and action. It would seem, then, that Metzinger is correct: 'For all scientific and philosophical purposes, the notion of a self—as a theoretical entity—can be safely eliminated' (2003, p. 563).

Of course, matters are not so simple. As Tom McClelland (2019) points out, the *Mismatch Argument* as formulated above is straightforwardly invalid. From the facts that (a) we represent a given entity as having a particular set of properties, and (b) no real entity has that set of properties, it does not follow that (c) the entity in question is not real. That is just one possibility that is consistent with the premises. Another is that the entity in question is real, but is radically misrepresented by us. Compare: if everyone on the planet came to believe that Donald Trump was a very stable genius, the man himself would continue to exist, despite this flagrant misrepresentation. Moreover, the discovery that our sun is a huge ball of flaming gas, rather than (say) a divinity, did not support eliminativism about the sun, but rather a dramatic revision of our beliefs about the kind of entity it is and the properties that it bears.

Thus, McClelland argues, the apparently dramatic mismatch between (a) our pretheoretic conception of the self, and (b) the kinds of entities to be found in reality, does not license eliminativism about selves; it may simply require a revision of our beliefs about what kinds of things selves are. He also offers positive reasons to prefer such revisionism. Specifically, he appeals to the idea that our self-representations are *de se* representations: on his gloss, representations that refer to whatever it is that bears them. Since these representations are, in fact, borne by something—such as the brain or the organism—whatever that thing is should be regarded as the referent of the self-model. On this view, the pretheoretic error that requires correction is not belief in the existence of selves. The error, rather, is a deep-seated misconception about the *kinds of things* that selves are: the reflexive assumption that they are Cartesian substances, rather than complex biological systems or processes.

One possible response on behalf of the no-self theory would be to hold that the mismatch is too great for identification to be on the cards. In other words, biological systems are so different from the kinds of things we pretheoretically take selves to be that it is more reasonable to eliminate the latter from our ontology than to identify them with the former. This is the line taken by Letheby and Gerrans (2017), who draw a comparison to the elimination of caloric in the mechanical theory of heat. However, as McClelland points out, it is very difficult to determine a quantitative threshold for how great a mismatch can be before revisionism is ruled out: many actual cases (such as that of the sun) suggest that any such threshold must be very high. Sometimes, even an extremely drastic misrepresentation of an entity leads us to a revisionary, not an eliminative, conclusion.

Another approach would be to highlight certain properties as necessary or essential to the concept of a self. This line is also taken by Letheby and Gerrans: 'The pretheoretic concept of SELF has sufficiently *central* and *defining* metaphysical commitments that it ... merits ... eliminative treatment' (2017, p. 8; my emphasis). But, as McClelland points out, it is very difficult to establish, in a principled, non-question-begging way, what properties are necessary or essential to a contested concept like SELF.

It would be possible to pursue these issues further. One strategy would be to analyse the differences between revisionary and eliminative responses to mismatch cases, to see if there is any principled way to decide which response is warranted in a given case. Another would be to scrutinise McClelland's claims about the nature of *de se* representations, or his potentially ambiguous claim that all mental representations must have a 'bearer'. (What is a 'bearer', in the relevant sense? Is it simply a substrate of some sort, or something more like a subject?) Once again, however, this would take us too far afield from our primary concerns.

For now, let us simply assume that McClelland is correct: the Mismatch Argument for anti-realism about the self fails. In this case, can psychedelic evidence tell us anything about the metaphysics of the self? Yes, it can. It can tell us that, if the self does exist, then it is something very different from what we automatically and unthinkingly take it (i.e., ourselves) to be: that the kind of thing we automatically and unthinkingly take ourselves to be simply does not exist. These are genuine insights that may not sloganise easily (à la 'the self does not exist') but are no less profound for all that.

If the predictive self-binding account is on the right track, then each of us, whether we are introspectively aware of it or not, experiences ourself as a Cartesian substance: a simple, indivisible, and persistent mental entity that undergoes experiences, thinks thoughts, feels feelings, and authors actions. But no such entity exists. Moreover, that which we habitually take for our own immediate unproblematic existence is no more than a virtual simulacrum or 'phenomenal avatar' (Gerrans 2015, p. 2) conjured by the brain for purposes of prediction and control. When a high degree of opacity is introduced into the phenomenal self-model by psychedelics or other means, there is something real that we learn. It may not be, exactly, that the self does not exist. But what we learn, at least, is that the experience we have been *mistaking* for our very being is no more than a contingent and fragile mental construction. Self qua Cartesian substance does not exist; self qua mental subject whose existence is immediately (non-representationally) apparent to consciousness does not exist; and self qua witnessing entity, necessarily experientially present in all conscious states, does not exist. The existential shock that often attends such realisations attests to our intuitive convictions to the contrary.

7.9 Conclusion

We have covered quite a bit of ground in this chapter and the last. The main take-home messages, however, are these: the epistemic risks of psychedelic therapy, given naturalism, are smaller than they might initially appear. This conclusion, already supported by the arguments of Chapter 4, is underscored by the positive picture of psychedelic therapy developed in these two chapters. Psychedelic therapy does not work mainly by inducing compelling metaphysical hallucinations and non-naturalistic metaphysical beliefs. Such ideations are sometimes involved in the process, but they are neither inevitable nor necessary. Rather, psychedelic therapy works mainly by undermining our fundamental assumptions about ourselves, our lives, and our relations to the world, facilitating the beneficial revision of these assumptions. This explains why there are so many reports from patients or volunteers who have experienced therapeutic benefits but do not emphasise non-naturalistic metaphysical apprehensions, focusing instead on feelings of psychological insight, new perspectives, emotional catharsis, connectedness, and acceptance. It also explains the quantitative findings reviewed in Chapter 5 that implicate (i) psychological insight, (ii) mindfulness-related capacities, and (iii) modulation of self-related neurocognitive systems (the DMN and SN) in the therapeutic process.

In this chapter, I have repeatedly discussed the phenomenal opacity induced by psychedelics in terms of important and genuine, albeit oft-misinterpreted, *insights*: insights into the constructed nature of the sense of self and the availability of other forms of self-modelling. This lays the groundwork for the second premise of my response to the Comforting Delusion Objection: that the epistemic benefits of psychedelic therapy, given naturalism, are greater than they initially appear. Arguing for this conclusion explicitly is the task of Chapter 8.

8
Epistemology

To be a poet is to have a soul so quick to discern, that no shade of quality escapes it, and so quick to feel, that discernment is but a hand playing with finely-ordered variety on the chords of emotion—a soul in which knowledge passes instantaneously into feeling, and feeling flashes back as a new organ of knowledge.

George Eliot, *Middlemarch*.

8.1 Introduction

If naturalism is true, then the use of psychedelics, even under controlled circumstances, carries epistemic risks. The upshot of the preceding chapters is that those risks are less than one might suppose. Metaphysical hallucinations of a Joyous Cosmology are neither the central mechanism, nor an inevitable concomitant, of psychedelic therapy. And even when they do occur, they need not be believed uncritically.

Nevertheless, the risks are real. Some psychedelic users claim sincerely to encounter genuinely existing disembodied entities, spirit realms, and transcendent Grounds of Being. On principled philosophical grounds, naturalists reject these claims as arising from compelling drug-induced hallucinations—misrepresentations of reality. Why not reject *all* claims to psychedelic-assisted epistemic benefit wholesale? We already know that some psychedelic-induced feelings of knowledge acquisition are erroneous; should we not assume, parsimoniously, that all are?

In this chapter, I argue that the answer is no. Some claims to psychedelic-assisted epistemic benefit are accurate. The key to understanding the epistemic profile of the psychedelic state comes from Andy Clark's dictum that prior knowledge in the predictive brain is 'always both constraining and enabling' (2016, p. 288). By weakening the influence of high-level priors, psychedelics both unconstrain and disable: certain epistemic benefits available in the sober state become unavailable, such as rational and critical thought and the ability to deploy much prior knowledge, while others unavailable in the sober state become available—principally, the opportunity to access information otherwise filtered out by overweighted priors, as well as the ability to represent certain kinds of information in novel and epistemically useful formats.

However, in our travels through the landscape of psychedelic epistemology, a second guiding principle comes from Jennifer Windt's observation that 'phenomenal certainty—the experience of persuasion or knowing—is not the same as epistemic justification' (2011, p. 246). Having a psychedelic experience in which some proposition P seems true, accompanied by a strong phenomenal feeling of certainty, does not constitute sufficient justification for believing that P is true. The phenomenal feeling of certainty is no different, in principle, from the phenomenal feelings of familiarity and salience, which are erroneously amplified in déjà vu and psychosis, as well as in some psychedelic states: having a psychedelic experience in which some place feels familiar or some stimulus seems important does not entail that one has visited the place before or that the stimulus is important. The feelings of certainty, familiarity, and salience[1] are just more components of the controlled hallucination that is conscious experience: 'designed' by evolution to track important higher-order properties of stimuli; good enough at the job under normal conditions, but fallible and susceptible to disruption and error. Of course, it can be difficult for those who undergo intense noetic feelings to take this sceptical stance seriously, because this is *precisely the function* of the phenomenal feeling of certainty: to instil confidence in some item or source of information.

I begin the chapter by criticising some general arguments that purport to demonstrate the impossibility of psychedelic-facilitated epistemic benefit. To my mind, such arguments are unpersuasive: the question whether psychedelics can facilitate epistemic benefits cannot be decided in the abstract. Instead, we must consider individual proposals about specific types of epistemic benefits on their own merits (Letheby 2019).

With these caveats in mind, what sorts of epistemic benefits might typical psychedelic experiences in modern clinical contexts afford? When it comes to gaining factual or propositional knowledge, the most plausible candidate is insight into one's previously unconscious mental states: psychodynamic insight into hidden desires, motivations, and the like. In section 8.3, I consider whether psychedelics can facilitate genuine insights of this kind. I argue that they probably can, but may also facilitate erroneous but beneficial 'placebo insights' (Jopling 2001). Apparent insights under the influence should be taken seriously, but in determining their veracity there is no substitute for subsequent sober evaluation.

In section 8.4, I argue that psychedelics can facilitate the acquisition of ability knowledge, or 'knowledge how'. Empirical findings on commonalities between the psychedelic state and mindfulness meditation suggest that psychedelic subjects can learn how to pay attention and relate to their inner experience in novel and beneficial ways that result from disruptions to self-binding mechanisms. The consolidation of these attentional skills may be an important part of the therapeutic process, at least in some cases.

---

[1] Analogous remarks apply to the sense of reality. The phenomenal feeling that the putative realities encountered in psychedelic experience are 'more real than real', or more real than those encountered in waking life, is of limited evidential value in itself. The sense of reality is yet another component of the controlled hallucination that is conscious experience. It is known to be modulated, for instance, in pathologies such as depersonalisation disorder (Varga 2012) as well as in psychedelic states.

In sections 8.5 and 8.6, I propose that several important epistemic benefits of psychedelics fall under the rubrics of *knowledge by acquaintance* and *new knowledge of old facts*. By collapsing the predictive processing (PP) hierarchy and opening up novel modes of neurocognitive function, psychedelics allow users to become (more-or-less) directly acquainted with certain facts that otherwise are accessible only indirectly or inferentially: facts about the potential of the mind and the constructed, mutable nature of the sense of self (Letheby 2015). This knowledge by acquaintance is the epistemic aspect of the phenomenal opacity involved in the therapeutic process. Psychedelics also facilitate the apprehension of otherwise-knowable facts in new 'modes of presentation': what previously was knowable only as a mere intellectual proposition can be experienced as a vividly embodied, affective, perceptual reality.

In section 8.7, I argue that transformative psychedelic experiences can yield numerous indirect epistemic benefits, which come via their psychosocial benefits: boosting psychosocial functioning often boosts epistemic functioning as well (Bortolotti 2015). The conclusion is that, by temporarily weakening the influence of prior beliefs and reconfiguring the brain's processing hierarchy, psychedelics make available significant epistemic benefits that are consistent with naturalism and often unavailable by any alternative means. Finally, in section 8.8, I conclude that many psychedelic states are, in Lisa Bortolotti's parlance, *epistemically innocent* (Letheby 2016). This means that, despite having real epistemic flaws, they also have significant epistemic benefits that are not available by any alternative means. In sum, psychedelics' overall epistemic profile is neither as dire as some sceptical naturalists might assume, nor as pristine as some entheogenic enthusiasts would like.

8.2 Psychopharmacology and epistemology

Suppose that your friend, let us call her Maria,[2] has volunteered and been selected to take part in a scientific trial of psilocybin. Maria is excited about this opportunity because, despite being an academic expert in the mind and brain sciences and thoroughly conversant with the literature on psychedelics, she has never taken a psychedelic herself. The day after her first psilocybin session, you visit Maria at her home. She seems peaceful, serene, but brimming with energy, and reports that the psychedelic experience was deeply transformative: not only are her mood and sense of well-being greatly elevated, but, moreover, she claims to have *learned* a lot from the experience— to have gained significant epistemic benefits by undergoing a drug-induced state of consciousness. Perhaps, like others before her, she claims to have learned more about her own mind in one afternoon than in years of psychotherapy or academic training.

---

[2] With apologies to Frank Jackson (1982) and Miri Albahari (2014), and in honour of Maria Estevez (2013) and the late María Sabina.

Perhaps she even claims to have gained deep insights into the human condition or the nature of reality.

If you are a sceptically minded analytic philosopher, you might press Maria—tactfully, one hopes—on the plausibility of her claim:

> Maria, are you sure this was *real* knowledge that you gained? After all, you were on drugs. You're a highly educated, critically minded person: You have to consider the possibility that you were just hallucinating. After all, these specific drugs are *called* 'hallucinogens'!

Perhaps, in the back of your mind, you might even be formulating an argument for the falsity of Maria's claim to have derived epistemic benefit from her psychedelic experience. The argument might go something like this:

1. Psychedelics are drugs
2. It is impossible to gain epistemic benefits by taking a drug
3. Therefore, it is impossible to gain epistemic benefits by taking psychedelics[3]

This *Argument from Drug Use* is valid: the premises entail the conclusion. However, it is unsound: as Maria will no doubt point out, the second premise is patently false. This is made clear by the old saw that a mathematician is a device for turning coffee into theorems,[4] as well as by neuroethical debates over the permissibility of 'pharmacological cognitive enhancement' (Sahakian and Morein-Zamir 2015) in which its *efficacy* is taken for granted. It obviously is possible to gain non-trivial epistemic benefits by the judicious ingestion of psychoactive substances. Whether psychedelics are among those substances or not is another question. But this question cannot be decided simply by noting that they *are* psychoactive substances.

At this juncture, if your scepticism persists, you might be tempted to venture another argument. You might say to Maria:

> Of course, *some* drugs can help you gain knowledge—but not *these* drugs! It's totally absurd to suggest that you learned anything by taking *hallucinogens*. I mean, it's right there in the name. Everyone knows that these drugs cause you to see things that aren't there and that their basic effect is to distort your perception of reality.

This is similar to an argument given by G.T. Roche (2010, p. 36) against the claim that psychedelic experiences can have epistemic benefits. We might gloss this argument as follows:

---

[3] I am deeply indebted to Ole Martin Moen for reminding me of the value of good old-fashioned syllogisms in thinking clearly about these (and many other) issues.
[4] Which apparently is due to the mathematician Alfréd Rényi (Kucharski 2013).

1. Psychedelics impair the mechanisms whereby the brain generates accurate representations of reality
2. It is impossible to gain epistemic benefits by impairing the mechanisms whereby the brain generates accurate representations of reality
3. Therefore, it is impossible to gain epistemic benefits by taking psychedelics

This new *Argument from Impairment* is valid, too, on the face of it. But, if Maria is in the mood to argue, she might find fault with both premises. The first premise is ambiguous: it might mean that impairing reality-representing mechanisms is *one* effect of psychedelics, or that it is their *only* effect. Clearly, on the second interpretation, this premise would beg the question against Maria. She will no doubt concede that psychedelics' effects include the impairment of some reality-representing mechanisms. She is well aware, for instance, that psychedelics can cause people to see actually stationary objects as moving, or to perceive spatial distances and temporal durations less accurately. She is also aware that they are known to promote suggestibility (Carhart-Harris et al. 2015), at least during their acute effects. Nonetheless, she is claiming that, in addition to their undeniably impairing effects, psychedelics can *also* have distinct, epistemically beneficial effects.

In order not to be question-begging, then, the first premise must be understood merely as saying that impairment is *one* effect of psychedelics; but on this reading, the argument is invalid. Even if one effect of psychedelics is the impairment of reality-representing mechanisms, and this is no way to gain epistemic benefits, it may still be possible to gain epistemic benefits by taking psychedelics—the benefits would just have to come via some of their other effects. On this weaker interpretation, the argument becomes analogous to the following: eating vindaloo stimulates capsaicin receptors; it is impossible to nourish oneself by stimulating capsaicin receptors; therefore, it is impossible to nourish oneself by eating vindaloo.[5]

Even if Maria were to grant the first premise in its strong, question-begging form, she might still find fault with the second premise. Being a student of the mind and brain sciences, she might even quote to you Clark's dictum that prior knowledge in the predictive brain is always both constraining and enabling. On the PP model of psychedelic action outlined in the preceding chapters, the maintenance of the high-level priors that psychedelics disrupt is a central part of the mechanism whereby the brain normally generates more-or-less accurate representations of (a certain slice of) reality—namely, prediction error-driven updating of a hierarchical generative model. But this is consistent with the idea that 'impairing' (or, more neutrally, disrupting) that mechanism by decreasing the precision-weighting of those priors might have epistemic benefits—for instance, by increasing the influence and availability of bottom-up information previously filtered out by those priors (Carhart-Harris and

---

[5] Of course, notwithstanding its undeniable nutritional content, a diet consisting mainly of vindaloo, like that of Dave Lister on the sci-fi sitcom *Red Dwarf*, would be no healthier than an epistemic diet consisting mainly of psychedelic experience.

Friston 2019). Recall the Hollow Mask Illusion, in which a mask presented in the concave orientation is perceived as convex. According to unpublished data, psychedelics decrease healthy subjects' susceptibility to this illusion (Passie unpublished, cited in Millière et al. 2018, p. 9). A simple explanation is as follows: by relaxing the prior belief that *all human faces are convex*, psychedelics afford greater influence to bottom-up sensory information that would otherwise be filtered out. They thereby facilitate veridical perception of the mask's orientation. So long as our reality-representing mechanisms are imperfect and partial, there is a real possibility that some epistemic benefit might be gained by impairing them temporarily.

If your intuitive resistance to Maria's claim of psychedelic-assisted epistemic benefit is sufficiently strong, you might hazard another argument at this point. This third argument focuses not on the fact that psychedelics are drugs, nor on claims about their cognitive effects, but on the fact that their putative epistemic benefits come via an *altered state of consciousness* (ASC). It takes the form of a dilemma:

1. For any putative item of knowledge gained during an ASC, either one has ASC-independent justification or one does not.
2. If one has ASC-independent justification, then the ASC is superfluous and is not, strictly speaking, responsible for the knowledge gain.
3. If one does not have ASC-independent justification, then the putative item of knowledge cannot be trusted (it may well be merely hallucination, illusion, or confabulation), so no knowledge gain has occurred.
4. Therefore, it is impossible to gain knowledge from an ASC (cf. Roche 2010, p. 36).

There are several ways Maria might respond to this *Argument from Alterity*. She might appeal to the distinction, pioneered in the philosophy of science, between the contexts of discovery and justification (Hoyningen-Huene 1987), insisting that her psychedelic experiences conferred genuine insights that she would never otherwise have had, while conceding that the justification for *accepting* these insights only came afterwards, from sober critical reflection on their plausibility. She might say, as many psychedelically treated patients do, that the epistemic benefits of her psychedelic session were not so much about learning new, previously unknown *facts*, but rather about coming to understand or grasp already known facts in a new and deeper way. Here she might invoke the philosophical idea of 'new knowledge of old facts', drawn from debates over Frank Jackson's (1982, 1986) Knowledge Argument[6] against physicalism. Or she might hold that theoretical considerations—perhaps drawn from PP—provide independent reason for trusting certain deliverances of the psychedelic state, such as putative psychodynamic insights. On this view, these theoretical considerations,

---

[6] My presentation of the issues in this chapter is heavily influenced by the debate that has sprung up around Jackson's argument and the corresponding thought experiment *Mary's Room* (Jackson 1982, 1986), both of which will come up again in section 8.5.

despite providing independent justification, would not render the ASC superfluous, because the latter would still be required to gain the specific insights themselves. The gist of this last response is that we might have independent justification for trusting some method of belief-formation, even though the source of that justification is not a *substitute* for that method (Letheby 2019). All three of these responses can be understood as challenges to premise 2. (Premise 1 would seem to be a logical truth; determining the plausibility of premise 3 is left as an exercise for the reader.)

Regardless of Maria's specific response to this new sceptical argument, the moral by now should be clear: the question cannot be decided in the abstract. General considerations will not suffice to determine the truth or falsity of Maria's (or anyone's) claim to have gained epistemic benefits by taking psychedelics. More information is required. All that we can do is to consider specific claims about specific types of epistemic benefits allegedly derived from psychedelic use, independently and on their own merits.

8.3 Knowledge that

Having grasped the futility of seeking a general answer to the question of psychedelic epistemology, at this point you may do what, perhaps, you ought to have done all along: ask Maria about the nature of the epistemic benefit(s) in question, and suspend judgement until you have more information. If you do so, there are many possible answers that she might give. We can classify these answers in accordance with standard epistemological categories. The type of epistemic benefit most often discussed in recent epistemology is the acquisition of *propositional knowledge*, also known as 'knowledge that' or 'factual knowledge'.

Propositional knowledge amounts, minimally, to *justified true belief*. According to philosophical consensus, knowing some proposition P entails (a) believing that P, where (b) P is true, and (c) one is justified (roughly, possessed of sufficient reasons or evidence[7]) in believing that P.[8] Paradigmatic examples include believing truly that the cat is on the mat, on the basis of normally functioning visual perception, and believing truly that Paris is the capital of France, due to reading a trustworthy encyclopaedia. Can psychedelics reliably facilitate the acquisition of knowledge of this kind?

---

[7] In adopting this intuitive understanding, I am deliberately sidestepping extensive controversies over the nature of epistemic justification.

[8] While the conditions of justification, truth, and belief are widely (although not universally) agreed to be necessary for propositional knowledge, they are also widely held to be insufficient, since the publication of Gettier's (1963) seminal article 'Is justified true belief knowledge?' Gettier presents cases in which subjects have justified true belief but intuitively lack knowledge. In light of this *Gettier Problem*, one of the most-discussed questions in recent epistemology concerns what fourth condition, if any, is required for knowledge.

Here I will ignore this complication. In my view, if we could show that psychedelics reliably facilitate the acquisition of justified true beliefs, that would be achievement enough. I also ignore this complication because it is far from clear, in any case, that propositional knowledge is the type most relevant to psychedelics' epistemic benefits.

Can controlled administration of lysergic acid diethylamide (LSD), psilocybin, or ayahuasca be the means whereby someone acquires a true belief *and* sufficient epistemic justification for it?

The most obvious candidate from a naturalistic standpoint concerns *psychodynamic insight* into one's previously unconscious or hidden mental states. Perhaps by disintegrating the self-model and loosening ego boundaries, psychedelics allow patients to make genuine discoveries about their own memories, desires, beliefs, and values. Their putative ability to do this was the justification for the *psycholytic* form of therapy practised in continental Europe in the 1960s, in which low doses of psychedelics were given as an adjunct or enhancer to repeated sessions of talk therapy. We encountered a description of this kind of insight in Chapter 7, from a patient with treatment-resistant depression who received psilocybin-assisted therapy in a recent trial:

[This patient] reported:

> [I] became myself at age 7, after my [grandparent] had died. I totally was back there, so vivid, so real, I had the emotions that I would have felt at the time: fearful, why did this happen, the naivety, the shock and confusion. I was getting overly upset and my parents were saying 'boys don't cry'.

This helped him realize how his unhealthy emotional habits as an adult developed.

> I saw that it's not [a] weakness to be emotional, that's an unhealthy attitude.
> **(Watts et al. 2017, p. 539)**

Quantitative evidence is scarce, but clinicians and patients reported that psychedelics did reliably increase access to unconscious material, and that clinical benefits resulted from this increased access (Eisner and Cohen 1958, Grof 1975). This coheres with recent findings that psychological insight predicts clinical benefits, given that such insights often concern psychological factors believed to underlie symptomatology (e.g., Malone et al. 2018, p. 5). One terminal patient who received LSD-assisted psychotherapy commented:

> I had the strong impression that things can be seen, which usually rest under the surface ... a lot of emotions were hidden for a long time that are usually not noticed at all became very, very present in that state when you have a break-through somehow.
> **(Gasser et al. 2015, p. 61).**

Assuming that such experiences do contribute causally to symptom reduction, a simple explanation is that the putative insights are genuine (Metzinger 2003, p. 249). Users of psychedelics in non-clinical contexts also report psychological insights, sometimes claiming to learn more about their own mind in a few hours than in years of therapy or academic training (Shanon 2002, 2010, Leary 1990, quoted in Pollan 2018, p. 187).

However, there is another explanation: the apparent insights induced by psychedelics might be psychologically beneficial *confabulations* (cf. Bortolotti 2018). Psychedelics sometimes induce false or implausible beliefs about the external world, accompanied by subjective feelings of certainty; why should they not do the same regarding the internal world? When we consider putative insights of the kind described above, there are at least two elements that might be mistaken: first, the re-lived memory might be inaccurate in some respect; second, even if the memory is accurate, the patient's belief about how the remembered episode affected their psychological functioning might be inaccurate. The key point is this: even if putative psychodynamic insights could be *proven* to underlie clinical improvements, this would not conclusively demonstrate their accuracy (cf. Carhart-Harris and Friston 2019). They might be cases of what Jopling (2001) calls 'placebo insight': apparent insight that causes psychological benefits despite being spurious. As Jopling says:

> the mere acquisition of [apparent] insight is not a guarantee that the insight is true ... the client's level of conviction about the validity and authenticity of a newly won insight is not a guarantee that the insight is true ... the therapist's conviction about the authenticity of the client's explorations, and the truth-value of the client's insight, is not a guarantee of the truth of the insight ... [and] the occurrence of therapeutic change following the acquisition of insight is not a guarantee of the insight's truth.
>
> (2001, pp. 23–24).

Of course, adequate epistemic justification does not require a *guarantee*—just sufficient evidence. The question then becomes: do we have any strong, positive grounds for thinking that psychedelic-facilitated apparent psychodynamic insights are genuine, besides (a) their apparent therapeutic benefits, and (b) patients' and therapists' confidence in their accuracy? Discussing whether or not psychedelic-induced insights are trustworthy, Carhart-Harris and Friston suggest that:

> the philosophical rabbit hole dissolves further in the face of the free-energy principle. This follows because the free-energy principle maintains that there is no absolute truth that is knowable absolutely—there is only evidence for a set of plausible hypotheses. In other words, the best beliefs or models are simply those with the greatest evidence—or minimum free energy.
>
> (2019, p. 335).

However, from a philosophical standpoint, this does not follow. Even if our knowledge of the world is fallible and our perception of it indirect, we can still rationally debate the truth of propositions, and often reach justified (if tentative) conclusions. If A emerges from psychedelic experience with a newfound conviction that the pursuit of material success alone does not beget happiness (Swift et al. 2017, p. 506), and B with a new-found conviction that he can communicate with aliens by building a floating pyramid on the Amazon (Mann 2011), we can reasonably conclude that A's belief is probably true and B's probably false—even if B's belief is 'best' or has 'the greatest evidence' in the sense that it minimises overall free energy or prediction error for B, given his total psychological situation. Of course, many real cases are harder to decide. However, the example simply illustrates a general point: the question of the veridicality of putative insights does not dissolve in the face of epistemological fallibilism (Cohen 1988) and an 'indirect' or, at any rate, inferentialist view of perception (Hohwy 2013).

It is important to emphasise that this philosophical point need not have any direct implications for clinical practice. Doubtless in many cases the best practical policy is to maintain 'clinical equipoise' and remain agnostic on the veridicality of putative insights (Carhart-Harris et al. 2018b, p. 404). However, here we are pursuing an *epistemological* evaluation of putative psychodynamic insights gained in the psychedelic state. Thus, we return to the question: are there any strong, positive grounds for trusting such putative insights?

An obvious place to look, per section 8.2 above, is to theoretical arguments. Perhaps there is something about how psychedelics act on the brain that makes them likely to facilitate genuine, rather than spurious, psychodynamic insights (cf. Letheby 2019). Indeed, when we consider the account of psychedelic therapy developed in this book, it seems to support this idea.

Recall Clark's Dictum: *prior knowledge is always both constraining and enabling.* Suppose that Maria, prior to her psilocybin session, had a fairly accurate, heavily weighted prior belief that she was a generous and selfless person. This model would enable her to apprehend many genuine higher-order patterns in her thoughts, feelings, and behaviour, but may constrain her self-knowledge in other ways—for instance, by filtering out evidence that she sometimes acts from irrational jealousy or selfish motives. I suggested in section 8.2 that temporary psychedelic inoculation against the Hollow Mask Illusion provides a proof of concept: it shows how relaxation of priors might facilitate more accurate perception by removing the constraint imposed by those priors. Similarly, relaxation of self-related priors might facilitate more accurate or comprehensive self-perception. With the filter that is her self-model weakened, Maria can apprehend accurately the irrational jealousy and selfishness that drive certain of her behaviours.

I have no doubt that this sort of thing happens. If the REBUS model ('RElaxed Beliefs Under pSychedelics'; Carhart-Harris and Friston 2019) and the predictive self-binding theory are on the right track, then it is plausible that psychedelics often facilitate veridical psychodynamic insights by weakening the filtering and constraining influence of high-level self-related priors. The argument for this conclusion would run as follows:

1. Decreasing the weighting of self-related priors can increase the probability of accurately apprehending certain facts about oneself (from general PP theory).

2. Psychedelic administration temporarily decreases the weighting of self-related priors (from the REBUS model and the predictive self-binding theory).
3. Therefore, psychedelic administration can increase the probability of accurately apprehending certain facts about oneself.

This case can be bolstered further by appealing to the connections between psychedelics and mindfulness meditation. We have seen that psychedelics both acutely and sub-acutely promote capacities for taking an open, accepting, non-reactive stance toward inner experience. On the face of it, this seems likely to promote accurate apprehension of one's own mental states by fostering a less egoically biased, reactive, and defensive mode of introspection. This contention receives further support from evidence concerning (i) commonalities between psychedelic states and meditative practices, and (ii) potential introspective benefits of the latter.

On the first count, sub-acute increases in decentring and lasting increases in self-transcendence, induced by ayahuasca, both correlate with modulation of the posterior cingulate cortex (PCC) (Sampedro et al. 2017, Bouso et al. 2015)—a region strongly implicated in the decentred stance characteristic of 'open awareness' meditation and related practices (Brewer et al. 2013, Millière et al. 2018, Winter et al. 2020). Altered PCC function has also been observed during open awareness practice after a psilocybin-assisted Zen retreat (Smigielski et al. 2019b).

On the second count, meditation experience has been found to predict greater introspective accuracy (Fox et al. 2012). Drawing on a range of evidence, Davis and Thompson (2015) offer a possible explanation for this effect in terms of increases in alertness and attentional capacity, and reductions in cognitive and affective biases. In terms congenial to the account developed here, Albahari (2019b) suggests that such biases are fundamentally bound up with self-modelling processes. She argues, on this basis, that safe and controlled downregulation of self-representation is likely to improve the accuracy of introspection.

Of course, there is no suggestion that typical psychedelic experiences and typical results of mindfulness training are precisely identical. Charting their exact similarities and differences is an important ongoing research project (Millière et al 2018, Heuschkel and Kuypers 2020). However, the evidence just reviewed sits well with the following claim: by unbinding mental contents from the self-model, promoting decentred and less defensive introspection, psychedelics often facilitate the acquisition of genuine psychodynamic insights unavailable in the ordinary waking state. We can thus formulate another argument, this time from analogy:

1. Meditation promotes introspective accuracy (Fox et al. 2012).
2. Meditation and psychedelic administration are similar in many respects relevant to the promotion of introspective accuracy (e.g., weakening self-related priors and related cognitive and affective biases; increasing the breadth of attention and decreasing its coupling to representations of self-related goals and concerns; and promoting mindfulness-related capacities such as decentring and acceptance).

3. Therefore, psychedelic administration probably promotes introspective accuracy too.

Both arguments are suggestive but, in my view, it would be premature to regard them as conclusive. Moreover, it is important to note that their conclusions are compatible with the idea that psychedelics sometimes induce placebo insights. Very few people would claim that *all* putative insights facilitated by psychedelics (or meditation) are veridical: psychedelic-assisted introspection is at least fallible. The evidence marshalled here provides tentative, but as yet inadequate, support for the conclusion that such putative insights are *usually* accurate. Any such putative insight still falls victim to the dilemma outlined in section 8.2: absent at least *some* ASC-independent reason(s) for trusting its veracity, there is insufficient evidence to conclude that it is a real insight rather than a placebo insight.

To make things more concrete, let us return to the example quoted on p. 167, of the patient who recalled being a young child grieving the death of his grandparent, and being told by his parents that 'boys don't cry'. What seems to have happened here is this: under the influence of psilocybin, the patient has relived genuine memories of formative early-life experiences and thereby arrived at a pivotal causal-explanatory insight: that his unhealthy emotional habits as an adult resulted, at least in part, from his internalisation of attitudes conveyed by his parents—attitudes such as *it is a weakness to be emotional*. But is it true that the childhood internalisation of such attitudes was causally responsible for this patient's development of unhealthy emotional habits? And is it true that these habits contributed causally to his depressive symptoms, such that psychedelic-facilitated awareness of the habits and their origins provided the opportunity to change them and decrease the probability of future depressive symptoms?

This may well be true. It seems eminently plausible. But, of course, it may well be false in some respect or other. And neither its accompaniment by a phenomenal feeling of knowing, nor its leading to clinical improvements, constitutes conclusive evidence of its truth. Psychedelic-facilitated psychodynamic insight almost certainly happens, but so too does psychedelic-facilitated psychodynamic *placebo* insight. There is no alternative but for the patient and the therapist to sort the wheat from the chaff together during the post-session integration period. Notwithstanding their overwhelming feeling of rightness, putative insights gained during the psychedelic state must be scrutinised for plausibility in just the same way as putative insights gained by any other means, such as the various talk therapies.

The somewhat unsatisfying conclusion, then, is that, when it comes to propositional knowledge about one's own mind, psychedelics facilitate both genuine insights and placebo insights, and there is no general formula for telling the two apart. Each putative insight must be scrutinised for plausibility after the session. There is tentative evidence that many such putative insights are genuine, but this evidence is inconclusive. More research is required on the commonalities between psychedelics and meditation, and how they affect the reliability of introspection.

For now, I conclude that psychedelics are undeniably useful for enhancing the *context of discovery* (i.e., the generation of promising new ideas). They do this not just in a random fashion, by injecting noise or entropy into the system, but in a principled manner: by decreasing the constraining influence of prior knowledge, they enable subjects to 'think outside the box' and access usually inaccessible possibilities. Psychedelic experience even contributes to the *context of justification*, in which ideas and hypotheses are scrutinised for plausibility, due to the evidence that it often facilitates accurate insights. However, the context of justification must also encompass critical, sober reflection during the post-session period. The combination of psychedelic experience and sober scrutiny will always provide greater justification for accepting any putative insight than the experience alone. As Bertrand Russell put it: 'insight, untested and unsupported, is an insufficient guarantee of truth, in spite of the fact that much of the most important truth is first suggested by its means' (Russell 1917).

From a philosophical standpoint, if Maria claims to have gained new *propositional* knowledge from her psychedelic experience, then her claim, once again, cannot be evaluated in the abstract. It can neither be accepted nor rejected uncritically. Its plausibility depends on the details of the proposition in question and the psychedelic-independent justification that is available. However, assuming that Maria—as is her wont—has given careful, sober thought to the accuracy or otherwise of the insight in question, and has ultimately come down in its favour, then it is reasonable to conclude that she has indeed gained new propositional knowledge by undergoing *and subsequently reflecting on* a psychedelic experience.

8.4 Knowledge how

Perhaps, however, propositional knowledge is not the (only) type of knowledge that Maria claims to have gained. Another type of knowledge that may be at issue is *ability knowledge*, or 'knowledge how' (Ryle 1945). Paradigmatic examples include knowing how to ride a bicycle, how to change a tyre, or how to program a computer. Is it possible that psychedelic experiences reliably facilitate the acquisition of new skills or abilities?

Benny Shanon makes some proposals along these lines in his discussion of epistemic benefits of the ayahuasca experience. Some of his candidates concern apparent enhancements to artistic performance and creativity during the psychedelic state:

> Under the intoxication, it is very common for people to feel that they are endowed with more stamina, are more in touch with their bodies, better tuned, and in a state of higher overall existential harmony. These inner sensations, in turn, may lead to a superior flowing of overt behavior, both bodily and social ... The heightened bodily energy afforded by ayahuasca is publicly observable in rituals of the Church of Santo Daime ... participants engage in vigorous, strictly structured communal dancing that [lasts] as much as 11 or 12 h. The dance demands perseverance,

inter-personal coordination, and adherence to established order. Clearly, this kind of performance could not be achieved and maintained under conditions of ordinary states of mind. Well balanced and tuned performance may be extended from the physical domain to the behavioral one. Many times, I have observed that during the ayahuasca inebriation I, like many others, manifested a remarkable level of *bon ton*: easy going gentility, effortlessly uttering of the right words at the right time, flowing interpersonal dynamics ... the intoxication induced a better performance in the 'dance of life'. Furthermore, the well-balanced, harmonious comportment is likely to render behavior, individual and inter-personal alike, more proper.

(Shanon 2010, pp. 270–271).

There are two points to make about this. The first is that a certain degree of scepticism is warranted concerning whether people on psychedelics are, in fact, reliably better performers in the 'dance of life'. The by-now familiar point applies: from the mere fact that they *feel* as though they are, it does not follow that they actually are. Masters and Houston (1966, pp. 104–108) recount some amusing and sobering[9] instances of psychedelic subjects feeling utterly in sync with other people present, and having experiences as of effortless non-verbal communication, when subsequent debriefing revealed that the two people had completely misunderstood each other and failed to communicate.[10] This note of caution is bolstered by empirical findings suggesting that psychedelics acutely impair the ability to recognise emotional facial expressions displayed on a screen (reviewed by Rocha et al. 2019, Preller and Vollenweider 2019). Of course, these findings do not conclusively refute Shanon's claim. There are obvious differences between viewing static, disembodied face images and interacting with real, embodied human beings (Letheby 2019). Also, these findings do not concern ayahuasca specifically. However, on at least some occasions, the feeling of being 'in sync' with others and behaving in a socially graceful manner under psychedelics may be entirely illusory.

The second point concerns the performance enhancements Shanon describes in the physical domain: enhanced stamina, coordination, and bodily skill. These phenomena lend themselves to objective verification more readily than their counterparts in the social domain. However, one might wonder whether they are *epistemic*. Is subjects' *knowledge how* to perform these activities really being increased, rather than their mere ability to perform them being transiently elevated? Compare: the performance of elite athletes is enhanced by steroids, but we would not necessarily conceptualise this in terms of knowledge how. Unless there is evidence that these heightened abilities outlast the ayahuasca experience, they might seem more like transient

---

[9] Pun intended.

[10] Masters and Houston insist, however, that such examples 'should not be isolated and then used as weapons against the psychedelic drug experience' because '[important] authentic communication also takes place' (1966, p. 108).

performance enhancements than epistemic benefits (Letheby 2019). Of course, it depends how one defines knowledge how: on some accounts, mere ability may be sufficient (Fantl 2017). We will return to this point momentarily.

Shanon's most interesting proposal concerning knowledge how initially sounds somewhat trivial. He suggests that, by drinking ayahuasca repeatedly, one learns how to participate skilfully in the drinking of ayahuasca:

> Longitudinally, consuming ayahuasca people may eventually become accomplished in the very art of drinking ayahuasca ... partaking of ayahuasca is not a one shot affair, but rather it is a long term course of study, a school. The knowledge acquired in this schooling involves not only the objects of knowing ... but also the vehicle of knowing ... drinking ayahuasca is an artful skill in its own right, and as such has to be mastered.
>
> **(Shanon 2010, pp. 272–273).**

At first, this might sound like the sort of ability knowledge that is of little use except to those determined to undergo the 'long term course of study' involved in repeated ritual ayahuasca consumption. It certainly sounds a far cry from the sort of knowledge or skills that might be gained in one or two clinically supervised psilocybin or LSD sessions—the sort of phenomenon that is my main concern in this book. However, this putative skill demands further analysis. What abilities, exactly, are exercised in the 'art of drinking ayahuasca'?

Some intriguing clues come from clinical wisdom about the type of mental 'set' that tends to promote beneficial and rewarding psychedelic experiences. Patients and subjects are routinely encouraged to adopt a specific attitude towards the unusual, sometimes confronting mental contents that arise under psychedelics: a mental posture of curiosity, acceptance, and non-resistance. They are instructed to 'Trust, Let go, and Be open' (Richards 2017, p. 324), and it is widely held that success in following these instructions promotes positive and beneficial experiences. This view is borne out by the findings of Russ et al. (2019a, 2019b) that a psychological state of 'surrender' at the time of ingestion predicts positive experiences under psilocybin. This also brings to mind the observations of Smigielski et al., in relation to their study of a psilocybin-assisted mindfulness retreat, that meditation practice:

> seems to enhance psilocybin's positive effects while countering possible dysphoric responses ... [highlighting] the interactions between non-pharmacological and pharmacological factors, and the role of emotion/attention regulation in shaping the experiential quality of psychedelic states ...
>
> **(2019a, p. 1).**

All of this suggests a simple but striking idea: perhaps at least part of what it is to become skilled in the 'art' of drinking ayahuasca is to learn how to maintain an open, curious, non-reactive attentional stance, while undergoing a variety of intense and unusual experiences. Perhaps the skill set that Shanon is describing includes, inter alia, knowing how to pay attention and relate to one's mental contents in decentred, psychologically flexible ways of the kind cultivated in mindfulness meditation (Letheby 2019). One subject's description of her third supervised psilocybin session is suggestive of this idea:

> Now there was a familiarity to this inner space, and I found I was able to navigate much more easily than during the previous sessions. I felt no fear and was able to keep an even keel emotionally and psychologically, and to largely maintain the role of observer. I told [one of the supervising therapists] it was like learning to ride a bicycle and leaning into the turns.
>
> (Estevez 2013, p. 128).

There is also quantitative evidence for this hypothesis, in the form of empirical studies, reviewed in section 5.2.2, showing lasting elevations in mindfulness-related capacities and psychological flexibility following psychedelic intake.

Here, then, is an argument for the claim that psychedelic intake reliably facilitates the acquisition, or increase, of a kind of knowledge how:

1. The sorts of attentional skills cultivated in mindfulness meditation amount to a kind of knowledge how.
2. Psychedelic intake reliably facilitates the acquisition, or increase, of the sorts of attentional skills cultivated in mindfulness meditation.
3. Therefore, psychedelic intake reliably facilitates the acquisition, or increase, of a kind of knowledge how.

This is one kind of epistemic benefit that Maria may have gained during her psilocybin session. Suppose that she is a dedicated practitioner of mindfulness meditation who has attended several retreats, but never had any strongly self-transcendent experiences. Under the influence of psilocybin, she had an intense episode of ego dissolution and, since the drug effects ended, she has found practising meditation a very different experience than it was before. She reports that she now *knows* how to 'let go' of thoughts and feelings as they arise in the mind. Whereas previously she had found her teachers' instructions to do so somewhat mysterious, now it is as though she has been shown where the 'mental muscle' is that is responsible for clinging to or identifying with thoughts,[11] and she knows how to relax that muscle because she knows what it feels like when that muscle is relaxed and when it is activated.[12] Such claims cohere with the remarks of Smigielski et al. (2019b) on their finding that the degree of

---

[11] Perhaps part of it is in the PCC (Brewer et al. 2013).
[12] This description is adapted from a real description, given to me by a friend, of the change in their own meditation practice after a psychedelic-induced mystical-type experience. I am grateful to this person for giving me permission to use an adapted and anonymised account of their experience here.

ego dissolution experienced under psilocybin predicted the degree of Default Mode Network (DMN) disintegration during subsequent open awareness practice:

> The psilocybin experience of [ego dissolution] might increase the meditators' capability of down-regulating DMN integration during [open awareness] practice, representing a neural mechanism frequently found during states of self-transcendence.
>
> **(Smigielski et al. 2019b, p. 213).**

Even if she has no prior interest in or experience of meditation, Maria may still describe having learned to pay attention to her thoughts and feelings in the open, accepting, non-reactive manner characteristic of mindfulness practice. She might give a report similar to the following, from a patient who received psilocybin-assisted therapy for treatment-resistant depression:

> I saw negative patterns in my life where if something bad happens, I used to just put it [to the back of my mind]. Afterwards, I allowed myself to experience everything—even if it is sadness. Now *I know how to deal with my feelings* rather than repress them.
>
> **(Watts et al. 2017, p. 541; my emphasis).**

On this view, one important epistemic benefit of psychedelic experiences is that they offer 'paradigms of a sort of attention' (Diamond 1982, p. 32)—a sort of attention that can result when the constraining influence of the self-model is reduced in conducive circumstances.

Can we conclude, then, that psychedelics promote a kind of knowledge how? The argument above is valid, and both premises seem plausible. The idea that the kinds of attentional skills cultivated in mindfulness meditation amount to a form of knowledge how is intuitive. The whole notion of meditation *training* is predicated on the idea that trainees learn how to do something with their minds that non-meditators do not know how to do. And a large body of evidence demonstrating neural and cognitive changes resulting from meditation practice suggests that they are, indeed, learning how to do *something* (Tang et al. 2015). Of course, the plausibility of this premise might vary depending on the details of specific philosophical accounts of knowledge how, which I will not delve into here. Two prominent approaches are to define knowledge how in terms of abilities or in terms of dispositions (Fantl 2017); on both approaches, it seems likely that mindfulness-related attentional skills will qualify.

Might there be any problem with the second premise? On the face of it, this premise seems like a relatively uncontroversial summary of the scientific evidence: assuming that the findings discussed in section 5.2.2 replicate, it will simply be a robust experimental finding that psychedelics reliably promote the relevant kinds of attentional skills.

There is an objection that might be raised, however, and it can be summarised as follows: perhaps psychedelics do not promote the *skills* cultivated in mindfulness practice, but instead offer a different causal pathway to the typical *effects* of those skills. After all, the various psychometric scales used to quantify mindfulness-related capacities measure how people tend to relate to their thoughts and feelings, but are neutral with respect to the underlying causes of these psychological tendencies. A given person's psychometric score for decentring or non-judging might reflect the results of deliberate, explicit learning, or it might simply reflect an innate psychological trait. The person may report having no idea how she is able to view her thoughts and feelings with such calm non-attachment, perhaps saying 'that's just the way I've always been!' This would stand in stark contrast to a long-term meditation practitioner who has gained some measure of mental calm and detachment by studious repeated training, and can describe (at least to some extent) *how* she avoids getting totally overwhelmed by, or 'caught up in', intense and distressing mental contents (Brewer et al. 2013).

The objection, then, runs as follows: we cannot infer from the psychometric evidence that psychedelics promote mindfulness-related attentional *skills*, because the evidence only demonstrates changes in attentional *dispositions*, and is neutral regarding whether those changes result from the exercise of skills or from some 'brute causal' process, such as 're-wiring' a person's attentional dispositions via mechanisms unavailable to introspection. The contrast being drawn is similar to an intuitive contrast between the antidepressant mechanisms of selective serotonin reuptake inhibitors (SSRIs) and those of cognitive behavioural therapy: both treatments can remediate emotional processing biases characteristic of depression but, from a phenomenological standpoint, it seems that one treatment achieves this by teaching patients skills of cognitive reappraisal whereas the other achieves the same result by pharmacological modulation of relevant mechanisms outside conscious awareness (Gerrans and Scherer 2013).

A satisfactory response to this objection would require delving into issues surrounding levels of explanation more deeply than I have done in this book. For now, I will simply note two things. The first is that, if the arguments I gave in Chapters 4–7 are on the right track, then psychedelic therapy is a personal-level process. I argued there that the bulk of the therapeutic and transformative work is done by conscious experiences that change how a subject sees the world, and subsequent, introspectable consolidation of these new ways of seeing and attending. So, if that account is roughly correct, then the present objection fails—the persistence of mindfulness-related capacities beyond the acute psychedelic state is indeed due to a conscious learning of attentional skills.

The second thing to note is that phenomenological reports support this idea. Subjects describe consciously learning attentional strategies during the psychedelic experience and its aftermath. We have seen a couple of these reports already—one on p. 175 from a healthy subject and one on p. 176 from a patient with treatment-resistant depression, both of whom received psilocybin. Here is a patient who received psilocybin treatment for distress relating to terminal illness:

[Brenda's] data also showed an increase in spirituality, as illustrated in her follow-up interview ... After the trial, Brenda became interested in pursuing her relationship with this new aspect of herself, and began seeking out opportunities to recollect and re-experience elements of the experience through meditation. She said:

> I've been exploring whether I can bring back other sensations from it ... I have been able to, and I've been doing a lot of meditating. I got into meditating afterward because it was like, 'I just don't want to lose this', ... I really felt like there was a real connection with Buddhism and meditation and the psilocybin experience for me. And I've been doing that everyday.
>
> **(Malone et al. 2018, p. 5).**

And a patient who received psilocybin treatment for tobacco addiction :

> Yesterday was kinda cloudy and a little overcast, and I was driving home and there was this one small patch of clouds that was lit up bright by the sun, and it was all surrounded by these dark clouds. And I was like, 'that's amazing' ... And then I caught that, because prior to the psilocybin I probably would never have noticed that. But, *I'm always on the lookout for those kinds of things*. So yeah, that's a pretty good example of me being more aware.
>
> **(Noorani et al. 2018, p. 763; my emphasis).**

Reports like these provide support for the idea that psychedelic-induced changes in attentional dispositions are, in fact, caused by the conscious acquisition of skills and techniques, rather than by a non-experiential process of 're-wiring'. An even more direct way to approach this question would be via follow-up interviews with expert meditators, in studies such as the one conducted by Smigielski et al. (2019a). It would be interesting to ask such participants about their perceptions of how the psychedelic experience affected their subsequent meditation practice. I predict that a majority would report gaining, through the psychedelic experience itself, some kind of increased *knowledge* or *understanding* of how to perform certain meditative practices, access certain modes of attention, or enter certain states of mind.

My conclusion, then, is that transformative psychedelic experiences often involve not just learning *to* let go (Wolff et al. 2020; cf. Stolaroff 1999) but also learning *how* to let go: learning how to attend openly and non-reactively to inner experience, and accept what arises. There is an obvious connection between this conclusion and the arguments of the previous section concerning knowledge that. Both kinds of knowledge acquisition arise from the same basic mechanism: the unbinding of mental contents from the self-model, promoting disidentification with those contents and conferring on them a degree of phenomenal opacity. This induces a decentred mode of introspection, allowing subjects to both (i) make specific discoveries about the contents of their minds during the experience, and (ii) get a taste of an alternative way of relating to their minds, which can be practised after the experience subsides.

8.5 Knowledge by acquaintance

A third type of knowledge discussed in epistemology is *knowledge by acquaintance*. The term is due to Bertrand Russell (1910) and is intended to contrast with 'knowledge by description', which might be acquired via testimony or by reading books. On an intuitive level, the idea is simple enough: there are many ways you can learn about Paris—by reading guidebooks and websites, by talking to people who have been there, by watching movies, and so forth. Or you can go to Paris and see it for yourself. Rather than being limited to indirect inferential or testimonial knowledge, you can gain direct, first-hand knowledge of Paris: you can become *acquainted* with it. In so doing, you come to know Paris in a new, distinctive, and more direct manner. At a first pass, knowledge by acquaintance is the kind of knowledge we are talking about when we speak of knowing *someone*, rather than knowing how to do something, or knowing that something is the case (Fantl 2017). One of the types of epistemic benefits that Maria is most likely to mention, or at least one of the types for which we have the strongest evidence, is the acquisition of knowledge by acquaintance with certain important facts (Letheby 2015).

The idea of knowledge by acquaintance figures prominently in debates over Frank Jackson's (1982, 1986) seminal thought experiment known as 'Mary's Room'. In the thought experiment, Mary is a super-neuroscientist who is raised inside a black and white room, at a future time when scientific knowledge is complete. In her monochrome environment, Mary masters the entirety of scientific knowledge (she is a *super*-neuroscientist, after all), with a particular focus on the neuroscience of colour vision. She possesses all the 'physical information' (i.e., third-personal, objective, scientific information) about what happens in someone's body and brain when they see something red—but she herself has never seen something red.

The pivotal point of the thought experiment occurs when Mary leaves her room for the first time and sees something red.[13] The intuition we are invited to share is that she will learn something new at this point, something previously unknown (and unknowable) to her on the basis of physical information alone: she will learn *what it is like to see red*. Jackson uses this intuition as the basis for an argument against physicalism, which he defines as the thesis that that 'all (correct) information is physical information' (1982, p. 127). The argument goes as follows: pre-release, Mary had all the physical information about colour vision, but lacked some (correct) information about colour vision: information about what it is like to see red. Hence, some correct information is not physical information; therefore, physicalism is false.

Many philosophers share the intuition that Mary gains some kind of knowledge when she first sees red, while remaining unpersuaded that this *Knowledge Argument* refutes physicalism. Consequently, much ink has been spilled on trying to articulate

---

[13] Obviously any other colour, or perhaps any basic sensory quality, would serve just as well to make the point.

(i) what sort of knowledge Mary gains, and (ii) how it is compatible with physicalism. One prominent suggestion is that, prior to her release, Mary has only indirect knowledge by description of red-experience, but upon release, she gains *knowledge by acquaintance* with red-experience (Conee 1994).

A possible problem for this view is that Russell defined knowledge by acquaintance as *direct* knowledge, with no representational mediation between the mind and the object of knowledge—but it is not clear that this ever happens. Indeed, on many modern views of cognition, including the computational view that I sketched in Chapter 5, section 5.4, the idea does not make sense: to have knowledge of something *just is* to harbour (the right kinds of) mental representations of it. Of course, it may not be helpful to think of representations as *mediating* knowledge, because this suggests a homuncular picture on which mental representations are interposed between objects of knowledge and a distinct, non-representational knowing subject (whose existence I deny). Still, the problem stands: if knowledge by acquaintance is non-representational, then it is incompatible with the basic view of cognition that I am assuming.

However, in responding to Jackson's argument, Conee adopts a more liberal definition of knowledge by acquaintance. For him, this kind of knowledge amounts to '[being] familiar with the known entity in the most direct way that it is possible for a person to be aware of that thing' (1994, p. 144).[14] The kind of knowledge of red-experiences one gets by *having* them is the most direct kind possible—certainly more direct than the theoretical knowledge Mary gains in her black-and-white room—and so constitutes knowledge by acquaintance. To have knowledge by acquaintance with a type of experience, on Conee's account, it is necessary for one to instantiate or undergo an experience of that type. Clearly, a mind can know about an experiential property more directly by instantiating it than by inferring that others instantiate it.

Adopting Conee's definition, we can formulate an argument for the claim that psychedelic use reliably causes the acquisition of knowledge by acquaintance with important facts:[15]

1. To have knowledge by acquaintance with some fact is to be familiar with that fact in the most direct way that it is possible for a person to be aware of that fact.
2. There are important facts such that psychedelic use reliably causes people to become familiar with those facts in the most direct way that it is possible for a person to be aware of those facts.

---

[14] Strictly speaking, Conee (1994, p. 141) holds knowledge by acquaintance with a phenomenal property requires both (a) experiencing the property and (b) noticing that one has experienced it. For him, these conditions are individually necessary and jointly sufficient. In the cases that I will discuss, it is fairly clear that subjects not only enjoy a 'maximally direct cognitive relation' (Conee 1994, p. 136) to the putative object of acquaintance knowledge, but also *notice* that they have enjoyed this relation.

[15] I am assuming that Conee's definition generalises, *mutatis mutandis*, to facts as opposed to entities or things.

3. Therefore, there are important facts such that psychedelic use reliably causes the acquisition of knowledge by acquaintance with those facts.

The argument is valid, and premise 1 is purely definitional, so all the work is going to be in justifying premise 2. Which specific facts are at issue, and what evidence is there that psychedelics reliably cause the acquisition of maximally direct familiarity with those facts?

On the first count, those sympathetic to Buddhist ideas might be tempted to propose the following two candidates: (1) that the self does not exist, and (2) that there can be totally selfless states of phenomenal consciousness. However, for reasons outlined in Chapter 7, we should be cautious about the claim that psychedelic experience can involve acquaintance with *those* facts. Perhaps it can, but more work is required to establish this claim. There are two facts in their vicinity, however, with which these experiences certainly can involve acquaintance: (1) that the human mind has vast, normally unrealised potential, and (2) that the ordinary sense of self is contingent, constructed, and mutable (Letheby 2015). I take these in turn.

On the first count, neuroscientific evidence speaks to the fact that the brain on psychedelics occupies many modes or configurations unavailable in the ordinary waking state—it explores a larger range of functional connectivity patterns or 'motifs', some of which are not seen outside of the psychedelic state (Tagliazucchi et al. 2014, Atasoy et al. 2017). Phenomenological evidence coheres with this observation. Indeed, I argued at length in Chapter 7 that, during the psychedelic experience, subjects discover novel and beneficial ways of seeing themselves and relating to their experiences, and the subsequent consolidation of these neurocognitive and attentional paradigms is central to the therapeutic mechanism. Walter Pahnke eloquently describes this discovery, as it is made by terminal cancer patients administered psychedelics in a therapeutic context:

> At this point, unless the patient previously had experienced mystical consciousness spontaneously, he becomes intensely aware of completely new dimensions of experience which he might never before have imagined possible. From his own personal experience, he now knows that there is more to the potential range of human consciousness than we ordinarily realize. This profound and awe-inspiring insight sometimes is experienced as if a veil had been lifted and can transform attitudes and behaviour.
>
> **(Pahnke 1969, p. 15).**

In a similar vein, a healthy psychedelic-naïve subject who received mescaline concluded that the most important outcome of his session was 'the knowledge and certainty I now have that it is truly possible to attain to a sense of harmony with all creatures and things' (Masters & Houston, 1966, p. 12).

The language here is certainly suggestive of something like knowledge by acquaintance. However, referring to the specifics of the definition that we are working with, why should we think that psychedelic subjects become familiar in the most direct way possible with the fact that their minds have vast, normally unrealised potential?

The basic reason has to do with the type of fact that this is. In philosophical parlance, it is a *modal* fact—in other words, a fact about what is necessary, possible, impossible, and so on. What makes it true that the mind has vast, normally unrealised potential is that (a) there are many ways that it is *possible* for the mind to be, such that (b) normally it is *not* those ways. Now, it is quite easy to gain knowledge by *description* of the vast, normally unrealised potential of one's mind by reading the mystical literature of the world's religions or the phenomenological literature on the psychedelic state. Having penned his classic *The Perennial Philosophy*, Aldous Huxley (1945) clearly had such knowledge prior to his first fateful exposure to mescaline in 1952. Having read the preceding chapters of this book, you have such knowledge too—assuming that you truly and justifiedly believe your own mind to be capable of the sorts of experiences described throughout. But when one comes to know the relevant modal fact in this manner, inductive inferences are involved: first one infers, from others' testimony, that their minds have such potential; then one infers that, since their minds have such potential and are relevantly similar to one's own mind, one's own mind must have such potential too.

By contrast, when one becomes familiar with the potential of one's mind under psychedelics, at most a single, trivial, deductive inference is involved: from actuality to possibility. One of the basic principles of modal logic is that what is actual must therefore be possible. When the normally unrealised potential of one's mind becomes manifest, the object and the vehicle of knowledge are one, or pretty close to it. By having the direct experience of one's mind occupying many extraordinary states, some of which are felt to be extremely valuable or deeply meaningful, a modal property of the mind becomes instantiated, giving rise to the conviction described by Pahnke and the mescaline subject quoted above. There is no more direct way for a human mind to become familiar with its own unrealised potential than by the temporary realisation of that very potential in that very mind. In some cases, this insight can change lives dramatically—for instance, by inspiring people to dedicate themselves to meditative disciplines that aim at the lasting realisation of this potential (Dass 2005, Osto 2016).

Similar considerations apply to the second fact I mentioned: that the ordinary sense of self is contingent, constructed, and mutable. As we have seen, the default mode of waking consciousness is permeated by the ubiquitous phenomenal self, around which its contents are organised and through which they are filtered. While phenomenal transparency reigns, there is an air of unquestioned necessity to all this: the self appears, phenomenologically, as a substantial entity that simply exists, not as the contents of a mental model. Our self-bound patterns of attention are so ubiquitous as to be invisible. They are the air that we breathe, the water in which the proverbial fish swims.

Under psychedelics, the discovery that our minds can be otherwise is inextricable from the discovery that *we* can be otherwise, which is inextricable from the phenomenal opacity that comes from unbinding the self-model. By experiencing radically different forms of self-modelling, we come to see vividly that the previously unquestioned sense of *who I am* is just a story, and can be told otherwise. It is not given, but constructed by a malleable modelling process. The fact with which we become acquainted is one that anxious, depressed, and addicted people may know intellectually but struggle to access experientially: that things can be otherwise. There are other ways I can be, other ways I can see, and other ways I can parse experience. These ways are not dim theoretical possibilities, but genuinely available to me. If the self were as solid and fixed as it normally appears, this would not be so.

In earlier work, I argued that psychedelic subjects gain knowledge by acquaintance with 'the metaphysical nature of the self' (Letheby 2015, p. 186); but, as we have seen, this claim is fraught with difficulties. On the other hand, the contingency and mutability of the ordinary *sense* of self is a modal fact with which psychedelic subjects plausibly do gain knowledge by acquaintance. This contingency and mutability is just the fact that it is *possible* for this ordinary sense to be radically altered, or absent from experience altogether—and psychedelics certainly facilitate dramatic discoveries of this fact. Here is how one such discovery played out for Michael Pollan, while on psilocybin:

> I was present to reality but as something other than my self. And although there was no self left to feel, exactly, there was a feeling tone, which was calm, unburdened, content. There was life after the death of the ego. This was big news…
>
> Nothing in my experience led me to believe this novel form of consciousness originated outside me; it seems just as plausible, and surely more parsimonious, to assume it was a product of my brain, just like the ego it supplanted. Yet this by itself strikes me as a remarkable gift: that we can let go of so much—the desires, fears, and defenses of a lifetime!—without suffering complete annihilation. This might not come as a surprise to Buddhists, transcendentalists, or experienced meditators, but it was sure news to me, who has never felt anything but identical to my ego. Could it be there is another ground on which to plant our feet?
>
> **(2018, pp. 264–265).**

Such discoveries are all apiece with the phenomenal opacity that psychedelics often introduce to the self-model. To discover that the sense of self can be absent or altered is to discover its status as constructed and virtual, and to see it as constructed and virtual is ipso facto to grasp the possibility of its revision. Psychedelic-induced knowledge of this modal fact constitutes knowledge by acquaintance for the same reasons as in the earlier case (indeed, the two cases are not cleanly distinct): there is no more direct way to become familiar with the possibility of one's sense of self being absent or radically altered than to experience a state of consciousness in which one's sense of self is actually absent or radically altered.

My conclusion, then, is that psychedelic use reliably causes the acquisition of knowledge by acquaintance with important facts, including (but probably not limited to) two *modal* facts about one's own mind: that it has vast, normally unrealised potential, and that its ordinary sense of self is contingent, constructed, and mutable.

According to the arguments of Chapter 7, these two epistemic benefits are intimately bound up with a key part of the therapeutic mechanism of psychedelics: the induction of phenomenal opacity into the self-model. This claim has empirical import. On its basis, I would predict a fairly strong correlation between (a) lasting psychological benefits of psychedelics, such as symptom reduction and increased well-being, and (b) increases in the degree of assent to such statements as these:

(i) I know from first-hand experience that my mind has vast potential that normally goes unrealised.

(ii) My ordinary sense of who I am is, in part, a story, and it is possible for me to change this story.

I would also expect increased assent to such statements to correlate with increases in psychological flexibility and mindfulness-related capacities, given the connections between these notions and the phenomenal opacity that comes from unbinding self-narratives. Thus, once again, there is a strong connection between gaining knowledge by acquaintance with these facts, and gaining the kinds of epistemic benefits outlined in sections 8.3 and 8.4. All of these benefits come via the unbinding of the self-model and the temporary diminution of its usual constraining influence on cognition and consciousness.

8.6 New knowledge of old facts

The arguments of this chapter so far suggest that, in her supervised psilocybin session and its immediate aftermath, Maria may well have gained new propositional knowledge about her own previously unknown mental states, although there is a real possibility that she has instead gained placebo insights. There is a good chance that she has gained knowledge how to pay attention to mental contents in certain beneficial ways related to mindfulness skills. And there is a very good chance that she has gained knowledge by acquaintance with important modal facts about her own mind, facts of which her academic studies had previously given her mere knowledge by description: the vast, normally unrealised potential of her mind, and the contingency and mutability of her ordinary sense of self.

There is a fourth type of epistemic benefit that she might claim, plausibly, to have gained. This type of benefit, like knowledge by acquaintance, is less about *what* one knows than about *how* one knows it. It is a type of benefit that is described in the literature on Jackson's Knowledge Argument as *new knowledge of old facts* (Burston 2017).

On some accounts, it comes about by gaining the ability to represent those old facts under a new and different *mode of presentation*. The basic idea is articulated clearly by a terminal patient reflecting on her experiences under psilocybin:

> Chrissy experienced significantly decreased anxiety, depression, death anxiety, hopelessness, demoralization, and increased purpose in life, spirituality, and death transcendence ... When prompted on a follow-up questionnaire whether her religious or spiritual beliefs had changed since her psilocybin session, she replied, '[The psilocybin experience] *brought my beliefs to life, made them real, something tangible and true*—it made my beliefs *more than something to think about*, really something to lean on and look forward to.'
>
> **(Malone et al. 2018, p. 4; my emphasis).**

This suggests that, prior to her psilocybin experience, Chrissy's religious or spiritual beliefs were merely 'something to think about', whereas under psilocybin they became something more than this: they were, as she puts it, brought to life, made (phenomenologically) real, tangible, and true. Pre-psilocybin, these beliefs were (re-)presented to her in the mode of a mere belief; under psilocybin, they were (re-)presented to her in the mode of a vividly experienced reality (Shanon 2010, pp. 274–275). Once again, Benny Shanon has proposed something like this in his seminal paper on epistemic benefits of the ayahuasca experience:

> The information gained may be banal but its mode of appreciation might be experienced as special ... The following example of my own happened during an ayahuasca session held in a hut, in the midst of the Amazonian forest, early in the morning. I was looking at the leaves of plants observing how they were directed towards the rays of the sun. I felt I was actually seeing the nurturing sustenance of the solar light. Have I obtained any 'information' I had not known beforehand? I doubt it. But I was open to see the world in a new light, perhaps in the manner a poet or an artist may.
>
> **(Shanon 2010, p. 268).**

This sort of thing happens quite often under psychedelics. One important and common example concerns the undeniable fact that we human beings are profoundly interconnected with, and not ultimately distinct from, the natural world. It is easy enough to gain a justified true belief in this proposition on the basis of argument and evidence, but our individual and collective behaviour toward the biosphere suggests that it is much more difficult to bring these beliefs to life—to make them real, tangible, and true. Often they remain merely 'something to think about', whose motivational impotence has increasingly tragic consequences.

When psychedelics weaken the boundaries of the phenomenal self, however, this psychological situation can change dramatically, as the following reports make clear:

'Before I enjoyed nature, now I feel part of it. Before I was looking at it as a thing, like TV or a painting. [But] you're part of it, there's no separation or distinction, you *are* it.' [Patient 1]

'I felt like sunshine twinkling through leaves, I *was* nature.' [Patient 8]

(Watts et al. 2017, p. 534; emphasis original).

During the psilocybin session, one cancer patient experienced feelings of 'being connected to everything, I mean, everything in nature ... and it wasn't like talking about it, which makes it an idea. It was experiential.'

(Swift et al. 2017, p. 497).

In the words of George Eliot, these subjects are:

passing through one of those rare moments of experience when we feel the truth of a commonplace, which is as different from what we call knowing it, as the vision of waters upon the earth is different from the delirious vision of the water which cannot be had to cool the burning tongue.

(Eliot 1871, p. 350).

Quantitative evidence suggests that such changes can have behavioural consequences. In a large-scale population study, Forstmann and Sagioglou found that lifetime experience with psychedelics 'uniquely predicted self-reported engagement in pro-environmental behaviours, and that this relationship was statistically explained by people's degree of self-identification with nature' (2017, p. 975). Similarly, Nour et al. (2017) reported that lifetime psychedelic experience was significantly correlated with nature-relatedness, which also correlated with the degree of ego dissolution during the respondent's most intense psychedelic experience. Psilocybin therapy for treatment-resistant depression significantly increased nature-relatedness for up to 12 months (Lyons and Carhart-Harris 2018a). Recently, a prospective survey study found that a single psychedelic experience significantly increased nature-relatedness for up to two years, correlating with the degree of ego dissolution and the self-reported influence of natural surroundings during the experience (Kettner et al. 2019). The authors of this study describe nature-relatedness as a strong predictor of 'pro-environmental awareness, attitudes, and behaviour ... outperforming all other variables tested as a single construct' (Kettner et al. 2019, p. 2).

Our present question is whether such changes amount to genuinely epistemic benefits. I believe they do. According to the New Knowledge/Old Fact response to Jackson's Knowledge Argument, Mary gains new factual knowledge upon release, but not of a fact previously unknown to her: rather, she gains a new type or item of knowledge about a fact of which she already had another type or item of knowledge. What then is the difference between her pre-release knowledge of red experience and her post-release knowledge? One answer is that they both represent the same fact, but under a different mode (Nida-Rümelin and O'Conaill 2019).

The notion of a mode of presentation is due originally to Frege (1948) and has many technical uses in the philosophy of language. However, on an intuitive level, it is simple enough. How is it possible to 'know that water is splashing but not know that H_2O molecules are moving, [or] vice versa'? (Lycan 2019). How is it possible to know that Buffy Summers is present but not know that the Slayer is present, or vice versa? The answer in each case is that, while there may only be one objective fact at issue, it is possible to represent that fact under multiple different modes. Moreover, since different modes of presentation typically reveal or highlight distinct aspects or properties, coming to know an already-known fact under a new mode of presentation can be genuinely informative, vindicating the intuition that Mary gains some substantive new knowledge on her release. If one already knows that Clark Kent works for the Daily Planet, but subsequently learns that Superman works for the Daily Planet, then one gains new knowledge of an old fact, by representing the same objective state of affairs under a new and different mode of presentation.

The precise nature of modes of presentation is controversial. However, the basic idea as I have sketched it has been used to do a lot of interesting work in the philosophy of mind and epistemology. One example relevant to our concerns is James Baillie's discussion of what he calls *the recognition of nothingness*—the 'existential shock' that attends the vivid apprehension of one's own mortality. Baillie describes his own experience of this existential shock as follows:

> Last night I entered into a state of mind unlike anything I had experienced before. I realized that I will die. It may be tomorrow, it may be in 50 years' time, but one way or another it is inevitable and utterly non-negotiable. I no longer just knew this theoretically, but knew it in my bones. The knowledge of my death was real to me, as if for the first time (in a way that it no longer is as I write these words). It was as if I had been given a glimpse of an aspect of reality that had previously been closed to me. It was as if the blinders had been removed, and I was the only person to have woken up from a collective dream to grasp the terror of the situation. It was to be defenseless against this fact, and without the possibility of defense. This new awareness was completely out of my control. I have no idea how it came about. All attempts to turn my attention to other matters failed completely. I could only wait, traumatized, in the hope that it would pass. I was in this state for the longest 10 min of my life.
>
> **(Baillie 2013, p. 187).**

According to Baillie, while each of us would readily assent to the proposition that 'I am mortal', there is nonetheless an important 'sense in which we, ordinary people in ordinary circumstances, don't really believe that we will die' (2019, p. 3). We spend most of our lives:

in the grip of deeply entrenched patterns of thought and feeling that prevent the knowledge of our mortality from being fully assimilated. Rather, we merely 'pay lip service' to the facts of our mortality … existential shock involves a distinctive *mode of presentation of oneself as a mortal being*, in a way that cuts through subtle layers of denial that govern our lives.

(Baillie 2019, p. 1; my emphasis).

Baillie holds that existential shock, however it may be precipitated, temporarily cuts through our ordinary 'dissociated condition of believing-while-not-believing that [we] will die' (Baillie 2019, p. 3; cf. Dor-Ziderman et al. 2019). This is reminiscent of Miri Albahari's epistemic analysis of *insight knowledge* into no-self arising from Buddhist meditation practice. According to Albahari, a central epistemic benefit gained by the practitioner who realises insight knowledge is the uprooting of a false 'action-based belief' in the existence of a self, which had conflicted with the practitioner's 'reflective belief' in the doctrine of no-self. This uprooting increases the coherence of the agent's mental economy, and facilitates 'subsequent doxastic integration of action-based with 'reflective' belief' (2014, p. 4). In both cases, there is a proposition that we believe intellectually, but we harbour other mental representations whose contents are inconsistent with that proposition, creating a condition of incoherence or dissociation in which we know something to be true but do not, as we might say, *really* believe it deep down (on the levels of processing, and in the representational formats, that inform motivation and action). While she does not put it in these terms, it seems plausible that Buddhist insight knowledge, as Albahari describes it, involves apprehending the putative fact of no-self under a novel phenomenal mode of presentation.

The similarity to the psychedelic examples above, concerning religious or spiritual beliefs and interconnectedness with nature, is obvious. Moreover, there are important similarities between the idea of gaining knowledge by acquaintance under psychedelics, and the idea of gaining new knowledge of old facts via novel modes of presentation. Both ideas involve coming to know something already known or otherwise knowable, in a new and more vivid way. They are, however, distinct phenomena. One reason is that it is possible to represent something under a different mode of presentation without acquiring maximally direct familiarity with it—indeed, without increasing the directness of one's familiarity with it at all.

Suppose, for example, that Maria has long accepted the quintessentially Buddhist proposition that everything in the universe is profoundly interconnected. While on psilocybin, she came to experience this interconnectedness as a vivid sensory, affective, phenomenal reality. As such, she came to know this old fact in a new and important way. But there is no real sense in which she became more *directly acquainted* with that fact than before. It *felt* to her as though she did, because her experiential world was transformed such that interconnectedness became a reality rather than a thin abstraction. Rather than some objective fact 'out there', her knowledge of which was mediated by a propositional belief, it seemed as though interconnectedness had 'come into' her experiential world. The experience was one *as of* going from indirect knowledge by description to direct knowledge by acquaintance. But Maria herself is no more closely acquainted with the objective fact of interconnectedness than previously: not, at any rate, if phenomenal states are thoroughly intracranial and representational. Her knowledge of the fact did not cease to be 'mediated' by representations: there was simply a change in the kinds of representations and their contents. She came to grasp or appreciate the old fact more fully and deeply by apprehending it under a vivid phenomenal mode of presentation.[16]

Similar remarks apply to many other facts that we are capable of believing intellectually on the basis of argument and evidence, but can grasp or appreciate more fully or deeply when they are presented to us experientially during psychedelic states or other ASCs. Consider, for example, the following claims by Aldous Huxley about the epistemic benefits of spiritual experience, induced by psychedelics or otherwise:

> Useful analytical knowledge about the world is replaced by some kind of biologically inessential but spiritually enlightening acquaintance with the world. For example, there can be direct aesthetic acquaintance with the world as beauty. Or there can be direct acquaintance with the intrinsic strangeness of existence, its wild implausibility. And finally there can be direct acquaintance with the world's unity.
>
> **(Huxley 1963).**

To each of these examples, the foregoing considerations apply: psychedelics may induce experiences *as of* becoming more directly acquainted with the beauty, strangeness, or unity of the world, but they do not lead people to actually become more directly acquainted with these properties or facts. Rather, they represent these facts under new modes of presentation, allowing people to *appreciate* them more deeply or *grasp* them more fully. Interestingly, what seems to happen to some of our beliefs under psychedelics is the polar opposite of the move from transparency to opacity: whereas some of our mental representations may cease to appear as reality itself, and instead be experienced as mere stories or mental constructions, other representations may cease to appear as mere beliefs and instead be experienced as tangible, palpable features of our phenomenal worlds. We then apprehend the contents of these beliefs 'with that distinctness which is no longer reflection but feeling—*an idea wrought back to the directness of sense*, like the solidity of objects' (Eliot 1871, p. 176; my emphasis).

---

[16] This is similar in spirit to Kenneth Tupper's (2003) proposal that psychedelics make available phylogenetically ancient 'mythic' and 'somatic' modes of understanding, which in turn connects with the proposal of Carhart-Harris et al. (2014) that psychedelics induce a regression to a primitive state of 'primary consciousness' (cf. Kraehenmann et al. 2017a). It has recently been suggested that psychedelics' capacity to induce the representation of information in pre-verbal sensory modes could play an important role in their therapeutic effects (Császár-Nagy et al. 2019). While the details remain to be worked out, this idea is broadly consistent with the account I have developed here. As we have seen, autobiographical insights under psychedelics often take the form of visions whose vivid sensory contents make them salient and memorable.

The same principle applies as with propositional knowledge: critical, sober scrutiny is essential. The psychedelic state will allow one to represent many different putative facts in new and vivid modes. For example, on psilocybin, Huston Smith (2000, p. 11) had a vivid and convincing experience as of the non-naturalistic metaphysical scheme known as 'emanationism'. Moreover, as we have seen, many subjects have vivid experiences as of theistic, idealistic, or otherwise non-naturalistic metaphysical facts. The fact that psychedelics induce a vivid phenomenal simulation of some view does not entail that the view is true. Its truth or otherwise must be determined by argument and evidence. However, when the view *is* true, psychedelics can afford the epistemic benefit of allowing one to grasp, understand, or appreciate its truth more deeply and fully, by facilitating access to new modes of presentation.

This principle is illustrated nicely by the findings of Pokorny et al. (2017) that psilocybin acutely increases emotional, but not cognitive, empathy (cf. Dolder et al. 2016). In other words, the psychedelic state does not necessarily make people any better at determining what others are actually feeling—at discovering new facts about the objective external world. But given some independent ability to learn about those facts, the state allows people to feel their significance more fully, by representing them in a vivid affective mode of presentation.

Part of the mechanism underlying this phenomenon may involve the desegregation of resting-state networks (i.e., increases in inter-network connectivity) that has been observed under psychedelics (Carhart-Harris 2019). Tagliazucchi et al. speculate that this increased cross-talk might represent:

> a collapse in the normal hierarchical organization of the brain … such that the boundaries between lower-level systems anchored to the external world and higher-level systems operating more autonomously from sensory information become blurred.
>
> **(2016, p. 1048).**

Perhaps by increasing connectivity or cross-talk between (a) mnemonic and affective systems, and (b) perceptual systems, psychedelics facilitate increased influence of the former on the latter. Thus, mnemonic and affective information might shape the content of perceptual representations more strongly, leading (inter alia) to the symbolic dramatisations and parables that sometimes characterise psychedelic-induced visual hallucinations (Carhart-Harris 2007). In this vein, it is interesting to note the finding of Kaelen et al. (2016) that enhanced visual imagery under LSD correlated with increased functional connectivity between parahippocampal and visual cortex, and increased information flow from the former to the latter, during music listening. Similarly, Carhart-Harris et al. (2012a) found that vivid recall of autobiographical memories under psilocybin were associated with increased activation in sensory cortical areas, including visual cortex—a pattern not observed when participants recalled such memories under placebo. It seems likely that psychedelics facilitate the representation of old facts in new modes by disrupting the brain's functional architecture, inducing unusual patterns of information flow between distinct neurocognitive systems.

For the sake of completeness, I will formulate an explicit argument for the claim that psychedelics often facilitate the acquisition of new knowledge of old facts:

1. Psychedelics often facilitate the apprehension of already known facts under new and distinctive modes of presentation.
2. If one apprehends an already known fact under a new and distinctive mode of presentation, then one thereby acquires new knowledge of an old fact.
3. Therefore, psychedelics often facilitate the acquisition of new knowledge of old facts.

Premise 2 is intended to be purely definitional; premise 1 is intended to be justified by the evidence reviewed in this section and in earlier chapters.

8.7 Indirect epistemic benefits

So far, we have focused on the possibility that Maria gained some significant epistemic benefit during her psychedelic experience itself and its immediate aftermath—that is, her post-session debrief with the supervising clinicians and her own reflections later that evening. After all, you are visiting her on the day immediately following her psilocybin session. However, it is possible that she will gain further, *indirect* epistemic benefits from the psychedelic experience as the days and weeks unfold—benefits that are caused not by the experience itself but by its after-effects.

This idea is partly inspired by Lisa Bortolotti's work on epistemic benefits of pathological or epistemically flawed cognitive states such as clinical delusions. Bortolotti (2015, 2020) begins with existing arguments that some delusional beliefs might have *psychological* benefits. One example is delusions that have been called 'motivated' or 'defensive', on the grounds that motivational factors may play a role in their formation or that they themselves may play a defensive psychological role. For instance, *anosognosia*, the denial of illness, might have a defensive function: someone who has suddenly acquired an extremely debilitating illness may succumb to utter despair if they were to confront the horrific reality of their situation in its totality. Thus, a delusory failure to acknowledge the terrible truth might confer psychological benefits by preserving some minimal level of functionality and staving off crippling depression.

Of course, this is not to say that such delusions are psychologically *harmless*—only that they may have psychological benefits as well as harms. Bortolotti's novel contribution is to suggest that a similar complexity might characterise the *epistemic* profiles of such mental states. Granted, for example, that defensive delusions do have psychological benefits, it would be tempting to assume a straightforward 'trade-off' view, according to which these psychological benefits are purchased with epistemic costs. On such a view, ignorance is bliss: to avoid utter misery, the deluded sacrifice knowledge of reality.[17] According to Bortolotti, this trade-off view is overly simplistic. In addition to (a) their undeniable psychological and epistemic harms, and (b) their putative psychological benefits, she suggests that such mental states might also have (c) significant *epistemic* benefits not available by any other means.

The idea that clinical delusions might have epistemic benefits sounds strange at first. Bortolotti's argument for the claim is predicated on the idea that psychological and epistemic functionality in humans are deeply intertwined. Take, for example, the case of anosognosia and assume that this delusion does indeed play a defensive psychological role for some patients. Given this assumption, if those same patients had *failed* to develop anosognosia in the wake of their illness, they would ex hypothesi have experienced a significant loss of psychosocial functioning: they would have succumbed to despair or depression, leading to adverse behavioural consequences and probable social withdrawal. However, because those patients do develop anosognosia, they are protected from those undesirable consequences.

Bortolotti's point is that such undesirable psychosocial consequences plausibly have undesirable *epistemic* consequences. As social creatures, one of the main ways that we gain information about the world around us, and expose our own beliefs to scrutiny, is by interacting with others. Moreover, we learn about the world by exploring it and engaging with it with some measure of curiosity. All of these behaviours decrease in the despairing and the depressed. Thus, insofar as defensive delusions protect against psychosocial catastrophe, they carry non-trivial epistemic benefits because they help to preserve the psychosocial functioning on which much of our epistemic functioning depends. If a person who has acquired a serious illness believes that she is, in fact, perfectly healthy, then she has suffered an undeniable epistemic harm—she is out of touch with the truth of her situation. But if this delusion helps her to cope and keep functioning in the world on some level, then this epistemic harm is offset by an epistemic benefit: the person is in a condition to keep acquiring reliable information and true beliefs about many topics other than her health status.

If Bortolotti is correct that the preservation of psychosocial functionality by defensive delusions has epistemic benefits, then the same point applies to the therapeutic use of psychedelics, for the simple reason that psychedelic therapy often restores or improves psychosocial functionality. To the extent that the depressed, the anxious, or the addicted experience durable symptom remission following a psychedelic session, they are likely to engage with other people and the world around them more, leading to precisely the epistemic benefits that Bortolotti describes. The same is true of healthy volunteers whose Openness to Experience is durably elevated following a psychedelic session (MacLean et al. 2011, Lebedev et al. 2016). People who score

---

[17] Despite the wording, the suggestion is not that this is a conscious decision.

higher in Openness exhibit greater curiosity, undergo more novel experiences, and seek out more new sources of information—all epistemic benefits.

In earlier work, I suggested another type of epistemic benefit that might result from therapeutic psychedelic use—rejuvenated capacities for the acquisition of *modal* knowledge consequent on the alleviation of depressive symptoms:

> People suffering from depression, for instance, have difficulty imagining other ways that they could be or certain courses of action they could take. Part of the rigidity [characteristic of such pathologies] is imaginative rigidity . . . the [cognitive] system is trapped in a narrow region of state space and tends not to envision creative solutions to problems or novel behavioural strategies. This seems straightforwardly to be a state of impoverished modal knowledge. There are possibilities available, but the suffering subject is unable to imagine these possibilities and thus unable to know of their availability. In this light, consider the [Entropic Brain] model of psychedelic therapy: the system is temporarily unconstrained, conferring a degree of freedom and flexibility, some measure of which outlasts the acute experience. One way this greater flexibility could manifest is as an increased ability to imagine possibilities. And a greater ability to imagine possibilities is, at least, a higher level of access to putative modal truths about oneself and one's life.
>
> **(Letheby 2015, p. 188).**

This suggestion has since been borne out by empirical findings. Psychedelic therapy can indeed have this kind of epistemic benefit for depressed patients. Lyons and Carhart-Harris (2018b) found that patients who responded successfully to psilocybin-assisted therapy for treatment-resistant depression became more accurate at estimating the probability that specific events would occur in their lives. There was no change in the accuracy with which they forecasted negative events; but, post-treatment, they became more accurate at forecasting *positive* events. While depressed, they had systematically underestimated the probability of positive events occurring in their lives during the coming month. After successful treatment, this bias was corrected somewhat and their estimations became more accurate. It is plausible that this change results from the sorts of changes to self-modelling described in Chapter 7.

Thus, there are at least two kinds of indirect epistemic benefits that can plausibly result from supervised psychedelic sessions:

(i) Improved epistemic functionality consequent on improved psycho-social functionality (the latter coming via symptom reduction or positive personality change).

(ii) Increased capacity to gain modal knowledge consequent on remediation of cognitive biases characteristic of pathology.

Together with the direct epistemic benefits canvassed earlier in this chapter, this adds up to a considerable range of epistemic benefits, consistent with naturalism, that may often result from the successful therapeutic or transformative use of psychedelics.

8.8 Epistemic innocence

In her discussion of motivated delusions, Bortolotti argues not only that such 'imperfect cognitions' can sometimes have significant epistemic benefits but also that these benefits are often not available to the subject at that time, by any other (less epistemically costly) means. The target of her broader research programme here is imperfect cognitions (i.e., those with clear epistemic costs) that nonetheless satisfy these two conditions: (i) they confer a significant epistemic benefit to the agent, and (ii) at the time, there is no alternative cognition available that would deliver the same epistemic benefit without the corresponding epistemic costs. She has coined the term 'epistemic innocence' to capture the complex epistemic status of imperfect cognitions that satisfy these two criteria (Bortolotti 2015).

The epistemic innocence project can be contrasted with the arguments of Flanagan and Graham (2017) concerning metaphysical hallucinations, positive illusions, and spiritual delusions. Like Bortolotti, these philosophers want to contest the reflexive pathologisation and dismissal of such cognitions on grounds of epistemic imperfection. However, they take a different approach. Flanagan and Graham's strategy is to question the idea that there is anything especially bad—or, at least, anything necessarily pathological—about inaccurate, implausible, or epistemically deficient mental states:

> The project of living a good and meaningful life is an extraordinarily high-stakes project and may well require states or conditions of mind and ways of being a person that are transgressive, even, a bit, as they used to say, mad or crazy. We describe [and defend] certain states of mind or, better, ways of normal worldmaking, which are sometimes pathologized but which are, from other perspectives, experientially enjoyable, beautiful, and truth seeking. They are at the epistemic edge, sometimes beyond that edge, but existentially inspiring and morally uplifting.
>
> **(Flanagan and Graham 2017, p. 294).**

I am inclined to agree with Flanagan and Graham's contention that there is no 'clear, precise, and firm link' (2017, p. 293) between epistemic accuracy and mental health. Having significant epistemic flaws, or carrying significant epistemic risks, is neither necessary nor sufficient for being pathological. However, pathologisation is not directly at issue in the Comforting Delusion Objection to psychedelic therapy. This objection does not allege that psychedelic therapy should be eschewed because it involves delusions in a literal, clinical sense, but simply because (i) its overall epistemic profile is (allegedly) quite bad, and (ii) there is some general disvalue, independent of pathological status, in epistemically poor mental states.

For reasons I outlined in Chapter 2, I am sympathetic to the claim that there is something problematic about deliberately purchasing well-being with substantial epistemic costs. Thus, my approach to defusing the naturalistic suspicion of psychedelic therapy is closer to Bortolotti's project than to Flanagan and Graham's. Rather than contesting the evaluative claim that epistemically bad cognitions are bad simpliciter, I have been contesting the descriptive claim that psychedelic states are, on the whole, epistemically bad cognitions. From a naturalistic standpoint, there is no denying that they carry epistemic risks; but, as I argued in earlier chapters, these risks are not absolute. In this chapter, I have tried to show that these risks are also offset by significant epistemic *benefits*, both direct and indirect.

Moreover, psychedelics facilitate uniquely rapid and reliable access to the specific, highly unusual states of consciousness that beget these benefits. Thus, in most if not all cases, there will be no alternative, less epistemically risky cognition that offers an equally reliable route to the same epistemic benefits at the same time. Per Clark's Dictum, the epistemic benefits that come from unconstraining the predictive brain cannot be accessed without partially disabling it. As such, most (if not all) psychedelic experiences induced under modern clinical conditions are epistemically innocent imperfect cognitions (Letheby 2016).

9
Spirituality

> Will not a tiny speck very close to our vision blot out the glory of the world, and leave only a margin by which we see the blot? I know no speck so troublesome as self.
>
> **George Eliot, *Middlemarch*.**

9.1 Introduction

My conclusion that the Comforting Delusion Objection fails depends on two premises: (i) that the epistemic risks of psychedelic therapy, given naturalism, are fairly small, and (ii) that its epistemic benefits, given naturalism, are fairly large. Conjointly, these refute a central assumption underlying the Objection: that the overall epistemic status of psychedelic therapy, given naturalism, is poor. The arguments of Chapter 8 conclude my case for these two premises, so the bulk of our substantive work is done.

However, there is one final matter to address. My goal is not merely to defend psychedelic therapy against naturalistic objections. It is also, more positively, to offer a conceptual framework for thinking about psychedelics' beneficial effects—a framework consistent with naturalism, but richer than narrowly 'psychotomimetic' or 'hallucinogenic' conceptions. As such, I said in Chapter 2 that in the course of answering the Comforting Delusion Objection I would also be attempting to naturalise the *Entheogenic Conception* of psychedelics. And the Entheogenic Conception, as I have defined it, sees psychedelics as agents not only of epistemic benefit but also of authentic *spiritual* experience and transformation. This is the final matter to be addressed: to show how a view of psychedelics as spirituality promoting agents can be understood and defended within a naturalistic framework.

There are at least two reasons why the putatively spiritual aspects of psychedelic experience are important for a natural philosophy of psychedelics. The first is that these aspects seem of overriding importance to many psychedelic subjects, perhaps even more so than epistemic aspects. The second reason is that the putatively spiritual aspects seem especially resistant to naturalisation, perhaps even more so than epistemic aspects. The claim that psychedelics can have epistemic benefits consistent with naturalism may seem, at most, highly implausible (albeit perhaps less so in light of Chapter 8). But the claim that psychedelics can have *spiritual* benefits consistent with naturalism is liable to seem downright incoherent. Surely, one might think, this claim is self-contradictory. Surely spirituality and naturalism are opposed by definition, naturalism being nothing more than the denial of the non-natural and the supernatural—of which *spirits* and *the spiritual* would seem to be paradigmatic examples.

Recently, however, several philosophers have argued that this apparent inconsistency is *merely* apparent: that the term 'spiritual' does not refer only to practices or experiences that involve non-naturalistic ideations. They contend that there are practices and experiences that can legitimately be called 'spiritual', but do not depend on any such ideations. These philosophers have been arguing, in other words, for the possibility of a *naturalised spirituality*. In this chapter, I argue that psychedelic evidence supports their contention: psychedelic research shows that there are genuine forms of spirituality that do not rely on non-naturalistic metaphysics.

I have made this argument at greater length elsewhere (Letheby 2017). Here I will simply outline briefly the psychedelic case for a naturalised spirituality. I begin, in section 9.2, by reviewing some recent philosophical work on naturalistic spirituality. Despite differences in detail, certain common themes emerge from this research. One of these is the idea that spirituality has to do with connection, aspiration, and asking the Big Questions. Another is that these are all forms of 'breaking through the narrow walls of the ego' (Stone 2012, p. 492).

In section 9.3, I argue that psychedelic research provides converging evidence for these claims. This evidence consists of three observations. First, transformative psychedelic experiences that people are moved to call 'spiritual' do not uniformly feature non-naturalistic metaphysical apprehensions. Second, such experiences typically do feature feelings of connection and aspiration, and attention to the Big Questions. Third, according to the account developed in this book, these all result primarily from breaking through the narrow walls of the ego. The concept of *unselfing*, introduced by the philosopher Iris Murdoch (1970), encapsulates the psychological processes that are at the heart of psychedelic spirituality, and that require, in themselves, no adherence to non-naturalistic metaphysics (cf. Kähönen 2020).

It is worth noting that there is considerable overlap between the psychological mechanisms underlying the epistemic benefits reviewed in Chapter 8 and those underlying the spiritual benefits that are the topic of the present chapter. Most obviously, the unbinding of the predictive self-model is central to both. However, the claim that such disruption can have epistemic benefits, and the claim that it can give rise to authentically spiritual experiences, are conceptually distinct and hence must be justified by different arguments.

9.2 Naturalising spirituality

The naturalising programme in philosophy attempts to show that various phenomena central to human life, such as moral truth, mental representation, and free will, are unmysterious parts of the natural world investigated and described by the sciences. Perhaps nothing seems a less promising target for this programme than spirituality. Of course, there is no problem in showing that the sorts of practices and experiences that people *call* 'spiritual' are wholly natural phenomena. But the idea that there might be practices that (i) can accurately be called 'spiritual', and that (ii) can be practised *sincerely* by those committed to naturalism and to intellectual honesty (Metzinger 2013a) sounds absurd. Surely the sincere practice of spirituality, by definition, requires belief in the spiritual—as opposed, metaphysically, to the natural.

Recently, however, increasing numbers of people have been self-identifying as 'spiritual but not religious' (Fuller 2001), demonstrating that the term 'spiritual' has acquired certain specific connotations. In particular, it seems often to connote an orientation that favours direct, experiential, and practical approaches to questions of meaning, purpose, and transcendence, in contradistinction to the mere dogma or belief frequently taken to characterise institutional religion. Given its connotations of experiential inquiry and practical transformation as opposed to blind faith and empty ritual, this raises the question whether spirituality really does require commitment to non-naturalistic metaphysical claims.

Several philosophers and philosophically inclined thinkers have answered in the negative. For example, Ursula Goodenough (1998, 2001) suggests that spirituality can involve reflective contemplation of nature, including scientific descriptions thereof, and of philosophical mysteries such as why there is something rather than nothing. Such contemplation involves expanding one's perspective beyond the cares and concerns of the individual self, and can evoke responses of wonder, awe, appreciation, and existential gratitude. However, it clearly does not depend on non-naturalistic metaphysical beliefs. Similarly, Robert Solomon (2002) holds that spirituality centrally involves developing broader perspectives by expanding attention beyond self-related concerns. Spirituality, for Solomon, also involves a sense of reverence and love of life, as well as feelings of existential gratitude grounded in an appreciation of the contingency of our own lives. Meanwhile, Sam Harris (2014), based in part on his own experiences practising Tibetan Buddhist Dzogchen meditation, reserves the term 'spirituality' for the gaining, and deepening, of direct experiential insight into the non-existence of the self. As we have seen, influential arguments for the no-self theory face considerable challenges. Nonetheless, this putative insight is clearly consistent with naturalism.

In an important review, Jerome Stone synthesises these and several other accounts of naturalistic spirituality, and extracts the following common core:

> We are spiritual, first, when our sense of connection is enlarged. Second, we are spiritual when we aspire to greater things, when we attempt to realize our ideals. Finally, we are spiritual when we ask the big questions. Note that these three—connection, aspiration, and reflection on profound questions—are all forms of enlarging our selves, of breaking through the narrow walls of the ego.
>
> (Stone 2012, p. 492).

Thinkers such as Goodenough, Solomon, and Harris, and others such as Owen Flanagan (2007) argue that the sincere practice of spirituality is compatible with a naturalistic worldview. They arrive at this conclusion by various routes: analysis of the concept of spirituality, reflective engagement in spiritual practices, and so forth. The renaissance of psychedelic research offers a golden opportunity for a distinctive approach: a *neurophilosophical* inquiry into naturalised spirituality (Letheby 2017). By 'neurophilosophical', I do not mean 'focused exclusively on brain scans and molecular pharmacology'. As outlined in Chapter 2, I simply mean an account that begins with the phenomena, and grounds philosophical conclusions in knowledge from the multidisciplinary mind and brain sciences—noting that an integrative psychedelic neuroscience needs qualitative research and psychometric data just as much as neuroimaging and neuropharmacology.

The golden opportunity arises from the fact that psychedelics reliably induce experiences that subjects feel moved to describe as 'spiritual'—even, in some cases, with no prior interest in or inclination towards spirituality (e.g., Fadiman 2005, Pollan 2018). This suggests that these experiences are *paradigmatically* spiritual: they consistently evoke the application of that term even by those with quite divergent beliefs about the subject. As such, the significance of the recent wave of psychedelic neuroscience is this: for the first time ever, scientists are in a position to safely, reliably, and repeatedly induce paradigmatically spiritual experiences in the laboratory (including the neuroimaging scanner) among diverse populations with differing prior beliefs and attitudes concerning spirituality. This gives us unprecedented access to high-quality evidence concerning the nature, causes, and consequences of paradigmatically spiritual experiences—evidence that is directly relevant to the question whether spirituality can be naturalised.

When we examine the evidence that has been gathered so far, we find a remarkable degree of convergence with the conclusions of philosophical inquiries. The findings from psychedelic research sit comfortably with the claim that we are spiritual 'when our sense of connection is enlarged ... when we aspire to greater things ... [and] when we ask the big questions', and with the idea that connection, aspiration, and reflection on big questions are all ways of 'breaking through the narrow walls of the ego' (Stone 2012, p. 492). Therefore, these findings also sit comfortably with the claim that authentic forms of naturalistic spirituality exist, because fostering such connection, aspiration, and reflection (by disrupting the default functioning of the self-model) does not require non-naturalistic metaphysical ideations. Let us now revisit some of these findings in light of philosophical concerns about naturalising spirituality.

9.3 Spirituality as unselfing

Reflecting on a psilocybin experience that we have encountered in earlier chapters, Michael Pollan writes:

I could easily confirm the 'fusion of [my] personal self into a larger whole', as well as the 'feeling that [I] experienced something profoundly sacred and holy' and 'of being at a spiritual height' and even the 'experience of unity with ultimate reality'. Yes, yes, yes, and yes—*provided, that is, my endorsement of those loaded adjectives doesn't imply any belief in a supernatural reality* ... something novel and profound had happened to me—something I am prepared to call spiritual, though only with an asterisk. I guess I've always assumed that spirituality implies a belief or faith I've never shared and from which it supposedly flows. But now I wondered, is this always or necessarily the case?

(2018, p. 284; my emphasis).

Here we find a fact of obvious significance for the current inquiry: that a psilocybin experience led a sceptically minded avowed naturalist to question, for the first time, whether spirituality necessarily requires 'belief' or 'faith'. What novel and profound episode led such a person to question his lifelong assumptions about the nature and entailments of spirituality? What kind of experience moved him to apply the term 'spiritual' (even if only 'with an asterisk') *despite* not tempting him to any belief in a supernatural reality?

Unsurprisingly, it was an experience of breaking through the narrow walls of the ego and feeling connected to something larger: in this case, the sounds of a Bach cello suite in which Pollan's altered consciousness sensed 'nothing less than the stream of human consciousness, something in which one might glean the very meaning of life and ... read life's last chapter'. This experience involved reflections, of a highly specific sort, on Big Questions, which had 'the unmistakeable effect of reconciling [Pollan] to death' (Pollan 2018, pp. 268–269).

The terms 'spiritual' and 'mystical' are not precisely synonymous, of course. However, of the many 'varieties of psychedelic experience' (Masters and Houston 1966), subjects tend, unsurprisingly, to regard the mystical-type experience as spiritual. Pollan's report provides one example of this. Another comes from the seminal study by Griffiths et al. (2008) in which healthy subjects received high-dose psilocybin. Subjects' willingness to count the experience among the five most 'spiritually significant' of their lives correlated with ratings of mystical-type experience, but not with other psychometric measures, such as ratings of the overall intensity of the experience. Given this relationship, some of the conclusions I drew earlier in this book about mystical-type experiences are directly relevant to psychedelic spirituality and its compatibility or otherwise with a naturalistic worldview.

Specifically: given the relationship between mystical-type experience and attributions of spiritual significance, the account of psychedelic therapy developed in this book supports the contention that spirituality can be naturalised. As we have seen, some mystical-type experiences feature non-naturalistic metaphysical epiphanies, while others do not. The common denominator, and the main factor that gives these experiences their transformative power, is the unbinding of the predictive self-model and the consequent liberation of attention from regulation and constraint by that model. What results, under conducive circumstances, is psychological insight, including the accessing of new, broader perspectives; seeing one's life within a wider context; emotional breakthroughs; and profound existential feelings of acceptance, embodiment, wonder, awe, and *connectedness*. We have seen that transformative psychedelic experiences often involve experiences of connection to something larger—the first of Stone's three pillars—and that many of these are independent of non-naturalistic metaphysics. Subjects report feelings of connectedness to their own minds, bodies, and emotions, to their values, to other people, to the biosphere and the cosmos at large. (And, in *some* cases, to a divine Reality, cosmic consciousness, or transcendent metaphysical principle.)

Another thing that often results, as Benny Shanon (2001, 2002) has pointed out, is philosophical reflection—reflection on the Big Questions. Irrespective of any prior interest or education in philosophy, many psychedelic subjects spontaneously begin exploring distinctively philosophical questions, and espousing recognisably philosophical views—about morality, the nature of consciousness and knowledge, the human condition, and so forth. The REBUS ('RElaxed Beliefs Under pSychedelics') model of Carhart-Harris and Friston (2019) provides an attractive explanation of this phenomenon. Philosophy and psychedelic experience both centrally involve exposing and scrutinising our most fundamental, usually unexamined, beliefs about self and world, rendering our foundational assumptions opaque, visible, and therefore dubitable. A key difference, of course, is that in modern academic philosophy this occurs in the medium of discursive rational reflection, whereas under psychedelics it occurs in the medium of our phenomenal models of reality (cf. Langlitz 2016). Here is how one patient described this experience after receiving psilocybin-assisted treatment for tobacco addiction:

> It was all about searching for answers to questions that are age-old. Maybe we have the answer to some of it, maybe we'll never have the answer to it. But none of it had to do with addiction to cigarettes. It all had to do with stretching space and time, and asking questions like, 'Why is there something rather than nothing?' And, 'What happened before the Big Bang?' ... All those things that had nothing, absolutely nothing—at least in the conscious thinking of it—with stopping smoking ... every time I think of a cigarette, it brings me back to the three sessions of the psilocybin trip, where you're trying to ask questions that there may not be answers to. So, that's more fun than smoking!
>
> (Noorani et al. 2018, p. 760).

This phenomenon constitutes another point of convergence between psychedelic use and mindfulness meditation. Here is the American Buddhist nun Pema Chödrön on the latter:

The path is a sense of wonder, becoming a two- or three-year-old child again, wanting to know all the unknowable things, beginning to question everything. We know we're never really going to find the answers, because these kinds of questions come from having a hunger and a passion for life—they have nothing to do with resolving anything or tying it all up into a neat little package. This kind of questioning is the journey itself. The fruition lies in beginning to realize our kinship with all humanity.

(Chödrön 1996, p. 11).

Stone's second pillar of spirituality is aspiration to greater things and the attempt to realise our ideals. Of the three, this is the one on which we have spent the least time in this book, but it sometimes emerges under the guise of psychological insight, when subjects report having epiphanies or realisations about their own values, priorities, and what matters to them. Sometimes this is described in terms of remembering, or reconnecting with, earlier versions of themselves, whose values are perceived as superior:

Participant 410 reflected,

Did I learn anything new? Have I done anything totally different than I ever did before? No! But I'm sort of going back into my … earlier life when I probably was a better person, to be honest with you.

Similarly, Participant 427 remarked,

I don't know if I really *learned*—it was more like letting back in stuff that I had blocked out? … I don't think I changed my values, just remembered more of them. Or just remembered to honour them more, or … *allow* them more.

(Noorani et al. 2018, p. 759).

The idea that psychedelic experiences can help subjects to (re-)connect with their values and aspirations is relevant to recent suggestions that psychedelics might be viable agents of *moral bioenhancement*—that, suitably used, they might constitute effective biotechnologies for improving individuals' moral character (Earp 2018; cf. Tennison 2012, Ahlskog 2017). It is also consistent with the finding that healthy subjects who undergo transformative psychedelic experiences report lasting increases in altruistic and prosocial behaviour—increases verified by community observers (Griffiths et al. 2006, 2008, 2011). At least part of the mechanism here may be an oft-described aspect of psychedelic experience that I, with my focus on epistemological issues, have under-emphasised: the experience of universal or boundless love. We encountered one patient's description of this experience earlier, in chapter 3. This description speaks directly to questions about naturalising the aspects of spiritual experience that sometimes evoke religious interpretations:

Just overcome with love and all the love that I have for my family and my friends. I felt that it was coming from them; also I felt that I was bathed in it. And if I were religious it definitely would have been a religious experience, I would have said bathed in God's love. And I don't think English really has a way to say this without using that word 'God', um maybe bathed in transcendent love. Bathed in universal love. It was such a strong feeling.

(Swift et al. 2017, p. 504).

Part of the mechanism leading to such experiences of universal love may well be that common core of mystical-type experience, the disruption and disintegration of the phenomenal self-model. It is a venerable idea, which awaits rigorous empirical investigation (Millière et al. 2018), that the experience of selfless consciousness might be a reliable means of promoting selflessness in the *moral* sense—i.e., decreased self-interested and increased altruistic motivation (Ahlskog 2017).[1] If this is true, then episodes of selfless consciousness (or self-unbinding) might have an important role to play in the moral life. One of the best-known articulations of this idea in recent Western philosophy is Iris Murdoch's notion of *unselfing*:

I am looking out of my window in an anxious and resentful state of mind, oblivious of my surroundings, brooding perhaps on some damage done to my prestige. Then suddenly I observe a hovering kestrel. In a moment everything is altered. The brooding self with its hurt vanity has disappeared. There is nothing now but kestrel. And when I return to thinking of the other matter it seems less important. And of course this is something which we may also do deliberately: give attention to nature in order to clear our minds of selfish care.

(Murdoch 1970, p. 84).

We can remain agnostic, for now, on whether unselfing really does promote virtuous *behaviour*, though there is intriguing preliminary evidence for this claim (cf. Kähönen 2020).[2] Considerable evidence shows that unselfing (understood as the unbinding of the self-model via disruption of its neuronal substrates) promotes other pillars of spirituality that require no non-naturalistic ideations: feelings of connectedness, aspiration, and reflection on the Big Questions. As Stone suggests, unselfing is indeed the core factor unifying the various elements of spirituality whose cultivation is consistent with a naturalistic outlook.

[1] Van Mulukom et al. (2020) report findings consistent with this hypothesis: an association between uncontrolled psychedelic experiences and decreased narcissistic tendencies. On the other hand, Pokorny et al. (2017) report some evidence that moral decision making, or a certain measure thereof, is unaltered during the acute psychedelic experience. (Of course this is consistent with the hypothesis that it is altered *after* the experience.)

[2] Juuso Kähönen and I converged independently on the idea of using Murdoch's concept of unselfing to analyse psychedelic experience.

Here, then, is a psychedelic argument for the claim that spirituality can be naturalised:

1. Unselfing and its typical effects, such as feelings of connection, aspiration, and reflection on Big Questions, are the features in virtue of which psychedelic experiences count as genuinely spiritual
2. Unselfing and these typical effects thereof do not require, and often occur in the absence of, any inclination towards non-naturalistic beliefs
3. Therefore, genuinely spiritual experiences do not require, and often occur in the absence of, any inclination towards non-naturalistic beliefs

Of course, an argument of this kind cannot be regarded as conclusive: terms such as 'spirituality' and their associated concepts are intrinsically contested. If someone adopts an understanding of spirituality on which it necessarily involves metaphysical beliefs in spirits or a spiritual realm, we cannot *demonstrate* that they are incorrect. There are doubtless legitimate senses of the term on which this entailment holds. However, I think that the considerations outlined here show that there is a real phenomenon, referred to by at least one legitimate sense of the term, on which the entailment fails: transformative practices and experiences of unselfing whose sincere undertaking requires no non-naturalistic ideations. Psychedelic evidence reveals a set of core features that move people to describe practices and experiences as 'spiritual' despite bearing no necessary connection to such ideations.

This concludes my case for the claim that the Entheogenic Conception of psychedelics can be naturalised. In the next and final chapter, I summarise the discussion and reflect on its implications, as well as suggesting some directions for future research.

10
Conclusion

> While fully developed mysticism seems to me mistaken, I yet believe that, by sufficient restraint, there is an element of wisdom to be learned from the mystical way of feeling, which does not seem to be attainable in any other manner. If this is the truth, mysticism is to be commended as an attitude towards life, not as a creed about the world.
>
> **Bertrand Russell, 'Mysticism and logic'.**

10.1 Testable predictions

In Chapter 2, I reviewed evidence for the safety, and therapeutic and transformative efficacy, of controlled psychedelic administration. I also reviewed evidence that psychedelics' lasting psychological benefits are mediated by mystical-type experiences. This latter evidence gives rise to the Comforting Delusion Objection. I outlined my plan for answering the Objection: assume that naturalism is true, and that the epistemic status of psychedelic therapy is important, and show that the Objection fails even on these assumptions. The strategy was to refute the third, originally suppressed, premise of the Objection: that if naturalism is true, then the overall epistemic status of psychedelic therapy is poor. In Chapter 3, I reviewed qualitative evidence and found initial, phenomenological clues that the lasting benefits of controlled psychedelic ingestion are not due primarily to non-naturalistic metaphysical ideations.

In Chapter 4, I argued that neither the induction of such ideations, nor the experience-independent stimulation of neuroplasticity, is the central mechanism of psychedelic therapy. The central mechanism is some genuinely psychological factor that correlates fairly well with the construct of a mystical-type experience, but is independent of non-naturalistic metaphysical ideations. In Chapter 5, I drew on both psychometric and neuroscientific evidence to argue that the relevant factor is the disruption and subsequent alteration of mental representations of the self (which is not necessarily equivalent to 'ego dissolution').

In Chapters 6 and 7, I outlined a neurocognitive theory of how this might work: the predictive self-binding account, based on predictive processing (PP) theory. I showed how the self-binding account can explain paradigmatic features of psychedelic therapy as described by patients. I also briefly considered the implications of this account for philosophical issues to do with self and self-consciousness. Collectively, the arguments of Chapters 4–7 show that the epistemic risks of psychedelics, given naturalism, are smaller than they initially appear.

In Chapters 8 and 9, I argued, on the basis of the predictive self-binding account, that psychedelic therapy has considerable epistemic and spiritual benefits that are consistent with naturalism. The epistemic benefits are often unavailable by any other, less epistemically costly means; thus, psychedelic therapy is epistemically innocent. And many of the spiritual benefits can be understood as forms of unselfing, which coheres with existing philosophical accounts of naturalistic spirituality.

What follows from these arguments? First, a series of testable predictions, which I outline in the current section. Second, some other possible avenues for future research, which I outline in section 10.2. Third, and finally, two important philosophical conclusions about psychedelic therapy: (i) the failure of the Comforting Delusion Objection, and (ii) the availability of a plausible naturalised Entheogenic Conception of psychedelics. I summarise these conclusions in section 10.3.

We begin with the testable predictions. In Chapter 4, I argued that increases in non-naturalistic metaphysical beliefs, while they sometimes occur and contribute to lasting benefits, are not the central mechanism of change in psychedelic therapy. Instead, the central mechanism is some other psychological factor that correlates with the construct of a mystical-type experience. If this is true, then it follows that ratings of acute mystical-type experience, and of increased non-naturalistic metaphysical belief, should each predict lasting benefits (e.g., symptom reduction, positive personality change, and increases in self-reported well-being). However, it follows that the former should be a *stronger* predictor, in virtue of the psychological factor with which I claim it correlates—namely, the disruption and revision of the self-model.

It must be acknowledged that the initial evidence does not look friendly to this prediction. Timmermann et al. (in preparation) have introduced the Metaphysical Belief Questionnaire (MBQ) to quantify changes in metaphysical beliefs resulting from psychedelic administration. In an online survey study, they administered the questionnaire to volunteers who independently planned to attend a psychedelic ceremony or retreat. At the time of writing, preliminary analyses of their findings suggest that psychedelic experiences in a ceremonial or retreat setting robustly increased non-naturalistic metaphysical beliefs, such as in mind–body dualism and the existence of supernatural realms, and that these increases strongly predicted lasting increases in well-being.

However, we cannot discount the possibility that various aspects of set and setting significantly influenced these outcomes: for example, the ceremonial setting itself, the prior beliefs of those inclined to seek out such settings, and the specific intentions that they had for their experiences. Also, importantly, Timmermann et al. did not report testing for correlations between increases in well-being and measures quantifying the acute experience, such as measures of mystical-type experience or psychological insight. Perhaps some such measure would have been a stronger predictor of increased well-being than the MBQ. The real test of my arguments in Chapter 4 will come when the MBQ, or a similar instrument, is administered in a double-blind clinical trial, along with such instruments as the Mystical Experience Questionnaire (MEQ), the Psychological Insight Questionnaire (PIQ), and the Emotional Breakthrough Inventory (EBI). Under these conditions, I would expect, not changes in MBQ scores, but some variable quantifying the acute experience--such as MEQ, PIQ, or EBI scores—to be the strongest predictor of lasting psychological benefits.

The other main argument of Chapter 4 was that the pure Molecular Neuroplasticity Theory of psychedelic therapy is false, on the grounds that (a) ratings of mystical-type experience and similar constructs are a robust dose-independent predictor of beneficial outcomes, and (b) this should not be the case, were the therapeutic benefits mediated primarily by some experience-independent causal process at the molecular level. This yields the prediction that attempts to mimic psychedelics' therapeutic effects with molecular variants that lack their phenomenological effects will fail, because those phenomenological effects (and their cognitive underpinnings) are the primary cause of the effects on well-being and symptomatology. Such attempts need not fail *utterly*: I accept that experience-independent pharmacological effects probably contribute somewhat to psychedelics' therapeutic effects. But any molecule that mimics only the experience-independent effects and not the phenomenological effects should not be as effective a therapeutic or transformative agent. If it turns out that psychedelics' therapeutic and transformative effects can be replicated fully by related molecules that lack their distinctive effects on consciousness, then the idea that psychedelic therapy is a personal-level process, and many of the other claims of this book, will be undermined.

In Chapter 5, I argued that changes to self-representation are the central causal factor in psychedelic therapy. This hypothesis yields the prediction that the sorts of findings reviewed in that chapter will replicate. Future studies examining psychological and neural correlates of therapeutic and transformative effects should continue to highlight such variables as (a) acute experiences of psychological insight and emotional breakthrough, (b) lasting increases in psychological flexibility and mindfulness-related capacities, and (c) acute, sub-acute, and long-term modulation of the Default Mode and Salience networks. In that chapter, I also argued that the PIQ is measuring the same basic phenomenon as the 'Insightfulness' sub-scale of the 11D-ASC (11 Dimensions of Altered States of Consciousness) scale. This entails the prediction that these two measures should be highly correlated—i.e., that the PIQ should show convergent validity with the Insightfulness sub-scale of the 11D-ASC.

The predictive self-binding account developed in Chapters 6 and 7 has empirical implications, too. Foremost among these is that, if more fine-grained instruments are developed to quantify the distinct varieties of ego dissolution experiences, these varieties should correlate differentially with specific neural changes: changes to the narrative self should correlate more strongly with modulation of the Default Mode Network (DMN) and changes to the minimal or embodied self with modulation of the Salience Network (SN).

One key claim of Chapters 7 and 8 was that the induction of phenomenal opacity into the self-model is part of the therapeutic mechanism. (Phenomenal opacity, recall, is the property that phenomenally conscious mental representations have when they are experienced *as* representations, rather than 'transparently' as reality itself.) Another claim was that this opacity is closely related to the gaining of knowledge by acquaintance with (a) the mind's vast unrealised potential and (b) the constructed, mutable nature of the sense of self. It follows that, if ways can be found to quantify this opacity and knowledge by acquaintance, they should be fairly robust predictors of lasting benefits. In section 8.5, I suggested that we might operationalise them by measuring increased assent to such statements as these:

(i) I know from first-hand experience that my mind has vast potential that normally goes unrealised.
(ii) My ordinary sense of who I am is, in part, a story, and it is possible for me to change this story.

I predict that increased assent to such statements after a psychedelic experience would correlate significantly with symptom reduction, positive personality change, and increases in well-being resulting from that experience.[1]

Another testable prediction comes from the ideas about knowledge how that I defended in Chapter 8. In section 8.4, I made a claim about the probable findings of qualitative interviews with expert meditators undergoing a similar protocol to that of Smigielski et al. (2019a, 2019b)—i.e., a psychedelic-assisted mindfulness retreat. My claim was that such practitioners would describe gaining some increased *knowledge* or *understanding*, during (or as a result of) their psychedelic-assisted meditation session, about how to perform certain meditative practices, or how to access certain attentional modes or states of mind. This prediction stems from my conjecture that the observed increases in mindfulness-related tendencies stem from a genuine process of conscious learning—an acquisition or increase of skills, rather than some brute unconscious mechanism whose outputs mimic the profile of such skills. I would predict similar results from a study in which two groups of novice meditators underwent a course of meditation training, with and without psychedelic assistance. I have in mind here something like the protocol of Griffiths et al. (2017), but with more formal and standardised meditation training—perhaps an eight-week Mindfulness Based Stress Reduction course, or something similar—and more explicit tests of meditative ability, perhaps incorporating neurofeedback tasks (e.g., Garrison et al. 2014).

Finally, in Chapter 9, I argued that the kind of spirituality exemplified by transformative psychedelic experiences can be naturalised. This argument was based partly on a correlation between (a) ratings of mystical-type experience, and (b) subjects' attributions of *spiritual significance* to the experience (Griffiths et al. 2008, 2016). Given this correlation, the relative independence of transformative mystical-type experiences from non-naturalistic metaphysical ideations suggests a corresponding

---

[1] Note that statement (ii) incorporates a fairly explicit expression of the opacity of the self-model.

independence of transformative *spiritual* experiences (as subjects understand that term) from such ideations. Thus, the account of naturalistic spirituality developed in that chapter yields the testable prediction that such findings should replicate: future research should continue to find robust correlations between ratings of mystical-type experience, and subjects' willingness to describe their experience as 'spiritual' or 'spiritually significant', if they are asked to interpret the latter terms as they see fit. Furthermore, if we were to compare ratings of mystical-type experience and non-naturalistic metaphysical ideations (measured by the MBQ or something similar), then the former should predict attributions of spiritual significance more strongly than the latter. This follows from my claim that unselfing, rather than non-naturalistic metaphysics, is at the heart of spirituality.

10.2 Future directions

Despite its somewhat presumptuous title, this book has barely scratched the surface of the fascinating issues that arise from a philosophical examination of psychedelic research. Before concluding the discussion, it is worth mentioning some (but only some!) of the outstanding questions in this emerging field of inquiry. In doing so, I will, of necessity, refer to specialised debates in various subfields of philosophy and the mind/brain sciences. Those unfamiliar with, or uninterested in, these debates can skip the present section without loss and proceed to section 10.3, in which I summarise the overarching conclusions of the book.

First, there are issues in the philosophy of mind pertaining to self and self-consciousness, which I discussed in passing at the end of Chapter 7. Does psychedelic evidence demonstrate the possibility of totally selfless consciousness? At first glance, the case looks compelling but, as we have seen, it faces numerous obstacles. Notably, there are several problems raised by Sebastián (2020). One concerns the possibility of cognitive bias in phenomenological reports. Another concerns the difficulty of discriminating between ego-elimination and ego-expansion interpretations of such reports. Yet another concerns whether such reports really describe experiences without *any* form of self-consciousness, including the putatively minimal form of self-consciousness described as 'for-me-ness' (Henriksen and Parnas 2019) or 'perspectival first-personal (PFP) awareness' Sebastián (2020). There is also Metzinger's (2003) argument that retrospective reports of totally selfless consciousness generate a performative contradiction.

Progress has been made on addressing these issues in a recent journal issue devoted to the topic of 'Radical disruptions of self-consciousness' (Millière and Metzinger 2020, Fink 2020, Letheby 2020, Millière 2020), but more work remains to be done. This work has conceptual, theoretical, and empirical aspects. Indeed, Sebastián (2020) has made some suggestions about future empirical tests of the hypothesis that PFP awareness is totally eliminated in some altered states. The detailed design of such tests could benefit from interdisciplinary collaboration between empirical researchers and philosophers who specialise in the analysis of such phenomenological notions. Given the numerous parallels between psychedelic experience and meditative states, it would also be interesting to see whether philosophical work on meditative traditions such as Buddhism could help to advance this debate. For example, in addition to notions such as 'for-me-ness', which is drawn from the phenomenological tradition, it might be fruitful to view psychedelic disruptions to self-consciousness in terms of Miri Albahari's (2006) distinction between 'personal' and 'perspectival' forms of mental ownership. Albahari's notion of perspectival ownership has clear similarities to Zahavi's for-me-ness (Albahari 2011). However, there may also be subtle differences that could shed new light on psychedelic phenomena. Similar remarks apply to other work on Buddhist philosophy, meditation practices, and self-consciousness (Millière et al. 2018).

The question whether psychedelic evidence supports metaphysical eliminativism about the self also remains open. The most obvious argument from the former to the latter is the Mismatch Argument, which I examined briefly in Chapter 7, section 7.8.2. This argument alleges that:

1. We represent the self as having a particular set of properties.
2. No real entity has that set of properties.
3. Therefore, the self is not real.

(McClelland 2019, p. 25).

According to the predictive self-binding account, psychedelic phenomenology provides support for premise 1, by providing an illuminating contrast between the ordinary (Cartesian) sense of self and certain states in which it is disrupted or lost. However, as we saw, the Mismatch Argument has been criticised by Tom McClelland (2019), who points out that it is invalid: an entity can still be real, even if we radically misrepresent its properties.

Several questions remain to be addressed here. It is worth asking whether there might be a stronger psychedelically informed argument for the no-self theory. On the other hand, McClelland's arguments themselves deserve further scrutiny. Recall: McClelland not only criticises the Mismatch Argument for the no-self theory, but also mounts a positive case for the 'illusion model' on which the self does exist but is misrepresented by us. The illusion model, rather than eliminating the self from our ontology, identifies it with the brain, or the body, or whatever is the *bearer* of our self-representations. This identification is motivated by two key claims. The first is that our self-representations purport to be *de se* representations, which McClelland defines as representations that refer to whatever bears them. The second is that there must be something that actually *is* the bearer of these representations, such as the brain or the body. This suggests to McClelland that this bearer should be regarded as the referent of our self-representations, and therefore as the self.

For the purposes of this book, I bracketed the issue of realism versus anti-realism about the self, noting that anti-realism about a certain *type* of self is still an important conclusion. But future work could address this issue head-on, in a manner perhaps informed by psychedelic evidence. Is it really true that all mental representations must have a 'bearer', in the sense required for the argument? Is this principle trivial and undeniable, or does it embody substantive and controversial assumptions? Also, is it true that our self-representations are *de se* representations, in that they refer to whatever bears them? Or do they rather purport to refer to a *specific type* of bearer—one, perhaps, to be found nowhere in reality? Detailed work on the phenomenology of self-consciousness and the content of our self-representations would be required to answer these questions, and this work might be informed by the study of psychedelic experience.

There are many other unaddressed questions at the border of psychedelic research, philosophy of mind and cognition, and theoretical cognitive neuroscience. For example, Benny Shanon (2002) argues that there are remarkable, highly specific cross-personal and cross-cultural commonalities in the contents of ayahuasca-induced visions. Some of these commonalities evoke Jungian ideas about archetypes. Indeed, Shanon suggests that:

> when attempting to account for cross-personal commonalities encountered with Ayahuasca, Jung's is the first theoretical approach that comes to mind. In fact, the scientific psychological literature seems to offer no other potential resource for explanation.
>
> **(Shanon 2002, p. 390).**

However, Shanon also notes that 'the nature of the Jungian archetypes is far from being clear' (Shanon 2002, p. 390). This theoretical argument deserves scrutiny. Has the existence of the alleged cross-personal and cross-cultural phenomenological commonalities been established securely, in a way that excludes prosaic explanations such as cultural transmission and interpretive bias? Are there any scientifically plausible, non-Jungian explanations of the existence of such 'cognitive universals'? (e.g., Winkelman 2017). If not, then how should the Jungian explanation be understood, and how does it relate to other theoretical frameworks such as PP?

A related question concerns autobiographically focused *psychodynamic* experiences under psychedelics: experiences in which subjects seem to gain insights about their own previously unconscious mental states. Classic examples of this kind of experience include the reliving of apparently repressed memories and the sudden awareness of apparently unconscious beliefs and desires. In Chapter 8, I mentioned one idea about how to explain such experiences in a PP framework: that they result from increased access to information previously filtered out by overweighted priors (cf. Carhart-Harris and Friston 2019). But this is just a thumbnail sketch, and leaves many questions unanswered. Notably, to explain such experiences, do we need to postulate a neurocognitive system that has many of the properties of the *dynamic unconscious* as described by Freud? (Carhart-Harris and Friston 2010). Or is the evidence better explained without such posits? (cf. O'Brien and Jureidini 2002a, 2002b).

Relatedly, is there explanatory value in linking psychedelic experience to Freud's notion of the *primary process* (Kraehenmann et al. 2017a), and is it accurate to describe psychedelic experience as involving a regression to a (phylogenetically and ontogenetically) 'primitive' mode of consciousness? (Carhart-Harris et al. 2014). What exactly are the similarities and differences between psychedelic experience and other states of consciousness, such as dreaming? (Kraehenmann 2017, Kraehenmann et al. 2017b). All of these questions would be interesting subjects for philosophical investigation.

There are also issues in the philosophy of science and medicine that arise in connection with psychedelic therapy. For instance, how can we make cogent *causal inferences* in psychedelic research—that is, inferences that this putative treatment really has certain causal effects? This question is prompted by the fact that effective double-blinding is very difficult in psychedelic clinical trials. The effects of the active treatment are so obvious and salient that it often becomes clear to a patient which group they are in. Thus, when a significant effect is found, how can we cogently infer that it was due to a treatment effect and not a placebo effect?

One possible way of addressing this issue is by means of ingenious experimental designs—for instance, designs that contrast various different doses of psychedelics, or that contrast psychedelics with 'active placebos' (active substances with some overlapping effects—for example, Griffiths et al. 2006). On the other hand, perhaps progress can be made by drawing on recent work on *mechanistic evidence* in the philosophy of medicine. Some philosophers have argued that not just correlational evidence from double-blind randomised controlled trials but also evidence about the mechanistic targets of drugs, can help to justify conclusions that a drug has a certain causal effect (Russo and Williamson 2011, Clarke et al. 2013, Landes et al. 2018). As Andrew Jones (2018) suggests, ideas from these debates could be useful in thinking about the unique methodological challenges of research into psychedelic therapy. Consider two facts, for instance: (i) psychedelics seem to target the functioning of brain network hubs whose functioning is altered in specific pathologies, and (ii) they seem to target, even in healthy subjects, psychological factors known to be altered in those pathologies (e.g., self-representation, salience attribution, and psychological flexibility). These facts surely constitute *some* evidence for the hypothesis that psychedelic therapy has a genuine causal effect on symptoms of those pathologies; but the strength of this evidence needs to be determined.

Issues concerning levels of explanation in psychedelic science also warrant further investigation. In this book, I have dealt with these issues in passing, to the extent that was necessary for my core arguments concerning the mechanisms of psychedelic therapy. I offered the framework of neurocognitive explanation as a way to link neurobiological and psychological levels of description, contending that the attribution of computational functions to neural structures is a viable way to explain psychological phenomena. But there is much more to be said, and an extensive body of work in the philosophy of biology and neuroscience has developed sophisticated conceptual tools for thinking about causal and explanatory relations between disciplines, subfields, and levels of explanation (e.g., Machamer et al. 2000, Craver 2007, Bechtel 2006, 2008, Craver and Darden 2013).

To take one example, Madsen et al. (2020) found that increases in mindfulness capacities three months after a single dose of psilocybin correlated negatively with changes in 5-HT2A receptor binding one week after the psychedelic experience. What exactly are the relations between these receptor-level changes and the psychological changes observed later? What, for that matter, are their relations to the psychological changes during the psychedelic experience itself and its immediate aftermath? Was the specific pattern of changes to receptor binding simply caused 'directly' at the pharmacological level, or was it partially 'mechanistically mediated' (Craver and Bechtel 2007) by specific patterns of macroscopic, systemic effects triggered by the initial pharmacological action of psilocin? More generally, does psychedelic therapy ever involve (innocent) forms of 'top-down causation' (Craver and Bechtel 2007) in which specific patterns of micro-level changes only occur via the mediation of such macroscopic, systemic effects? If so, how are such cases to be analysed? More empirical evidence is needed, of course. But, given the seemingly complex interactions between multiscale phenomena in psychedelic therapy, it provides, at the least, a valuable case study for philosophical ideas concerning inter-level explanatory relations and causal interactions.[2]

Psychedelic therapy also raises issues in the philosophy of psychiatry. Some have suggested that the advent of psychedelic therapy constitutes a 'new paradigm' in the study and treatment of psychiatric disorder (e.g., Nichols et al. 2017, Schenberg 2018, Inserra 2019). This claim merits scrutiny. Of course, I argued in Chapter 7 that psychedelic therapy involves something like a 'neurocognitive paradigm shift' in the mind/brain of the individual patient. But it is also worth asking whether the widespread adoption of psychedelic therapy would constitute a new paradigm in psychiatric research, in Kuhn's (1970) technical sense of 'paradigm'. If so, then what are the constituents of the old paradigm and of the new, and what are the intractable anomalies that have precipitated the current period of crisis (or 'extraordinary science') in psychiatry (Poland and Tekin 2017)? How exactly are the constituents of the new paradigm derived from the evidence concerning psychedelic therapy?

Another question is whether the evidence concerning psychedelic therapy has implications for *psychiatric nosology*, the taxonomy of mental disorder. Some have suggested that it does—for instance, its remarkable transdiagnostic efficacy might put pressure on the idea of anxiety, depression, and addiction as 'discrete nosological entities' (Schenberg 2018, p. 1) while suggesting new ways of explaining their characteristic symptoms. Issues in psychiatric nosology have received considerable philosophical attention in the past 30 years (e.g., Stein 1991, Radden 1994, Zachar and Kendler 2017). It could be illuminating to examine the putative nosological implications of psychedelic therapy through the lens of these debates.

---

[2] Another fascinating example of recent scientific work relevant to these issues is provided by Kringelbach et al. (2020).

A related but distinct question arises from the apparent commonalities between psychedelic therapy in patients and transformation in healthy subjects. If psychedelics do reduce psychiatric symptoms and promote well-being by a common mechanism, what implications, if any, does this have for the relationship between pathology and normality? Does it provide support for the 'continuity thesis' (Petrolini 2017) that psychopathological symptoms are deeply continuous with normal psychological tendencies found in the broader population? Relatedly, is it true, as some (e.g., Friedman 2006, Sessa 2014) have suggested, that psychedelic therapy, given its spiritual or transcendent aspects, is in tension with the so-called 'medical model' of psychiatry? The intuitive appeal of this claim is obvious. However, a considerable body of philosophical scholarship has examined what it might mean to view psychiatry as a branch of medicine (Murphy 2020). It would be interesting to examine psychedelic therapy through the lens of this work, in order to determine whether the tension is real or merely apparent.

Despite the obvious relevance of my arguments to ethical and policy discussions, I have not engaged in such discussions directly (apart from my brief attempt, in Chapter 2, to motivate the idea that the epistemic status of psychedelic therapy matters). However, there is an emerging body of literature that examines ethical dimensions of therapeutic and transformative psychedelic use. There are two distinct issues that arise here. First, there is the question whether psychedelics themselves can function as effective agents of moral enhancement—whether they can reliably improve individuals' moral character or cognition, and, if so, how. Second, there are ethical questions about the use of psychedelics, given their real risks: how should they be (permitted to be) used? By whom, under what circumstances, and for what purposes? On the first count, some authors have argued that psychedelics represent promising interventions for moral enhancement (Tennison 2012, Earp 2018), and others have speculated about *how* psychedelic experiences might improve moral cognition (Ahlskog 2017, Kähönen 2020). On the second count, it has been argued that the unique features of psychedelic therapy entail an ethical requirement for an 'enhanced consent process' beyond what is required for other psychiatric treatments (Smith and Sisti 2020). We will return to this idea shortly.

Mention of psychedelic moral enhancement brings us to the final set of outstanding issues that I want to canvass. These issues are epistemological. There are potential epistemic benefits and risks of psychedelics that I have not considered in this book. For example, one possible mechanism for psychedelics' putative moral enhancement effects is that they can facilitate the acquisition of *moral knowledge*. Juuso Kähönen (2020) has given a thoughtful account of how this might work within a naturalistic framework, invoking Murdoch's ideas about unselfing and its centrality to the moral life. This is a type of potential epistemic benefit that I have not considered in any detail (although it probably sometimes involves acquiring new knowledge of old facts). It would also be interesting to analyse, from an epistemological standpoint, claims about the *educational* value of psychedelic experiences (Tupper 2003, Roberts 2006) and their putative ability to enhance 'existential intelligence' (Tupper 2002).

There are doubtless other possible epistemic benefits of psychedelic use that I have not considered, and ingenious experimental methods for testing whether they in fact occur. As we have seen, there are studies examining psychedelics' effects on the perception of emotional facial expressions (Rocha et al. 2019) and on empathy (Dolder et al. 2016, Pokorny et al. 2017, Mason et al. 2019). Lyons and Carhart-Harris (2018b) have examined their effects on the accuracy of future life forecasting. Studies like these provide paradigms for experimental investigations into psychedelic epistemology. This is a fertile area for interaction between philosophical analysis and empirical research. There is also a body of research investigating the effects of psychedelics on creativity (e.g., Sessa 2008, Girn et al. 2020), which I have not examined. Clearly analysing this research would be relevant to a comprehensive epistemological evaluation of the psychedelic state. Future work on psychedelic epistemology could also benefit from fuller integration with work on epistemic benefits of meditation practice (e.g., Albahari 2014, 2019a, Davis and Thompson 2015, Lutz et al. 2019).

Finally, there are possible epistemic *risks* of psychedelic use that I have not considered. I have focused heavily on whether psychedelics promote non-naturalistic metaphysical beliefs. But of course, even if naturalism is true, there are other types of epistemic risks than this. This point is brought home by a thoughtful article by Greif and Šurkala (2020), published shortly before this book went to press, on the compassionate use of psychedelic therapy. These authors consider what I have been calling the Comforting Delusion Objection, and argue that it fails. However, their response has several facets, and does not fit neatly into the options that I canvassed in Chapter 2. They argue that there is no good evidence that the acquisition of non-naturalistic metaphysical beliefs actually takes place, and cite evidence that non-naturalistic metaphysical ideations are not part of the causal mechanism of psychedelic therapy. Thus far, this is essentially the approach that I have taken here. Greif and Šurkala are questioning the premise that, if naturalism is true, then the epistemic status of psychedelic therapy is poor.

But Greif and Šurkala also suggest that, even if there were compelling evidence that non-naturalistic ideations are typically acquired, this would not constitute a strong objection to psychedelic therapy. This is not because they think that naturalism is false. Their response is not that of those who accept the existence of a divine Reality or cosmic consciousness. Rather, Greif and Šurkala contend that naturalism, as a metaphysical position, is too controversial to have any business dictating medical practice. Philosophical metaphysics is a highly contested field with very little consensus. For Greif and Šurkala, this means that no position in this field is sufficiently well established, or securely known, to warrant serious scruples about a medical treatment that causes patients to disbelieve it. Since we do not, on their view, *know* that naturalism is true, we do not know that the induction of non-naturalistic beliefs amounts to epistemic harm. Thus, even if we knew that such beliefs were reliably induced by psychedelics, we would not thereby know that psychedelic administration is epistemically harmful.

This argument deserves fuller consideration than I can give it here. One might wonder whether naturalism is, indeed, as contentious or epistemically insecure as Greif and Šurkala suggest. However, suppose for now that these authors are correct, and epistemic scruples about metaphysical beliefs have no place in medical practice. Such considerations may still inform the decisions of individuals. Perhaps the arguments that undergoing psychedelic therapy is consistent with a naturalistic outlook are most useful, not to policymakers but to individuals deciding whether to undergo such therapy. Consider a naturalistic, atheistic terminal cancer patient who has been offered psilocybin-assisted therapy and is considering this decision. Elsewhere I have compared the choice apparently facing this person, on a naïve view of psychedelic therapy, to the choice posed by Pascal's Wager (Letheby 2016). Pascal infamously argued that we ought to believe in God for pragmatic reasons: belief has vast advantages if God exists but only moderate disadvantages if God does not exist, while disbelief has vast disadvantages if God exists but only moderate advantages if God does not exist. One classic objection to Pascal's argument alleges that it depends on the implausible thesis of *doxastic voluntarism*, the view that we can simply choose our beliefs. Psychedelic therapy might seem, prima facie, to offer a way around this difficulty (Saka 2021). But to a naturalist reluctant to buy peace of mind with a comforting delusion, this would be a bug, not a feature, of psychedelic therapy.

A different worry about Pascal's Wager is similar in spirit to Nozick's Experience Machine: that there is something intellectually dishonest or morally problematic about forming beliefs for pragmatic rather than epistemic reasons. This is exactly the sort of worry that an intellectually scrupulous, convinced naturalist might have about psychedelic therapy. Given the popular image of psychedelics and the sorts of beliefs and worldviews with which they have often been associated, this person might reasonably worry that they would be signing up to trade their critical faculties for happiness, volunteering to undergo an outlandish but overwhelmingly convincing experience that would lead them to embrace dubious beliefs about reality. And if that were the case, they might reasonably view this as a good reason not to sign up.

As I mentioned earlier, Smith and Sisti (2020) have argued that the unique features of psychedelic therapy require an 'enhanced consent' process, in which the distinctive and unusual mechanisms and possible side effects of this intervention are communicated in detail to prospective patients. One category of side effects that they mention includes changes to beliefs, values, and personality. They note that 'non-spiritual, agnostic or atheist patients may take the development of a newfound sense of spirituality or belief in God to be a loss if it is incongruent with their prior values or if it is disruptive to relationships with others' (Smith and Sisti 2020, p. 3).

Smith and Sisti note the obvious connections between their argument and the work of L.A. Paul (2014) on transformative experience. Paul defines a transformative experience as one that is both epistemically and personally transformative: it involves the acquisition of knowledge that could not have been acquired otherwise, and it changes personality in some deep and fundamental way. Clearly, many psychedelic experiences are paradigmatic examples. This is another important avenue for future research: considering the implications of Paul's analyses for the ethics and rationality of decisions to undergo psychedelic therapy (cf. Forstmann et al. 2020), and for the nature and content of such an enhanced consent process.

However, the arguments of this book are also clearly relevant to the content of such an enhanced consent process. If the evidence favoured the Metaphysical Belief Theory of psychedelic therapy, then it would be important to communicate to patients that the acquisition of non-naturalistic metaphysical beliefs was not just a possible side effect but an intrinsic part of the treatment modality and a sine qua non of its clinical benefits. But on the strength of my arguments here, we can paint a different picture—one perhaps more reassuring to sceptically minded naturalists who might benefit from psychedelic therapy. Non-naturalistic metaphysical ideations are not an inevitable part of the process and, even when they do occur, one remains capable of scrutinising them critically after the fact. The treatment is not centrally about inducing beliefs in God or divinity, but rather about coming to see oneself and one's life differently, which can involve genuine and profound insights that are consistent with naturalism. (Of course, beliefs in God or divinity are sometimes developed, and this fact needs to be communicated—but as a potential side-effect, not as an essential component). In Lisa Bortolotti's terms, psychedelic therapy does not involve a simple 'trade-off' between epistemic risks and psychological benefits: there are epistemic benefits involved, too.

However, in discussing the arguments of Greif and Šurkala, and the situation facing a naturalistic prospective psychedelic therapy patient, an important area for future investigation is revealed. We are not yet in a position to reassure such a patient, or even her critically minded, non-naturalistically inclined counterpart, about the *total* epistemic risk/benefit profile of psychedelic therapy, for the simple reason that a systematic investigation of this profile has not yet been undertaken. The ideas I have outlined here constitute the beginning, not the end, of this important conversation.

I have argued, on the basis of the current evidence, that the risks (as I deem them) of acquiring unshakeable, rationally impervious beliefs in a cosmic consciousness or divine Reality are reasonably small. Greif and Šurkala contend that these are not the sorts of epistemic risks that should worry us overmuch, even if they are large. But what of other epistemic risks? How confident can we be that psychedelic use rarely causes serious harm to one's critical faculties? There is anecdotal evidence that it *sometimes* does (cf. Marsella and Price-Williams 1974). Consider, for example, the case of Julian Haynes, who built a floating pyramid on the Amazon in order to communicate with aliens he had encountered in ayahuasca-induced visions (Mann 2011). Clearly psychedelic use does not always have such effects, and there is little evidence for such effects resulting from controlled use in recent clinical trials. But our understanding of its overall epistemic profile remains limited, and it has often been associated with occult, paranormal, or pseudoscientific beliefs (Carhart-Harris and Friston 2019, pp. 335–336).

In Chapter 2, I reviewed considerable evidence that long-term religious users of psychedelics have good psychological health relative to the broader population. Our knowledge of their epistemic health is more limited. This category of psychedelic effects deserves further investigation—not just in religious users but (prospectively) in volunteers for clinical trials. One possibility would be to administer psychometric measures of belief in conspiracy theories (e.g., Brotherton et al. 2013) or of generic critical thinking skills (e.g., Loo and Thorpe 1999). Of course, the results of such empirical measures will always require philosophical interpretation before normative epistemological conclusions can be drawn—and, as Greif and Šurkala emphasise, such interpretations will often be contentious.[3] But by combining such analysis with administration of measures like these, as well as the MBQ of Timmermann et al. (in preparation) and the life-forecasting measures used by Lyons and Carhart-Harris (2018a), we can hope to obtain a fuller and clearer picture of the range of epistemic risks and opportunities associated with controlled psychedelic administration.[4]

Perhaps the most important, if the least precise, philosophical question about psychedelics is this: what should we make of these enigmatic substances, and how should we regard the remarkable experiences that they induce—experiences that many count among the most important of their lives? I believe that I have made some progress toward answering this question. In the next section, I conclude the book by saying what that progress amounts to.

10.3 Naturalistic entheogenics

The Comforting Delusion Objection to psychedelic therapy holds that:

1. Naturalism is true.
2. If the epistemic status of psychedelic therapy is poor, then we should hesitate to recommend or prescribe it.
3. If naturalism is true, then the epistemic status of psychedelic therapy is poor.
4. Therefore, we should hesitate to recommend or prescribe psychedelic therapy.

If premise 1 is false, and there really is a cosmic consciousness, or spirit world, as some psychedelic researchers hold, then clearly the Objection fails. If premise 2 is false, and the epistemic status of psychedelic therapy is relatively unimportant, as Flanagan and Graham contend, then clearly the Objection fails.

I have tried to show that the Objection fails even if neither of those conditions holds—even if naturalism is true and the epistemic status of psychedelic therapy is

---

[3] When we are considering psychedelics' lasting effects on epistemically relevant psychological traits, a useful philosophical framework might be *virtue epistemology*, which emphasises the cognitive agent, rather than her individual beliefs, as the locus of epistemic evaluation (Battaly 2008). It would be interesting to view increases in Openness to Experience (MacLean et al. 2011), mindfulness-related capacities (Sampedro et al. 2017), and, more speculatively, awe-proneness (cf. Anderson et al. 2020) through this kind of lens.

[4] For interesting epistemological discussions of psychedelic use that I have not engaged with directly here, see Waters (1975) and Hales (2006).

very important. This shows that the Objection fails, whatever is the case. My grounds are simple: premise 3 is false. Even if naturalism is true, the epistemic status of psychedelic therapy is still reasonably good, according to our best current evidence.

My grounds for this claim, in turn, are twofold. First, the epistemic risks of psychedelic therapy, given naturalism, are not as great as they initially appear. Psychedelic therapy does not work mainly by inducing comforting metaphysical beliefs about the nature of reality, but by disintegrating and rewriting rigid and maladaptive self-models. Not every psychedelic subject who has a transformative 'mystical-type experience' in the psychometric sense has an experience as of non-naturalistic metaphysical realities; and even those who do have such experiences need not accept their deliverances uncritically. Second, the epistemic benefits of psychedelic therapy, given naturalism, are greater than they initially appear. Carefully conducted psychedelic sessions can afford myriad epistemic benefits, direct and indirect, many unavailable by any other means; thus, psychedelic therapy is epistemically innocent.

In the course of arguing for the negative conclusion that the Comforting Delusion Objection fails, I have also been arguing for a positive conclusion: that there exists a viable *naturalistic Entheogenic Conception* of psychedelics and their transformative effects. The Entheogenic Conception of psychedelics is the venerable conviction that these remarkable substances, used appropriately, are effective agents of transformative insight and spiritual experience. I have tried to show that there is a recognisable version of this conviction that is consistent with naturalism and plausible in light of current scientific knowledge. I will now outline the central contours of such a conception.

Contra the late Huston Smith, the basic message of the entheogens is not that there is another *metaphysical* Reality that puts this one in the shade. It is that there are other *phenomenological* Realities, many of which put our ordinary, default mode in the shade. Many of these other Realities, especially the salutary ones, result largely from a reduction in the constraining influence of the self-model. Induced by pharmacological or other means, in conducive circumstances, unselfed modes of consciousness show us what is possible in terms of feelings of wonder, awe, and connectedness with myriad aspects of the inner and outer worlds. Moreover, while there is no guarantee of this, many of these alternative phenomenal simulations depict reality more accurately, in important respects, than do our ordinary, default experiential worlds—or at least foreground important and real aspects of it that the latter marginalise or overlook.

The phenomenal opacity induced by psychedelics gives rise to knowledge by acquaintance with two important, conceptually distinguishable but practically inextricable facts:

1. That one's experience of self and world is profoundly contingent and constructed, and
2. That it can therefore be constructed otherwise.

Knowledge by acquaintance with the second fact takes both general and particular forms. Subjects become acquainted with the bare fact that their experience can be constructed otherwise, as well as with specific alternative ways in which it can be constructed. For certain modes of experience, this amounts to seeing the 'possibility and attractiveness' (Diamond 1982, p. 34) of specific ways of paying attention, and parsing and constructing the world. In seeing this, subjects also gain a certain amount of knowledge how: through the experience of paying attention in different ways, they get some clues about how they might continue to pay attention in order to foster modes of consciousness relevantly similar to the desirable ones they experience. This is a beginner's version of the sort of knowledge how cultivated in mindfulness meditation practice. This is why subjects deliberately attempt to practise new paradigms of attention in the integration period, through both formal and informal methods.

Induced skilfully, unselfed consciousness can be an ecstatic, radically transformative thing, revealing not the objective accuracy of a Joyous Cosmology but the subjective availability of a Joyous Phenomenology. Our default waking mode of consciousness is defined and constrained by ubiquitous and typically unnoticed existential feelings, often of isolation, disconnection, and meaninglessness, resulting from rigid and unconscious beliefs about the self and its relations to the rest of the world. Weakening these beliefs gives rise to vastly different modes of consciousness characterised by different patterns of existential feeling. When phenomenal reality is filtered and structured less strongly through the goals and preferences of a reified, essentialised self, we can experience wonder, awe, broader perspectives, and feelings of profound kinship with the entirety of manifest existence.

Moreover, this puts us in a position to gain genuine, otherwise unavailable knowledge. Metaphysical hallucinations and comforting delusions lurk in this quarter, and there is no substitute for subsequent sober analysis of the products of the psychedelic state. Nevertheless, this state makes available genuine and sometimes transformative insights into the nature and potential of our own subjectivity, revealing the constraining role of the self-model and the phenomenal possibilities that open up when this regulatory function is relaxed.

For those sympathetic to non-naturalistic approaches to consciousness, such as idealism and panpsychism, there is still an important message in the arguments of this book: that a great deal of the psychedelic experience and its existential significance can be accounted for without such posits. Put positively, there is a surprising amount of common ground between naturalistic and non-naturalistic accounts of the psychedelic state. The former can endorse many of the distinctive and typical claims of the latter, suitably interpreted. This is just to say that key pillars of the Entheogenic Conception can be naturalised.

Psychedelic therapy is neither a pure, low-level pharmacotherapy, nor a matter of changing explicit metaphysical convictions. Rather, it is a process of deconstructing and re-writing maladaptive, largely unconscious, abstract beliefs about self and world that structure our experience. It is neither a purely anti-epistemic matter of hallucination and delusion, nor an unquestionable fount of transcendental truth. Rather, it is a matter of temporarily weakening the simultaneously constraining and enabling influence of prior knowledge, thereby creating unique opportunities both for insight and for error. Charles Grob is correct, after all, to call psychedelic therapy an 'existential medicine'—even from a naturalistic standpoint—because it constitutively involves a transformative experiential re-appraisal of fundamental assumptions concerning the self, the wider world, and the relations between the two.

The dichotomy between pure neuroplasticity theories of psychedelic therapy, on one hand, and metaphysical belief/alief theories, on the other, is false: the truth lies somewhere in the middle. Likewise with the dichotomy between a wholly anti-epistemic, hallucinogenic conception of the drugs, on one hand, and a non-naturalistic, strongly entheogenic conception, on the other.

Unconstraining cognition by unselfing; revealing the vast potential of human consciousness by exposing the constructed nature of all experience, including the ordinary sense of self—this is the essence of psychedelic therapy, and it is perfectly consistent with a naturalistic worldview.

References

Aday, J.S., Davoli, C.C., and Bloesch, E.K., 2019a. 2018: A watershed year for psychedelic science. *Drug Science, Policy and Law, 5*, pp. 1–4.

Aday, J.S., Bloesch, E.K., and Davoli, C.C., 2019b. Can psychedelic drugs attenuate age-related changes in cognition and affect? *Journal of Cognitive Enhancement, 4*, pp. 219–227.

Aday, J.S., Mitzkovitz, C.M., Bloesch, E.K., Davoli, C.C., and Davis, A.K., 2020. Long-term effects of psychedelic drugs: A systematic review. *Neuroscience & Biobehavioral Reviews, 113*, pp. 179–189.

Addis, D.R., 2020. Mental time travel? A neurocognitive model of event simulation. *Review of Philosophy and Psychology, 11*, pp. 233–259.

Agin-Liebes, G.I., Malone, T., Yalch, M.M., Mennenga, S.E., Ponté, K.L., Guss, J., Bossis, A.P., Grigsby, J., Fischer, S., and Ross, S., 2020. Long-term follow-up of psilocybin-assisted psychotherapy for psychiatric and existential distress in patients with life-threatening cancer. *Journal of Psychopharmacology, 34*(2), pp. 155–166.

Ahlskog, R., 2017. Moral enhancement should target self-interest and cognitive capacity. *Neuroethics, 10*(3), pp. 363–373.

Ainsworth, P.M., 2010. What is ontic structural realism? *Studies in History and Philosophy of Science Part B: Studies in History and Philosophy of Modern Physics, 41*(1), pp. 50–57.

Albahari, M., 2006. *Analytical Buddhism: The Two-tiered Illusion of Self.* Houndmills: Palgrave Macmillan.

Albahari, M., 2011. Nirvana and ownerless consciousness. In Siderits, M., Thompson, E., and Zahavi, D. (eds) *Self, no self?: Perspectives from Analytical, Phenomenological, & Indian traditions*, pp. 79–113. Oxford University Press.

Albahari, M., 2014. Insight knowledge of no self in Buddhism: An epistemic analysis. *Philosophers' Imprint, 14*(21), pp. 1–30.

Albahari, M., 2019a. Perennial idealism: A mystical solution to the mind-body problem. *Philosophers Imprint, 19*(44), pp. 1–37.

Albahari, M., 2019b. The mystic and the metaphysician: Clarifying the role of meditation in the search for ultimate reality. *Journal of Consciousness Studies, 26*(7–8), pp. 12–36.

Almeida, R.N., Galvão, A.C.D.M., Da Silva, F.S., Silva, E.A.D.S., Palhano-Fontes, F., Maia-de-Oliveira, J.P., de Araujo, D.B., Lobão-Soares, B., and Galvão-Coelho, N., 2019. Modulation of serum brain-derived neurotrophic factor by a single dose of ayahuasca: Observation from a randomized controlled trial. *Frontiers in Psychology, 10*, p. 1234.

Amada, N., Lea, T., Letheby, C., and Shane, J., 2020. Psychedelic Experience and the Narrative Self: An Exploratory Qualitative Study. *Journal of Consciousness Studies, 27*(9–10), pp. 6–33.

Anderson, B.T., 2012. Ayahuasca as antidepressant? Psychedelics and styles of reasoning in psychiatry. *Anthropology of Consciousness, 23*(1), pp. 44–59.

Anderson, C.L., Dixson, D.D., Monroy, M., and Keltner, D., 2020. Are awe-prone people more curious? The relationship between dispositional awe, curiosity, and academic outcomes. *Journal of Personality, 88*(4), pp. 762–779.

Angel, L., 2002. Mystical naturalism. *Religious Studies, 38*(3), pp. 317–338.

Argento, E., Braschel, M., Walsh, Z., Socias, M.E., and Shannon, K., 2018. The moderating effect of psychedelics on the prospective relationship between prescription opioid use and suicide risk among marginalized women. *Journal of Psychopharmacology, 32*(12), pp. 1385–1391.

Argento, E., Capler, R., Thomas, G., Lucas, P., and Tupper, K.W., 2019. Exploring ayahuasca-assisted therapy for addiction: A qualitative analysis of preliminary findings among an indigenous community in Canada. *Drug and Alcohol Review*, 38, pp. 781–789.

Atasoy, S., Roseman, L., Kaelen, M., Kringelbach, M.L., Deco, G., and Carhart-Harris, R.L., 2017. Connectome-harmonic decomposition of human brain activity reveals dynamical repertoire re-organization under LSD. *Scientific Reports*, 7(1), p. 17661.

Audi, R., 2000. Philosophical naturalism at the turn of the century. *Journal of Philosophical Research*, 25, pp. 27–45.

Baer, R.A., Smith, G.T., Lykins, E., Button, D., Krietemeyer, J., Sauer, S., Walsh, E., Duggan, D., and Williams, J.M.G., 2008. Construct validity of the five facet mindfulness questionnaire in meditating and nonmeditating samples. *Assessment*, 15(3), pp. 329–342.

Baillie, J., 2013. The expectation of nothingness. *Philosophical Studies*, 166(1), pp. 185–203.

Baillie, J., 2019. The recognition of nothingness. *Philosophical Studies*. DOI: https://doi.org/10.1007/s11098-019-01329-6

Barbosa, P.C.R., Cazorla, I.M., Giglio, J.S., and Strassman, R., 2009. A six-month prospective evaluation of personality traits, psychiatric symptoms and quality of life in ayahuasca-naïve subjects. *Journal of Psychoactive Drugs*, 41(3), pp. 205–212.

Barbosa, P.C.R., Mizumoto, S., Bogenschutz, M.P., and Strassman, R.J., 2012. Health status of ayahuasca users. *Drug Testing and Analysis*, 4(7–8), pp. 601–609.

Barbosa, P.C.R., Strassman, R.J., da Silveira, D.X., Areco, K., Hoy, R., Pommy, J., Thoma, R., and Bogenschutz, M., 2016. Psychological and neuropsychological assessment of regular hoasca users. *Comprehensive Psychiatry*, 71, pp. 95–105.

Barrett, F.S., Bradstreet, M.P., Leoutsakos, J.M.S., Johnson, M.W., and Griffiths, R.R., 2016. The Challenging Experience Questionnaire: Characterization of challenging experiences with psilocybin mushrooms. *Journal of Psychopharmacology*, 30(12), pp. 1279–1295.

Battaly, H., 2008. Virtue epistemology. *Philosophy Compass*, 3(4), pp. 639–663.

Bayne, T., 2010. *The Unity of Consciousness*. Oxford: Oxford University Press.

Beauchamp, G., 1990. Island: Aldous Huxley's psychedelic utopia. *Utopian Studies*, 1(1), pp. 59–72.

Bechtel, W., 1998. Representations and cognitive explanations: Assessing the dynamicist's challenge in cognitive science. *Cognitive Science*, 22(3), pp. 295–317.

Bechtel, W., 2006. Reducing psychology while maintaining its autonomy via mechanistic explanation. In Schouten, M. and De Jong, H. L. (eds) *The Matter of the Mind: Philosophical Essays on Psychology, Neuroscience and Reduction*, pp. 172–198. Wiley-Blackwell.

Bechtel, W., 2008. *Mental Mechanisms: Philosophical Perspectives on Cognitive Neuroscience*. New York: Lawrence Erlbaum Associates.

Bechtel, W., 2013. The endogenously active brain: The need for an alternative cognitive architecture. *Philosophia Scientiæ*. DOI: https://doi.org/10.4000/philosophiascientiae.846

Bechtel, W. and McCauley, R.N., 1999. Heuristic identity theory (or back to the future): The mind-body problem against the background of research strategies in cognitive neuroscience. In Hahn, M. and Stoness, S.C. (eds) *Proceedings of the 21st Annual Meeting of the Cognitive Science Society*, pp. 67–72. Mahwah, NJ: Lawrence Erlbaum Associates.

Belser, A.B., Agin-Liebes, G., Swift, T.C., Terrana, S., Devenot, N., Friedman, H.L., Guss, J., Bossis, A., and Ross, S., 2017. Patient experiences of psilocybin-assisted psychotherapy: An interpretative phenomenological analysis. *Journal of Humanistic Psychology*, 57(4), pp. 354–388.

Bienemann, B., Ruschel, N.S., Campos, M.L., Negreiros, M.A., and Mograbi, D.C., 2020. Self-reported negative outcomes of psilocybin users: A quantitative textual analysis. *PLoS One*, 15(2), p. e0229067.

Billon, A., 2016. Making sense of the Cotard syndrome: Insights from the study of depersonalisation. *Mind & Language*, 31(3), pp. 356–391.

Billon, A., and Kriegel, U., 2015. Jaspers' dilemma: The psychopathological challenge to subjectivity theories of consciousness. In Gennaro, R.J. (ed.) *Disturbed Consciousness: New Essays on Psychopathology and Theories of Consciousness*, pp. 29–54. Cambridge, MA: MIT Press.

Blanke, O. and Metzinger, T., 2009. Full-body illusions and minimal phenomenal selfhood. *Trends in Cognitive Sciences*, *13*(1), pp. 7–13.

Blofeld, J., 1966. A high yogic experience achieved with mescaline. *Psychedelic Review*, *1*(7), pp. 28–32.

Bogenschutz, M.P. and Johnson, M.W., 2016. Classic hallucinogens in the treatment of addictions. *Progress in Neuro-Psychopharmacology and Biological Psychiatry*, *64*, pp. 250–258.

Bogenschutz, M.P. and Pommy, J.M., 2012. Therapeutic mechanisms of classic hallucinogens in the treatment of addictions: from indirect evidence to testable hypotheses. *Drug Testing and Analysis*, *4*(7–8), pp. 543–555.

Bogenschutz, M.P., Forcehimes, A.A., Pommy, J.A., Wilcox, C.E., Barbosa, P.C.R., and Strassman, R.J., 2015. Psilocybin-assisted treatment for alcohol dependence: a proof-of-concept study. *Journal of Psychopharmacology*, *29*(3), pp. 289–299.

Bogenschutz, M.P., Podrebarac, S.K., Duane, J.H., Amegadzie, S.S., Malone, T.C., Owens, L.T., Ross, S., and Mennenga, S.E., 2018. Clinical interpretations of patient experience in a trial of psilocybin-assisted psychotherapy for alcohol use disorder. *Frontiers in Pharmacology*, *9*, p. 100.

Bond, F.W., Hayes, S.C., Baer, R.A., Carpenter, K.M., Guenole, N., Orcutt, H.K., Waltz, T., and Zettle, R.D., 2011. Preliminary psychometric properties of the Acceptance and Action Questionnaire–II: A revised measure of psychological inflexibility and experiential avoidance. *Behavior Therapy*, *42*(4), pp. 676–688.

Boone, W. and Piccinini, G., 2016. The cognitive neuroscience revolution. *Synthese*, *193*(5), pp. 1509–1534.

Bortolotti, L., 2015. The epistemic innocence of motivated delusions. *Consciousness and Cognition*, *33*, pp. 490–499.

Bortolotti, L., 2018. Stranger than fiction: Costs and benefits of everyday confabulation. *Review of Philosophy and Psychology*, *9*(2), pp. 227–249.

Bortolotti, L., 2020. *The Epistemic Innocence of Irrational Beliefs*. Oxford: Oxford University Press.

Bouso, J.C., González, D., Fondevila, S., Cutchet, M., Fernández, X., Barbosa, P.C.R., Alcázar-Córcoles, M.Á., Araújo, W.S., Barbanoj, M.J., Fábregas, J.M., and Riba, J., 2012. Personality, psychopathology, life attitudes and neuropsychological performance among ritual users of ayahuasca: A longitudinal study. *PLoS One*, *7*(8), p. e42421.

Bouso, J.C., Fábregas, J.M., Antonijoan, R.M., Rodríguez-Fornells, A., and Riba, J., 2013. Acute effects of ayahuasca on neuropsychological performance: differences in executive function between experienced and occasional users. *Psychopharmacology*, *230*(3), pp. 415–424.

Bouso, J.C., Palhano-Fontes, F., Rodríguez-Fornells, A., Ribeiro, S., Sanches, R., Crippa, J.A.S., Hallak, J.E., de Araujo, D.B., and Riba, J., 2015. Long-term use of psychedelic drugs is associated with differences in brain structure and personality in humans. *European Neuropsychopharmacology*, *25*(4), pp. 483–492.

Bouso, J.C., dos Santos, R.G., Alcázar-Córcoles, M.Á., and Hallak, J.E., 2018. Serotonergic psychedelics and personality: a systematic review of contemporary research. *Neuroscience & Biobehavioral Reviews*, *87*, pp. 118–132.

Braga, R.M., Sharp, D.J., Leeson, C., Wise, R.J., and Leech, R., 2013. Echoes of the brain within default mode, association, and heteromodal cortices. *Journal of Neuroscience*, *33*(35), pp. 14031–14039.

Breeksema, J.J., Niemeijer, A.R., Krediet, E., Vermetten, E., and Schoevers, R.A., 2020. Psychedelic treatments for psychiatric disorders: A systematic review and thematic synthesis of patient experiences in qualitative studies. *CNS Drugs*, *34*, pp. 925–946.

Brewer, J.A. and Garrison, K.A., 2014. The posterior cingulate cortex as a plausible mechanistic target of meditation: Findings from neuroimaging. *Annals of the New York Academy of Sciences, 1307*(1), pp. 19–27.

Brewer, J., Garrison, K., and Whitfield-Gabrieli, S., 2013. What about the "self" is processed in the posterior cingulate cortex? *Frontiers in Human Neuroscience, 7*, p. 647.

Brotherton, R., French, C.C., and Pickering, A.D., 2013. Measuring belief in conspiracy theories: The generic conspiracist beliefs scale. *Frontiers in Psychology, 4*, p. 279.

Brown, K.W. and Ryan, R.M., 2003. The benefits of being present: Mindfulness and its role in psychological well-being. *Journal of Personality and Social Psychology, 84*(4), pp. 822–848.

Broyd, S.J., Demanuele, C., Debener, S., Helps, S.K., James, C.J., and Sonuga-Barke, E.J., 2009. Default-mode brain dysfunction in mental disorders: A systematic review. *Neuroscience & Biobehavioral Reviews, 33*(3), pp. 279–296.

Burston, E., 2017. On the nature of psychedelic substances, the profound experiences they engender, and the alleviation of neuroexistential angst. Honours thesis, University of Adelaide.

Burwick, T., 2014. The binding problem. *Wiley Interdisciplinary Reviews: Cognitive Science, 5*(3), pp. 305–315.

Carhart-Harris, R., 2007. Waves of the unconscious: The neurophysiology of dreamlike phenomena and its implications for the psychodynamic model of the mind. *Neuropsychoanalysis, 9*(2), pp. 183–211.

Carhart-Harris, R.L., 2018. The entropic brain—revisited. *Neuropharmacology, 142*, pp. 167–178.

Carhart-Harris, R.L., 2019. How do psychedelics work? *Current Opinion in Psychiatry, 32*(1), pp. 16–21.

Carhart-Harris, R.L. and Friston, K.J., 2010. The default-mode, ego-functions and free-energy: a neurobiological account of Freudian ideas. *Brain, 133*(4), pp. 1265–1283.

Carhart-Harris, R.L. and Friston, K.J., 2019. REBUS and the anarchic brain: Toward a unified model of the brain action of psychedelics. *Pharmacological Reviews, 71*(3), pp. 316–344.

Carhart-Harris, R.L. and Nutt, D.J., 2017. Serotonin and brain function: A tale of two receptors. *Journal of Psychopharmacology, 31*(9), pp. 1091–1120.

Carhart-Harris, R.L., Leech, R., Williams, T.M., Erritzoe, D., Abbasi, N., Bargiotas, T., Hobden, P., Sharp, D.J., Evans, J., Feilding, A., and Wise, R.G., 2012a. Implications for psychedelic-assisted psychotherapy: Functional magnetic resonance imaging study with psilocybin. *British Journal of Psychiatry, 200*(3), pp. 238–244.

Carhart-Harris, R.L., Erritzoe, D., Williams, T., Stone, J.M., Reed, L.J., Colasanti, A., Tyacke, R.J., Leech, R., Malizia, A.L., Murphy, K., and Hobden, P., 2012b. Neural correlates of the psychedelic state as determined by fMRI studies with psilocybin. *Proceedings of the National Academy of Sciences, 109*(6), pp. 2138–2143.

Carhart-Harris, R.L., Leech, R., Hellyer, P.J., Shanahan, M., Feilding, A., Tagliazucchi, E., Chialvo, D.R., and Nutt, D., 2014. The entropic brain: A theory of conscious states informed by neuroimaging research with psychedelic drugs. *Frontiers in Human Neuroscience, 8*, p. 20.

Carhart-Harris, R.L., Kaelen, M., Whalley, M.G., Bolstridge, M., Feilding, A., and Nutt, D.J., 2015. LSD enhances suggestibility in healthy volunteers. *Psychopharmacology, 232*(4), pp. 785–794.

Carhart-Harris, R.L., Kaelen, M., Bolstridge, M., Williams, T.M., Williams, L.T., Underwood, R., Feilding, A., and Nutt, D.J., 2016a. The paradoxical psychological effects of lysergic acid diethylamide (LSD). *Psychological Medicine, 46*(7), pp. 1379–1390.

Carhart-Harris, R.L., Bolstridge, M., Rucker, J., Day, C.M., Erritzoe, D., Kaelen, M., Bloomfield, M., Rickard, J.A., Forbes, B., Feilding, A., and Taylor, D., 2016b. Psilocybin with psychological support for treatment-resistant depression: an open-label feasibility study. *Lancet Psychiatry, 3*(7), pp. 619–627.

Carhart-Harris, R.L., Muthukumaraswamy, S., Roseman, L., Kaelen, M., Droog, W., Murphy, K., Tagliazucchi, E., Schenberg, E.E., Nest, T., Orban, C., and Leech, R., 2016c. Neural correlates of the LSD experience revealed by multimodal neuroimaging. *Proceedings of the National Academy of Sciences, 113*(17), pp. 4853–4858.

Carhart-Harris, R.L., Roseman, L., Bolstridge, M., Demetriou, L., Pannekoek, J.N., Wall, M.B., Tanner, M., Kaelen, M., McGonigle, J., Murphy, K., and Leech, R., 2017. Psilocybin for treatment-resistant depression: fMRI-measured brain mechanisms. *Scientific reports, 7*(1), p. 13187.

Carhart-Harris, R.L., Erritzoe, D., Haijen, E., Kaelen, M., and Watts, R., 2018a. Psychedelics and connectedness. *Psychopharmacology, 235*(2), pp. 547–550.

Carhart-Harris, R.L., Bolstridge, M., Day, C.M.J., Rucker, J., Watts, R., Erritzoe, D.E., Kaelen, M., Giribaldi, B., Bloomfield, M., Pilling, S., and Rickard, J.A., 2018b. Psilocybin with psychological support for treatment-resistant depression: Six-month follow-up. *Psychopharmacology, 235*(2), pp. 399–408.

Carruthers, G. and Schier, E., 2017. Why are we still being hornswoggled? Dissolving the hard problem of consciousness. *Topoi, 36*(1), pp. 67–79.

Chödrön, P., 1996. *Awakening Loving-Kindness*. Boston: Shambhala.

Chomsky, N., 1959. Verbal behavior by BF Skinner. *Language, 35*(1), pp. 26–58.

Churchland, P.S., 1989. *Neurophilosophy: Toward a Unified Science of the Mind-Brain*. Cambridge, MA: MIT Press.

Churchland, P.S., 1996. The hornswoggle problem. *Journal of Consciousness Studies, 3*(5–6), pp. 402–408.

Churchland, P.S., 2011. *Braintrust: What Neuroscience Tells Us about Morality*. Princeton University Press.

Clark, A., 2001. *Mindware: An Introduction to the Philosophy of Cognitive Science*. Oxford University Press.

Clark, A., 2013. Whatever next? Predictive brains, situated agents, and the future of cognitive science. *Behavioral and Brain Sciences, 36*(3), pp. 181–204.

Clark, A., 2016. *Surfing Uncertainty: Prediction, Action, and the Embodied Mind*. Oxford University Press.

Clarke, B., Gillies, D., Illari, P., Russo, F., and Williamson, J., 2013. The evidence that evidence-based medicine omits. *Preventive Medicine, 57*(6), pp. 745–747.

Close, J.B., Hajien, E.C., Watts, R., Roseman, L., and Carhart-Harris, R.L., 2020. Psychedelics and psychological flexibility—Results of a prospective web-survey using the Acceptance and Action Questionnaire II. *Journal of Contextual Behavioral Science, 16*, pp. 37–44.

Cohen, S., 1970. *Drugs of Hallucination: The LSD Story*. St. Albans: Paladin.

Cohen, S., 1988. How to be a fallibilist. *Philosophical Perspectives, 2*, pp. 91–123.

Conee, E., 1994. Phenomenal knowledge. *Australasian Journal of Philosophy, 72*(2), pp. 136–150.

Copeland, J., 1993. *Artificial Intelligence: A Philosophical Introduction*. Oxford: Blackwell.

Costantini, M. and Haggard, P., 2007. The rubber hand illusion: Sensitivity and reference frame for body ownership. *Consciousness and Cognition, 16*(2), pp. 229–240.

Craig, A.D., 2002. How do you feel? Interoception: The sense of the physiological condition of the body. *Nature Reviews Neuroscience, 3*(8), pp. 655–666.

Craig, A.D., 2009. How do you feel—now? The anterior insula and human awareness. *Nature Reviews Neuroscience, 10*, pp. 59–70.

Craighead, W.E. and Dunlop, B.W., 2014. Combination psychotherapy and antidepressant medication treatment for depression: For whom, when, and how. *Annual Review of Psychology, 65*, pp. 267–300.

Craver, C.F., 2007. *Explaining the Brain: Mechanisms and the Mosaic Unity of Neuroscience*. Oxford University Press.

Craver, C.F. and Bechtel, W., 2007. Top-down causation without top-down causes. *Biology & Philosophy, 22*(4), pp. 547–563.

Craver, C.F. and Darden, L., 2013. *In Search of Mechanisms: Discoveries Across the Life Sciences.* University of Chicago Press.

Creswell, J.D., 2017. Mindfulness interventions. *Annual Review of Psychology, 68*, pp. 491–516.

Császár-Nagy, N., Kapócs, G., and Bókkon, I., 2019. Classic psychedelics: The special role of the visual system. *Reviews in the Neurosciences, 30*(6), pp. 651–669.

Cuijpers, P., Noma, H., Karyotaki, E., Vinkers, C.H., Cipriani, A., and Furukawa, T.A., 2020. A network meta-analysis of the effects of psychotherapies, pharmacotherapies and their combination in the treatment of adult depression. *World Psychiatry, 19*(1), pp. 92–107.

Cummins, R., Roth, M., and Harmon, I., 2014. Why it doesn't matter to metaphysics what Mary learns. *Philosophical Studies, 167*(3), pp. 541–555.

Damasio A.R., 1994. *Descartes' Error: Emotion, Reason, and the Human Brain.* New York: Putnam's Sons.

Damasio, A., 1999. *The Feeling of What Happens: Body, Emotion and the Making of Consciousness.* Reprint, London: Vintage Books, 2000.

Dambrun, M. and Ricard, M., 2011. Self-centeredness and selflessness: A theory of self-based psychological functioning and its consequences for happiness. *Review of General Psychology, 15*(2), pp. 138–157.

DARPA, 2019. Structure-guided drug design could yield fast-acting remedies for complex neuropsychiatric conditions. DOI: https://www.darpa.mil/news-events/2019-09-11

Dass, R., 2005. Walking the path: Psychedelics and beyond. In Walsh, R. and Grob, C.S. (eds) *Higher Wisdom: Eminent Elders Explore the Continuing Impact of Psychedelics*, pp. 207–221. New York: SUNY Press.

Davey, C.J., Pujol, J., and Harrison, B.J., 2016. Mapping the self in the brain's default mode network. *Neuroimage, 132*, pp. 390–397.

Davey, C.G. and Harrison, B.J., 2018. The brain's center of gravity: How the default mode network helps us to understand the self. *World Psychiatry, 17*(3), pp. 278–279.

Davis, A.K., So, S., Lancelotta, R., Barsuglia, J.P., and Griffiths, R.R., 2019. 5-methoxy-N, N-dimethyltryptamine (5-MeO-DMT) used in a naturalistic group setting is associated with unintended improvements in depression and anxiety. *The American Journal of Drug and Alcohol Abuse, 45*(2), pp. 161–169.

Davis, A.K., Barrett, F.S., and Griffiths, R.R., 2020. Psychological flexibility mediates the relations between acute psychedelic effects and subjective decreases in depression and anxiety. *Journal of Contextual Behavioral Science, 15*, pp. 39–45.

Davis, J. and Thompson, E., 2015. Developing attention and decreasing affective bias: Towards a cross-cultural cognitive science of mindfulness. In Brown, K.W., Creswell, J.D., and Ryan, R.M. (eds) *Handbook of Mindfulness: Theory, Research, and Practice.* New York: The Guilford Press.

de Araujo, D.B., Ribeiro, S., Cecchi, G.A., Carvalho, F.M., Sanchez, T.A., Pinto, J.P., de Martinis, B.S., Crippa, J.A., Hallak, J.E., and Santos, A.C., 2012. Seeing with the eyes shut: neural basis of enhanced imagery following ayahuasca ingestion. *Human Brain Mapping, 33*(11), pp. 2550–2560.

Dennett, D.C., 1984. *Elbow Room: The Varieties of Free Will Worth Wanting.* Cambridge, MA: MIT Press.

Dennett, D.C., 1991. *Consciousness Explained.* Boston: Little, Brown and Co.

Dennett, D., 1992. The self as the center of narrative gravity. In Kessel, F. Cole, P., and Johnson, D. (eds) *Self and Consciousness: Multiple Perspectives.* Hillsdale, NJ: Lawrence Erlbaum.

Dennett, D., 2003. Who's on first? Heterophenomenology explained. *Journal of Consciousness Studies, 10*(9–10), pp. 19–30.

Devitt, M. and Sterelny, K., 1999. *Language and Reality: An Introduction to the Philosophy of Language.* Cambridge, MA: MIT Press.

Diamond, C., 1982. Anything but argument? *Philosophical Investigations*, 5(1), pp. 23–41.

Díaz, J.L., 2013. Salvia divinorum: A psychopharmacological riddle and a mind-body prospect. *Current Drug Abuse Reviews*, 6(1), pp. 43–53.

Digman, J.M., 1990. Personality structure: Emergence of the five-factor model. *Annual Review of Psychology*, 41(1), pp. 417–440.

Dittrich, A., 1998. The standardized psychometric assessment of altered states of consciousness (ASCs) in humans. *Pharmacopsychiatry*, 31(Supp. 2), pp. 80–84.

Doblin, R., 1991. Pahnke's "Good Friday Experiment": A long-term follow-up and methodological critique. *Journal of Transpersonal Psychology*, 23(1), pp. 1–28.

Doblin, R.E., Christiansen, M., Jerome, L., and Burge, B., 2019. The past and future of psychedelic science: An introduction to this issue. *Journal of Psychoactive Drugs*, 51(2), pp. 93–97.

Dolder, P.C., Schmid, Y., Müller, F., Borgwardt, S., and Liechti, M.E., 2016. LSD acutely impairs fear recognition and enhances emotional empathy and sociality. *Neuropsychopharmacology*, 41(11), pp. 2638–2646.

Dor-Ziderman, Y., Lutz, A., and Goldstein, A., 2019. Prediction-based neural mechanisms for shielding the self from existential threat. *NeuroImage*, 202, p. 116080.

dos Santos, R.G., 2014. Potential therapeutic effects of psilocybin/psilocin are minimized while possible adverse reactions are overrated. *Therapeutic Drug Monitoring*, 36(1), pp. 131–132.

dos Santos, R.G. and Hallak, J.E.C., 2020. Therapeutic use of serotoninergic hallucinogens: A review of the evidence and of the biological and psychological mechanisms. *Neuroscience & Biobehavioral Reviews*, 108, pp. 423–434.

dos Santos, R.G., Osório, F.L., Crippa, J.A.S., Riba, J., Zuardi, A.W., and Hallak, J.E., 2016a. Antidepressive, anxiolytic, and antiaddictive effects of ayahuasca, psilocybin and lysergic acid diethylamide (LSD): A systematic review of clinical trials published in the last 25 years. *Therapeutic Advances in Psychopharmacology*, 6(3), pp. 193–213.

dos Santos, R.G., Osório, F.L., Crippa, J.A.S., and Hallak, J.E., 2016b. Classical hallucinogens and neuroimaging: A systematic review of human studies: Hallucinogens and neuroimaging. *Neuroscience & Biobehavioral Reviews*, 71, pp. 715–728.

dos Santos, R.G., Bouso, J.C., Alcázar-Córcoles, M.Á., and Hallak, J.E., 2018a. Efficacy, tolerability, and safety of serotonergic psychedelics for the management of mood, anxiety, and substance-use disorders: A systematic review of systematic reviews. *Expert Review of Clinical Pharmacology*, 11(9), pp. 889–902.

dos Santos, R.G., Sanches, R.F., Osório, F.D.L., and Hallak, J.E., 2018b. Long-term effects of ayahuasca in patients with recurrent depression: A 5-year qualitative follow-up. *Archives of Clinical Psychiatry (São Paulo)*, 45(1), pp. 22–24.

Dretske, F.I., 1995. *Naturalizing the Mind*. Cambridge, MA: MIT Press.

Dunlap, J., 1961. *Exploring Inner Space: Personal Experiences under LSD-25*. New York: Harcourt, Brace & World.

Durr, R.A., 1970. *Poetic Vision and the Psychedelic Experience*. Syracuse University Press.

Dyck, E., 2010. *Psychedelic psychiatry: LSD from clinic to campus*. Johns Hopkins University Press.

Dyck, E., 2019. Psychedelics and dying care: A historical look at the relationship between psychedelics and palliative care. *Journal of Psychoactive Drugs*, 51(2), pp. 102–107.

Earp, B.D., 2018. Psychedelic moral enhancement. *Royal Institute of Philosophy Supplements*, 83, pp. 415–439.

Eisner, B.G. and Cohen, S., 1958. Psychotherapy with lysergic acid diethylamide. *Journal of Nervous and Mental Disease*, 127, pp. 528–539.

Eliot, G., 1871/1994. *Middlemarch*. Wordsworth Editions Limited.

Ellis, Havelock, 1897. A note on the phenomena of mescal intoxication. *Lancet*, 149, pp. 1540–1542.

Elsey, J.W., 2017. Psychedelic drug use in healthy individuals: A review of benefits, costs, and implications for drug policy. *Drug Science, Policy and Law, 3*, pp. 1–11.

Erritzoe, D., Roseman, L., Nour, M.M., MacLean, K., Kaelen, M., Nutt, D.J., and Carhart-Harris, R.L., 2018. Effects of psilocybin therapy on personality structure. *Acta Psychiatrica Scandinavica, 138*(5), pp. 368–378.

Erritzoe, D., Smith, J., Fisher, P.M., Carhart-Harris, R., Frokjaer, V.G., and Knudsen, G.M., 2019. Recreational use of psychedelics is associated with elevated personality trait openness: Exploration of associations with brain serotonin markers. *Journal of Psychopharmacology, 33*(9), pp. 1068–1075.

Estevez, M., 2013. *One Kind of Knowing: Reports from a Hallucinogen Research Volunteer.* Self-published.

Fadiman, J., 2005. Transpersonal transitions: The higher reaches of psyche and psychology. In Walsh, R. and Grob, C.S. (eds) *Higher Wisdom: Eminent Elders Explore the Continuing Impact of Psychedelics*, pp. 21–46. New York: SUNY Press.

Fadiman, J. and Korb, S., 2019. Might microdosing psychedelics be safe and beneficial? An initial exploration. *Journal of Psychoactive Drugs, 51*(2), pp. 118–122.

Faillace, L.A., 1966. Clinical use of psychotomimetic drugs. *Comprehensive Psychiatry, 7*(1), pp. 13–20.

Fantl, J., 2017. Knowledge how. In Zalta, E.N. (ed.), *The Stanford Encyclopedia of Philosophy* (Fall 2017 edition). DOI: https://plato.stanford.edu/archives/fall2017/entries/knowledge-how

Fasching, W., 2008. Consciousness, self-consciousness, and meditation. *Phenomenology and the Cognitive Sciences, 7*(4), pp. 463–483.

Fink, S. B., 2020. Look who's talking! Varieties of ego-dissolution without paradox. *Philosophy and the Mind Sciences, 1*(1), pp. 1–36.

Flanagan, O., 2007. *The Really Hard Problem: Meaning in a Material World.* Cambridge, MA: MIT Press.

Flanagan, O., 2018. Hallucinating oneness: Is oneness true or just a positive metaphysical illusion? In Ivanhoe, P.J. (ed.) *The Oneness Hypothesis: Beyond the Boundary of Self*, pp. 269–284. Columbia University Press.

Flanagan, O. and Graham, G., 2017. Truth and sanity: Positive illusions, spiritual delusions, and metaphysical hallucinations. In Poland, J. and Tekin, S. (eds) *Extraordinary Science and Psychiatry: Responses to the Crisis in Mental Health Research*, pp. 293–313. Cambridge, MA: MIT Press.

Forman, R.K., 1998. What does mysticism have to teach us about consciousness? *Journal of Consciousness Studies, 5*(2), pp. 185–201.

Forrest, B., 2000. Methodological naturalism and philosophical naturalism: Clarifying the connection. *Philo, 3*(2), pp. 7–29.

Forstmann, M. and Sagioglou, C., 2017. Lifetime experience with (classic) psychedelics predicts pro-environmental behavior through an increase in nature relatedness. *Journal of Psychopharmacology, 31*(8), pp. 975–988.

Forstmann, M., Yudkin, D.A., Prosser, A.M., Heller, S.M., and Crockett, M.J., 2020. Transformative experience and social connectedness mediate the mood-enhancing effects of psychedelic use in naturalistic settings. *Proceedings of the National Academy of Sciences, 117*(5), pp. 2338–2346.

Fox, K.C., Zakarauskas, P., Dixon, M., Ellamil, M., Thompson, E., and Christoff, K., 2012. Meditation experience predicts introspective accuracy. *PloS One, 7*(9), p. e45370.

Fox, K.C., Nijeboer, S., Dixon, M.L., Floman, J.L., Ellamil, M., Rumak, S.P., Sedlmeier, P., and Christoff, K., 2014. Is meditation associated with altered brain structure? A systematic review and meta-analysis of morphometric neuroimaging in meditation practitioners. *Neuroscience & Biobehavioral Reviews, 43*, pp. 48–73.

Fox, K.C., Dixon, M.L., Nijeboer, S., Girn, M., Floman, J.L., Lifshitz, M., Ellamil, M., Sedlmeier, P., and Christoff, K., 2016. Functional neuroanatomy of meditation: A review and meta-analysis of 78 functional neuroimaging investigations. *Neuroscience & Biobehavioral Reviews, 65*, pp. 208–228.

Fox, K.C., Girn, M., Parro, C.C., and Christoff, K., 2018. Functional neuroimaging of psychedelic experience: An overview of psychological and neural effects and their relevance to research on creativity, daydreaming, and dreaming. In Jung, R. E. and Vartanian, O. (eds) *The Cambridge Handbook of the Neuroscience of Creativity*, pp. 92–113. Cambridge University Press. DOI: https://doi.org/10.1017/9781316556238.007

Fox, M.D., Snyder, A.Z., Vincent, J.L., Corbetta, M., Van Essen, D.C., and Raichle, M.E., 2005. The human brain is intrinsically organized into dynamic, anticorrelated functional networks. *Proceedings of the National Academy of Sciences, 102*(27), pp. 9673–9678.

Fransson, P., 2006. How default is the default mode of brain function? Further evidence from intrinsic BOLD signal fluctuations. *Neuropsychologia, 44*(14), pp. 2836–2845.

Fransson, P. and Marrelec, G., 2008. The precuneus/posterior cingulate cortex plays a pivotal role in the default mode network: Evidence from a partial correlation network analysis. *Neuroimage, 42*(3), pp. 1178–1184.

Frege, G., 1948. Sense and reference. *The Philosophical Review, 57*(3), pp. 209–230.

Fresco, D.M., M.T. Moore, M.H.M. van Dulmen, Z.V. Segal, S.H. Ma, J.D. Teasdale, and J.M.G. Williams., 2007. Initial psychometric properties of the experiences questionnaire: Validation of a self-report measure of decentering. *Behavior Therapy, 38*(3), pp. 234–246.

Friedman, H., 2006. The renewal of psychedelic research: Implications for humanistic and transpersonal psychology. *The Humanistic Psychologist, 34*(1), pp. 39–58.

Fuller, R.C., 2001. *Spiritual, but not Religious: Understanding Unchurched America*. Oxford University Press.

Gaia, G., 2016. *Changa's Alchemy: Narratives of Transformation in Psychedelic Experiences*. Master's thesis. University Van Amsterdam. DOI: https://www.academia.edu/download/50397508/G.Gaia_Changas_Alchemy.pdf

Gallagher, S., 2000. Philosophical conceptions of the self: Implications for cognitive science. *Trends in Cognitive Sciences, 4*(1), pp. 14–21.

Gallimore, A.R., 2015. Restructuring consciousness—the psychedelic state in light of integrated information theory. *Frontiers in Human Neuroscience, 9*, p. 346.

Gandy, S., 2019. Psychedelics and potential benefits in "healthy normals": A review of the literature. *Journal of Psychedelic Studies, 3*(3), pp. 280–287.

Garcia-Campayo J, Navarro-Gil M, Andrés E, Montero-Marin J, López-Artal L, Demarzo MMP, 2014. Validation of the Spanish versions of the long (26 items) and short (12 items) forms of the Self-Compassion Scale (SCS). *Health and Quality of Life Outcomes, 12*(1), p. 4. DOI: https://doi.org/10.1186/1477-7525-12-4

Garcia-Romeu, A., Griffiths, R., and W Johnson, M., 2014. Psilocybin-occasioned mystical experiences in the treatment of tobacco addiction. *Current Drug Abuse Reviews, 7*(3), pp. 157–164.

Garcia-Romeu, A., Kersgaard, B., and Addy, P.H., 2016. Clinical applications of hallucinogens: A review. *Experimental and Clinical Psychopharmacology, 24*(4), pp. 229–268.

Garcia-Romeu, A., Davis, A.K., Erowid, F., Erowid, E., Griffiths, R.R., and Johnson, M.W., 2019. Cessation and reduction in alcohol consumption and misuse after psychedelic use. *Journal of Psychopharmacology, 33*(9), pp. 1088–1101.

Garcia-Romeu, A., Davis, A.K., Erowid, E., Griffiths, R.R., and Johnson, M.W., 2020. Persisting reductions in cannabis, opioid, and stimulant misuse after naturalistic psychedelic use: An online survey. *Frontiers in Psychiatry, 10*, p. 955.

Gasser, P., Holstein, D., Michel, Y., Doblin, R., Yazar-Klosinski, B., Passie, T., and Brenneisen, R., 2014. Safety and efficacy of lysergic acid diethylamide-assisted psychotherapy for anxiety associated with life-threatening diseases. *Journal of Nervous and Mental Disease, 202*(7), pp. 513–520.

Gasser, P., Kirchner, K., and Passie, T., 2015. LSD-assisted psychotherapy for anxiety associated with a life-threatening disease: A qualitative study of acute and sustained subjective effects. *Journal of Psychopharmacology, 29*(1), pp. 57–68.

Gendler, T.S., 2008. Alief and belief. *Journal of Philosophy, 105*(10), pp. 634–663.

Gerrans, P., 2014. *The Measure of Madness: Philosophy of Mind, Cognitive Neuroscience, and Delusional Thought.* Cambridge, MA: MIT Press.

Gerrans, P., 2015. All the self we need. In Metzinger, T. and Windt, J.M. (eds) *Open MIND*: 15(T). Frankfurt am Main: MIND Group. DOI: https://doi.org/10.15502/9783958570078

Gerrans, P., 2019. Depersonalization disorder, affective processing and predictive coding. *Review of Philosophy and Psychology, 10*(2), pp. 401–418.

Gerrans, P. and Scherer, K., 2013. Wired for despair: The neurochemistry of emotion and the phenomenology of depression. *Journal of Consciousness Studies, 20*(7–8), pp. 254–268.

Gettier, E.L., 1963. Is justified true belief knowledge? *Analysis, 23*(6), pp. 121–123.

Gill, K.S., 1981. Aldous Huxley: The quest for synthetic sainthood. *Modern Fiction Studies, 27*(4), pp. 601–612.

Girn, M. and Christoff, K., 2018. Expanding the scientific study of self-experience with psychedelics. *Journal of Consciousness Studies, 25*(11–12), pp. 131–154.

Girn, M., Mills, C., Roseman, L., Carhart-Harris, R.L., and Christoff, K., 2020. Updating the dynamic framework of thought: Creativity and psychedelics. *NeuroImage.* DOI: https://doi.org/10.1016/j.neuroimage.2020.116726

Gładziejewski, P., 2016. Predictive coding and representationalism. *Synthese, 193*(2), pp. 559–582.

Goff, P., 2019. *Galileo's Error: Foundations for a New Science of Consciousness.* Oxford University Press.

Gold, I. and Stoljar, D., 1999. A neuron doctrine in the philosophy of neuroscience. *Behavioral and Brain Sciences, 22*(5), pp. 809–830.

Goldberg, S.B., Tucker, R.P., Greene, P.A., Davidson, R.J., Wampold, B.E., Kearney, D.J., and Simpson, T.L., 2018. Mindfulness-based interventions for psychiatric disorders: A systematic review and meta-analysis. *Clinical Psychology Review, 59*, pp. 52–60.

Goldberg, S.B., Pace, B.T., Nicholas, C.R., Raison, C.L., and Hutson, P.R., 2020. The experimental effects of psilocybin on symptoms of anxiety and depression: A meta-analysis. *Psychiatry Research, 284*, p. 112749.

Goleman, D., 1972. The Buddha on meditation and states of consciousness, Part I: The teachings. *Journal of Transpersonal Psychology, 4*(1), pp. 1–44.

González, D., Carvalho, M., Cantillo, J., Aixalá, M., and Farré, M., 2019. Potential use of ayahuasca in grief therapy. *OMEGA-Journal of Death and Dying, 79*(3), pp. 260–285.

González, D., Cantillo, J., Pérez, I., Farré, M., Feilding, A., Obiols, J.E., and Bouso, J.C., 2020. Therapeutic potential of ayahuasca in grief: A prospective, observational study. *Psychopharmacology, 237*, pp. 1171–1182.

Goodenough, U., 1998. *The Sacred Depths of Nature.* Oxford University Press.

Goodenough, U., 2001. Vertical and horizontal transcendence. *Zygon®, 36*(1), pp. 21–31.

Goodwin, G.M., 2016. Psilocybin: Psychotherapy or drug. *Journal of Psychopharmacology, 30*(12), pp. 1201–1202.

Graham, G. and Stephens, G.L. (eds) 1994. *Philosophical Psychopathology.* Cambridge, MA: MIT Press.

Grant, J.E., Lust, K., and Chamberlain, S.R., 2019. Hallucinogen use is associated with mental health and addictive problems and impulsivity in university students. *Addictive Behaviors Reports, 10*, p. 100228. DOI: https://doi.org/10.1016/j.abrep.2019.100228

Greicius, M.D., Srivastava, G., Reiss, A.L., and Menon, V., 2004. Default-mode network activity distinguishes Alzheimer's disease from healthy aging: Evidence from functional MRI. *Proceedings of the National Academy of Sciences, 101*(13), pp. 4637–4642.

Greif, A. and Šurkala, M., 2020. Compassionate use of psychedelics. *Medicine, Health Care, and Philosophy.* DOI: http://dx.doi.org/10.1007/s11019-020-09958-z

Griffiths, R.R., Richards, W.A., McCann, U., and Jesse, R., 2006. Psilocybin can occasion mystical-type experiences having substantial and sustained personal meaning and spiritual significance. *Psychopharmacology, 187*(3), pp. 268–283.

Griffiths, R.R., Richards, W.A., Johnson, M.W., McCann, U.D., and Jesse, R., 2008. Mystical-type experiences occasioned by psilocybin mediate the attribution of personal meaning and spiritual significance 14 months later. *Journal of Psychopharmacology, 22*(6), pp. 621–632.

Griffiths, R.R., Johnson, M.W., Richards, W.A., Richards, B.D., McCann, U., and Jesse, R., 2011. Psilocybin occasioned mystical-type experiences: immediate and persisting dose-related effects. *Psychopharmacology, 218*(4), pp. 649–665.

Griffiths, R.R., Johnson, M.W., Carducci, M.A., Umbricht, A., Richards, W.A., Richards, B.D., Cosimano, M.P., and Klinedinst, M.A., 2016. Psilocybin produces substantial and sustained decreases in depression and anxiety in patients with life-threatening cancer: A randomized double-blind trial. *Journal of Psychopharmacology, 30*(12), pp. 1181–1197.

Griffiths, R.R., Johnson, M.W., Richards, W.A., Richards, B.D., Jesse, R., MacLean, K.A., Barrett, F.S., Cosimano, M.P., and Klinedinst, M.A., 2017. Psilocybin-occasioned mystical-type experience in combination with meditation and other spiritual practices produces enduring positive changes in psychological functioning and in trait measures of prosocial attitudes and behaviors. *Journal of Psychopharmacology, 32*(1), pp. 49–69.

Griffiths, R.R., Hurwitz, E.S., Davis, A.K., Johnson, M.W., and Jesse, R., 2019. Survey of subjective "God encounter experiences": Comparisons among naturally occurring experiences and those occasioned by the classic psychedelics psilocybin, LSD, ayahuasca, or DMT. *PloS One, 14*(4), p. e0214377. DOI: https://doi.org/10.1371/journal.pone.0214377

Grimm, O., Kraehenmann, R., Preller, K.H., Seifritz, E., and Vollenweider, F.X., 2018. Psilocybin modulates functional connectivity of the amygdala during emotional face discrimination. *European Neuropsychopharmacology, 28*(6), pp. 691–700.

Grinde, B. and Stewart, L., 2020. A global workspace, evolution-based model of the effect of psychedelics on consciousness. *Psychology of Consciousness: Theory, Research, and Practice.* DOI: https://doi.org/10.1037/cns0000234

Grinspoon, L. and Bakalar, J.B., 1979. *Psychedelic Drugs Reconsidered.* New York: Basic Books.

Grob, C.S., 2007. The use of psilocybin in patients with advanced cancer and existential anxiety. In Winkelman, M. and Roberts, T.B. (eds), *Psychedelic Medicine: New Evidence for Hallucinogenic Substances as Treatments,* pp. 205–216. Westport, CT: Praeger.

Grob, C.S., Danforth, A.L., Chopra, G.S., Hagerty, M., McKay, C.R., Halberstadt, A.L., and Greer, G.R., 2011. Pilot study of psilocybin treatment for anxiety in patients with advanced-stage cancer. *Archives of General Psychiatry, 68*(1), pp. 71–78.

Grof, S., 1975. *Realms of the Human Unconscious: Observations from LSD Psychotherapy.* New York: Viking.

Grof, S., 1980. *LSD Psychotherapy.* Pomona, CA: Hunter House.

Guillot, M., 2017. I me mine: On a confusion concerning the subjective character of experience. *Review of Philosophy and Psychology, 8*(1), pp. 23–53.

Gusnard, D.A., Akbudak, E., Shulman, G.L., and Raichle, M.E., 2001. Medial prefrontal cortex and self-referential mental activity: relation to a default mode of brain function. *Proceedings of the National Academy of Sciences, 98*(7), pp. 4259–4264.

Guttmann, E., 1936. Artificial psychoses produced by mescaline. *British Journal of Psychiatry, 82*(338), pp. 203–221.

Haack, S., 1999. Defending science-within reason. *Principia: An International Journal of Epistemology*, 3(2), pp. 187–212.

Haijen, E.C., Kaelen, M., Roseman, L., Timmermann, C., Kettner, H., Russ, S., Nutt, D., Daws, R.E., Hampshire, A.D., Lorenz, R., and Carhart-Harris, R.L., 2018. Predicting responses to psychedelics: A prospective study. *Frontiers in Pharmacology*, 9, p. 897.

Halberstadt, A.L., 2015. Recent advances in the neuropsychopharmacology of serotonergic hallucinogens. *Behavioural Brain Research*, 277, pp. 99–120.

Hales, S.D., 2006. *Relativism and the Foundations of Philosophy*. Cambridge, MA: MIT Press.

Halpern, J.H. and Pope Jr, H.G., 2003. Hallucinogen persisting perception disorder: What do we know after 50 years? *Drug and Alcohol Dependence*, 69(2), pp. 109–119.

Halpern, J.H., Sherwood, A.R., Hudson, J.I., Yurgelun-Todd, D., and Pope, H.G., 2005. Psychological and cognitive effects of long-term peyote use among Native Americans. *Biological Psychiatry*, 58(8), pp. 624–631.

Halpern, J.H., Sherwood, A.R., Passie, T., Blackwell, K.C., and Ruttenber, A.J., 2008. Evidence of health and safety in American members of a religion who use a hallucinogenic sacrament. *Medical Science Monitor*, 14(8), pp. SR15–SR22.

Hamilton, J.P., Farmer, M., Fogelman, P., and Gotlib, I.H., 2015. Depressive rumination, the default-mode network, and the dark matter of clinical neuroscience. *Biological Psychiatry*, 78(4), pp. 224–230.

Harman, W.W., 1963. The issue of the consciousness-expanding drugs. *Main Currents*, 20, pp. 5–14. DOI: http://www.hofmann.org/papers/IssueCED.htm

Harman, W.W., McKim, R.H., Mogar, R.E., Fadiman, J., and Stolaroff, M.J., 1966. Psychedelic agents in creative problem-solving: A pilot study. *Psychological Reports*, 19(1), pp. 211–227.

Harmer, C.J. and Cowen, P.J., 2013. "It's the way that you look at it"—A cognitive neuropsychological account of SSRI action in depression. *Philosophical Transactions of the Royal Society of London B: Biological Sciences*, 368(1615), p. 20120407.

Harris, S., 2014. *Waking Up: A Guide to Spirituality Without Religion*. New York: Simon and Schuster.

Hartogsohn, I., 2018. The meaning-enhancing properties of psychedelics and their mediator role in psychedelic therapy, spirituality, and creativity. *Frontiers in Neuroscience*, 12, p. 129.

Haugeland, J., 1985. *Artificial Intelligence: The Very Idea*. Cambridge, MA: MIT Press.

Hayes, S.C., 1984. Making sense of spirituality. *Behaviorism*, 12(2), pp. 99–110.

Hayes, S.C., Law, S., Malady, M., Zhu, Z., and Bai, X., 2020. The centrality of sense of self in psychological flexibility processes: What the neurobiological and psychological correlates of psychedelics suggest. *Journal of Contextual Behavioral Science*, 15, pp. 30–38.

Heifets, B.D. and Malenka, R.C., 2019. Disruptive psychopharmacology. *JAMA Psychiatry*, 76(8), pp. 775–776.

Hempel, C.G., 1980. Comments on Goodman's ways of worldmaking. *Synthese*, 45(2), pp. 193–199.

Hendricks, P.S., 2018. Awe: A putative mechanism underlying the effects of classic psychedelic-assisted psychotherapy. *International Review of Psychiatry*, 30(4), pp. 331–342.

Hendricks, P.S., Clark, C.B., Johnson, M.W., Fontaine, K.R., and Cropsey, K.L., 2014. Hallucinogen use predicts reduced recidivism among substance-involved offenders under community corrections supervision. *Journal of Psychopharmacology*, 28(1), pp. 62–66.

Hendricks, P.S., Thorne, C.B., Clark, C.B., Coombs, D.W., and Johnson, M.W., 2015a. Classic psychedelic use is associated with reduced psychological distress and suicidality in the United States adult population. *Journal of Psychopharmacology*, 29(3), pp. 280–288.

Hendricks, P.S., Johnson, M.W., and Griffiths, R.R., 2015b. Psilocybin, psychological distress, and suicidality. *Journal of Psychopharmacology*, 29(9), pp. 1041–1043.

Hendricks, P.S., Crawford, M.S., Cropsey, K.L., Copes, H., Sweat, N.W., Walsh, Z., and Pavela, G., 2018. The relationships of classic psychedelic use with criminal behavior in the United States adult population. *Journal of Psychopharmacology, 32*(1), pp. 37–48.

Henriksen, M.G. and Parnas, J.S.S., 2019. Experiences without for-me-ness? Reconsidering alleged counter examples from psychopathology and psychedelics. *Thaumazein, 7*, pp. 6–20.

Heuschkel, K. and Kuypers, K.P., 2020. Depression, mindfulness, and psilocybin: Possible complementary effects of mindfulness meditation and psilocybin in the treatment of depression. A review. *Frontiers in Psychiatry, 11*. DOI: https://doi.org/10.3389/fpsyt.2020.00224

Hill, H. and Bruce, V., 1993. Independent effects of lighting, orientation, and stereopsis on the hollow-face illusion. *Perception, 22*(8), pp. 887–897.

Ho, J.T., Preller, K.H., and Lenggenhager, B., 2020. Neuropharmacological modulation of the aberrant bodily self through psychedelics. *Neuroscience & Biobehavioral Reviews, 108*, pp. 526–541.

Hofmann, A., Frey, A., Ott, H., T ZILKA, P.E.T.R., and Troxler, F., 1958. Elucidation of the structure and the synthesis of psilocybin. *Experientia, 14*(11), pp. 397–399.

Hofmann, A., 1980. *LSD: My Problem Child. 1979.* Trans. Jonathan Ott. New York: McGraw.

Hohwy, J., 2007a. The sense of self in the phenomenology of agency and perception. *Psyche, 13*(1), pp. 1–20.

Hohwy, J., 2007b. Functional integration and the mind. *Synthese, 159*(3), pp. 315–328.

Hohwy, J., 2013. *The Predictive Mind.* Oxford University Press.

Hohwy, J. and Michael, J., 2017. Why should any body have a self? In de Vignemont, F. and Alsmith, A.J.T. (eds) *The Subject's Matter: Self-Consciousness and the Body*, pp. 363–392. Cambridge, MA: MIT Press.

Hohwy, J., Roepstorff, A., and Friston, K., 2008. Predictive coding explains binocular rivalry: An epistemological review. *Cognition, 108*(3), pp. 687–701.

Holoyda, B., 2020. The psychedelic renaissance and its forensic implications. *Journal of the American Academy of Psychiatry and the Law, 48*(1), pp. 87–97.

Horst, S., 2009. Naturalisms in philosophy of mind. *Philosophy Compass, 4*(1), pp. 219–254.

Hoyningen-Huene, P., 1987. On the varieties of the distinction between the context of discovery and the context of justification. *Studies in History and Philosophy of Science, 18*, pp. 501–515.

Hutto, D.D. and Myin, E., 2012. *Radicalizing Enactivism: Basic Minds without Content.* Cambridge, MA: MIT Press.

Huxley, A., 1945. *The Perennial Philosophy.* Reprint, New York: Harper Colophon Books, 1970.

Huxley, A., 1954. *The Doors of Perception.* Reprint, New York: HarperCollins, 2009.

Huxley, A., 1963. Culture and the individual. *Playboy.* DOI: https://www.erowid.org/culture/characters/huxley_aldous/huxley_aldous_article1.shtml

Huxley, A., 1965. *Letters of Aldous Huxley.* Ed. Grover Smith. London: Chatto & Windus.

Inserra, A., 2019. Current status of psychedelic therapy in Australia and New Zealand: Are we falling behind? *Australian & New Zealand Journal of Psychiatry, 53*(3), pp. 190–192.

Jackson, F., 1982. Epiphenomenal qualia. *Philosophical Quarterly, 32*(127), pp. 127–136.

Jackson, F., 1986. What Mary didn't know. *Journal of Philosophy, 83*(5), pp. 291–295.

Jiménez-Garrido, D.F., Gómez-Sousa, M., Ona, G., Dos Santos, R.G., Hallak, J.E., Alcázar-Córcoles, M.Á., and Bouso, J.C., 2020. Effects of ayahuasca on mental health and quality of life in naïve users: A longitudinal and cross-sectional study combination. *Scientific Reports, 10*, 4075. DOI: https://doi.org/10.1038/s41598-020-61169-x

Johansen, P.Ø. and Krebs, T.S., 2015. Psychedelics not linked to mental health problems or suicidal behavior: A population study. *Journal of Psychopharmacology, 29*(3), pp. 270–279.

Johnson, M.W., 2018. Psychiatry might need some psychedelic therapy. *International Review of Psychiatry, 30*, pp. 285–290.

Johnson, M.W., Sewell, R.A., and Griffiths, R.R., 2012. Psilocybin dose-dependently causes delayed, transient headaches in healthy volunteers. *Drug and Alcohol Dependence, 123*(1–3), pp. 132–140.

Johnson, M.W., Garcia-Romeu, A., Cosimano, M.P., and Griffiths, R.R., 2014. Pilot study of the 5-HT2AR agonist psilocybin in the treatment of tobacco addiction. *Journal of Psychopharmacology, 28*(11), pp. 983–992.

Johnson, M.W., Garcia-Romeu, A., and Griffiths, R.R., 2017. Long-term follow-up of psilocybin-facilitated smoking cessation. *American Journal of Drug and Alcohol Abuse, 43*(1), pp. 55–60.

Johnson, M.W., Richards, W.A., and Griffiths, R.R., 2008. Human hallucinogen research: Guidelines for safety. *Journal of Psychopharmacology, 22*(6), pp. 603–620.

Johnson, M.W., Hendricks, P.S., Barrett, F.S., and Griffiths, R.R., 2019. Classic psychedelics: An integrative review of epidemiology, mystical experience, brain network function, and therapeutics. *Pharmacology & Therapeutics, 197*, pp. 83–102.

Johnstad, P.G., 2018. Powerful substances in tiny amounts: An interview study of psychedelic microdosing. *Nordic Studies on Alcohol and Drugs, 35*(1), pp. 39–51.

Johnstad, P.G., 2020. A dangerous method? Psychedelic therapy at Modum Bad, Norway, 1961–76. *History of Psychiatry, 31*(2), pp. 217–226.

Jones, A., 2018. *Clarifying the Mechanisms by which Psychedelics Achieve Therapeutic Efficacy.* (Master's dissertation, University of British Columbia)

Jopling, D.A., 2001. Placebo insight: The rationality of insight-oriented psychotherapy. *Journal of Clinical Psychology, 57*(1), pp. 19–36.

Kabat-Zinn, J., 2013. *Full Catastrophe Living: Using the Wisdom of Your Body and Mind to Face Stress, Pain and Illness,* revised edition. London: Piatkus.

Kaboodvand, N., Bäckman, L., Nyberg, L., and Salami, A., 2018. The retrosplenial cortex: A memory gateway between the cortical default mode network and the medial temporal lobe. *Human Brain Mapping, 39*(5), pp. 2020–2034.

Kaelen, M., Barrett, F.S., Roseman, L., Lorenz, R., Family, N., Bolstridge, M., Curran, H.V., Feilding, A., Nutt, D.J., and Carhart-Harris, R.L., 2015. LSD enhances the emotional response to music. *Psychopharmacology, 232*(19), pp. 3607–3614.

Kaelen, M., Roseman, L., Kahan, J., Santos-Ribeiro, A., Orban, C., Lorenz, R., Barrett, F.S., Bolstridge, M., Williams, T., Williams, L., and Wall, M.B., 2016. LSD modulates music-induced imagery via changes in parahippocampal connectivity. *European Neuropsychopharmacology, 26*(7), pp. 1099–1109.

Kaelen, M., Giribaldi, B., Raine, J., Evans, L., Timmerman, C., Rodriguez, N., Roseman, L., Feilding, A., Nutt, D., and Carhart-Harris, R., 2018. The hidden therapist: Evidence for a central role of music in psychedelic therapy. *Psychopharmacology, 235*(2), pp. 505–519.

Kähönen, J., 2020. Psychedelic Unselfing and Moral Perception. Master's thesis, University of Helsinki.< https://helda.helsinki.fi/bitstream/handle/10138/315556/Kahonen_Kaytannollinen_Filosofia.pdf >. 2 July 2020.

Kelly, J.F., Stout, R.L., Magill, M., Tonigan, J.S., and Pagano, M.E., 2011. Spirituality in recovery: A lagged mediational analysis of Alcoholics Anonymous' principal theoretical mechanism of behavior change. *Alcoholism: Clinical and Experimental Research, 35*(3), pp. 454–463.

Kelly, J.R., Baker, A., Babiker, M., Burke, L., Brennan, C., and O'Keane, V., 2019. The psychedelic renaissance: The next trip for psychiatry? *Irish Journal of Psychological Medicine*, pp. 1–5. DOI: https://doi.org/10.1017/ipm.2019.39

Kettner, H., Gandy, S., Haijen, E.C., and Carhart-Harris, R.L., 2019. From egoism to ecoism: Psychedelics increase nature relatedness in a state-mediated and context-dependent manner. *International Journal of Environmental Research and Public Health, 16*(24), p. 5147.

Klee, G.D., 1963. Lysergic acid diethylamide (LSD-25) and ego functions. *Archives of General Psychiatry*, 8(5), pp. 461–474.

Klüver, H., 1926. Mescal visions and eidetic vision. *American Journal of Psychology*, 37(4), pp. 502–515.

Kometer, M., Pokorny, T., Seifritz, E., and Volleinweider, F.X., 2015. Psilocybin-induced spiritual experiences and insightfulness are associated with synchronization of neuronal oscillations. *Psychopharmacology*, 232(19), pp. 3663–3676.

Kornfield, J., 1979. Intensive insight meditation: A phenomenological study. *Journal of Transpersonal Psychology*, 11(1), p. 41.

Kraehenmann, R., 2017. Dreams and psychedelics: Neurophenomenological comparison and therapeutic implications. *Current Neuropharmacology*, 15(7), pp. 1032–1042.

Kraehenmann, R., Preller, K.H., Scheidegger, M., Pokorny, T., Bosch, O.G., Seifritz, E., and Vollenweider, F.X., 2015. Psilocybin-induced decrease in amygdala reactivity correlates with enhanced positive mood in healthy volunteers. *Biological Psychiatry*, 78(8), pp. 572–581.

Kraehenmann, R., Pokorny, D., Aicher, H., Preller, K.H., Pokorny, T., Bosch, O.G., Seifritz, E., and Vollenweider, F.X., 2017a. LSD increases primary process thinking via serotonin 2A receptor activation. *Frontiers in Pharmacology*, 8, p. 814.

Kraehenmann, R., Pokorny, D., Vollenweider, L., Preller, K.H., Pokorny, T., Seifritz, E., and Vollenweider, F.X., 2017b. Dreamlike effects of LSD on waking imagery in humans depend on serotonin 2A receptor activation. *Psychopharmacology*, 234(13), pp. 2031–2046.

Krebs, T.S., 2015. Protecting the human rights of people who use psychedelics. *Lancet Psychiatry*, 2(4), pp. 294–295.

Krebs, T.S. and Johansen, P.Ø., 2012. Lysergic acid diethylamide (LSD) for alcoholism: Meta-analysis of randomized controlled trials. *Journal of Psychopharmacology*, 26(7), pp. 994–1002.

Krebs, T.S. and Johansen, P.Ø., 2013. Psychedelics and mental health: A population study. *PloS One*, 8(8), p. e63972.

Kringelbach, M.L., Cruzat, J., Cabral, J., Knudsen, G.M., Carhart-Harris, R., Whybrow, P.C., Logothetis, N.K., and Deco, G., 2020. Dynamic coupling of whole-brain neuronal and neurotransmitter systems. *Proceedings of the National Academy of Sciences*, 117(17), pp. 9566–9576.

Krystal, J.H., Karper, L.P., Seibyl, J.P., Freeman, G.K., Delaney, R., Bremner, J.D., Heninger, G.R., Bowers, M.B., and Charney, D.S., 1994. Subanesthetic effects of the noncompetitive NMDA antagonist, ketamine, in humans: Psychotomimetic, perceptual, cognitive, and neuroendocrine responses. *Archives of General Psychiatry*, 51(3), pp. 199–214.

Kucharski, A., 2013. The man who turned coffee into theorems. <https://theconversation.com/the-man-who-turned-coffee-into-theorems-16008>. 23 June 2020.

Kuhn, T.S., 1970. *The Structure of Scientific Revolutions,* 2nd ed. Reprint: University of Chicago Press, 2012.

Landes, J., Osimani, B., and Poellinger, R., 2018. Epistemology of causal inference in pharmacology. *European Journal for Philosophy of Science*, 8(1), pp. 3–49.

Langlitz, N., 2013. *Neuropsychedelia: The Revival of Hallucinogen Research since the Decade of the Brain*. University of California Press.

Langlitz, N., 2016. Is there a place for psychedelics in philosophy? Fieldwork in neuro- and perennial philosophy. *Common Knowledge*, 22(3), pp. 373–384.

Lavazza, A., 2017. Ways of being well: Realistic and unrealistic well-being. In Taddio, L., and Molin, K.W. (eds) *New Perspectives on Realism*. Mimesis International.

Lazarus, R.S., 1991. *Emotion and Adaptation*. Oxford University Press.

Lea, T., Amada, N., and Jungaberle, H., 2020. Psychedelic microdosing: A subreddit analysis. *Journal of Psychoactive Drugs*, 52(2), pp. 101–112.

Leary, T., 1990. *Flashbacks: A Personal and Cultural History of an Era: An Autobiography.* New York: G. P. Putnam's Sons.

Leary, T., Alpert, R., and Metzner, R., 1964. *The Psychedelic Experience: A Manual Based on the Tibetan Book of the Dead.* New York: Citadel Press.

Lebedev, A.V., Lövdén, M., Rosenthal, G., Feilding, A., Nutt, D.J., and Carhart-Harris, R.L., 2015. Finding the self by losing the self: Neural correlates of ego-dissolution under psilocybin. *Human Brain Mapping, 36*(8), pp. 3137–3153.

Lebedev, A.V., Kaelen, M., Lövdén, M., Nilsson, J., Feilding, A., Nutt, D.J., and Carhart-Harris, R.L., 2016. LSD-induced entropic brain activity predicts subsequent personality change. *Human Brain Mapping, 37*(9), pp. 3203–3213.

Leech, R., Braga, R., and Sharp, D.J., 2012. Echoes of the brain within the posterior cingulate cortex. *Journal of Neuroscience, 32*(1), pp. 215–222.

Leech, R. and Sharp, D.J., 2014. The role of the posterior cingulate cortex in cognition and disease. *Brain, 137*(1), pp. 12–32.

Letheby, C., 2015. The philosophy of psychedelic transformation. *Journal of Consciousness Studies, 22*(9–10), pp. 170–193.

Letheby, C., 2016. The epistemic innocence of psychedelic states. *Consciousness and cognition, 39*, pp. 28–37.

Letheby, C., 2017. Naturalizing psychedelic spirituality. *Zygon, 52*(3), pp. 623–642.

Letheby, C. and Gerrans, P., 2017. Self unbound: Ego dissolution in psychedelic experience. *Neuroscience of Consciousness*, (1). DOI: https://doi.org/10.1093/nc/nix016

Letheby, C., 2019. The varieties of psychedelic epistemology. In Wyrd, N., Luke, D., Tollan, A., Adams, C., and King, D. (eds) *Psychedelicacies: More Food for Thought from Breaking Convention.* Strange Attractor Press.

Letheby, C., 2020. Being for no-one: Psychedelic experience and minimal subjectivity. *Philosophy and the Mind Sciences, 1*(I), pp. 1–26. DOI: https://doi.org/10.33735/phimisci.2020.I.47

Leuner, H., 1967. Present state of psycholytic therapy and its possibilities. In Abramson, H.A. (ed.) *The Use of LSD in Psychotherapy and Alcoholism*, pp. 101–116. Indianapolis: Bobbs-Merrill.

Levin, M.E., Hildebrandt, M.J., Lillis, J., and Hayes, S.C., 2012. The impact of treatment components suggested by the psychological flexibility model: A meta-analysis of laboratory-based component studies. *Behavior Therapy, 43*(4), pp. 741–756.

Lewis, C.R., Preller, K.H., Braden, B.B., Riecken, C., and Vollenweider, F.X., 2020. Rostral anterior cingulate thickness predicts the emotional psilocybin experience. *Biomedicines, 8*, p. 34. doi:10.3390/biomedicines8020034

Lewis, C.R., Preller, K.H., Kraehenmann, R., Michels, L., Staempfli, P., and Vollenweider, F.X., 2017. Two dose investigation of the 5-HT-agonist psilocybin on relative and global cerebral blood flow. *Neuroimage, 159*, pp. 70–78.

Loo, R. and Thorpe, K., 1999. A psychometric investigation of scores on the Watson-Glaser critical thinking appraisal new Form S. *Educational and Psychological Measurement, 59*(6), pp. 995–1003.

Lou, H.C., Changeux, J.P., and Rosenstand, A., 2017. Towards a cognitive neuroscience of self-awareness. *Neuroscience & Biobehavioral Reviews, 83*, pp. 765–773.

Luke, D. and Terhune, D.B., 2013. The induction of synaesthesia with chemical agents: A systematic review. *Frontiers in Psychology, 4*, p. 753.

Lutz, A., Mattout, J., and Pagnoni, G., 2019. The epistemic and pragmatic value of non-action: a predictive coding perspective on meditation. *Current Opinion in Psychology, 28*, pp. 166–171.

Ly, C., Greb, A.C., Cameron, L.P., Wong, J.M., Barragan, E.V., Wilson, P.C., Burbach, K.F., Zarandi, S.S., Sood, A., Paddy, M.R., and Duim, W.C., 2018. Psychedelics promote structural and functional neural plasticity. *Cell Reports, 23*(11), pp. 3170–3182.

Lycan, W., 2019. Representational theories of consciousness. In Zalta, E.N. (ed.) *The Stanford Encyclopedia of Philosophy* (Fall 2019 edition). DOI: https://plato.stanford.edu/archives/fall2019/entries/consciousness-representational

Lyons, T. and Carhart-Harris, R.L., 2018a. Increased nature relatedness and decreased authoritarian political views after psilocybin for treatment-resistant depression. *Journal of Psychopharmacology*, 32(7), pp. 811–819.

Lyons, T. and Carhart-Harris, R.L., 2018b. More realistic forecasting of future life events after psilocybin for treatment-resistant depression. *Frontiers in Psychology*, 9, p. 1721.

Machamer, P., Darden, L., and Craver, C.F., 2000. Thinking about mechanisms. *Philosophy of Science*, 67(1), pp. 1–25.

MacLean, K.A., Johnson, M.W., and Griffiths, R.R., 2011. Mystical experiences occasioned by the hallucinogen psilocybin lead to increases in the personality domain of openness. *Journal of Psychopharmacology*, 25(11), pp. 1453–1461.

MacLean, K.A., Leoutsakos, J.M.S., Johnson, M.W., and Griffiths, R.R., 2012. Factor analysis of the mystical experience questionnaire: A study of experiences occasioned by the hallucinogen psilocybin. *Journal for the Scientific Study of Religion*, 51(4), pp. 721–737.

Madsen, M.K., Fisher, P.M., Stenbæk, D.S., Kristiansen, S., Burmester, D., Lehel, S., Páleníček, T., Kuchař, M., Svarer, C., Ozenne, B., and Knudsen, G.M., 2020. A single psilocybin dose is associated with long-term increased mindfulness, preceded by a proportional change in neocortical 5-HT2A receptor binding. *European Neuropsychopharmacology*, 33, pp. 71–80.

Majić, T., Schmidt, T.T., and Gallinat, J., 2015. Peak experiences and the afterglow phenomenon: When and how do therapeutic effects of hallucinogens depend on psychedelic experiences? *Journal of Psychopharmacology*, 29(3), pp. 241–253.

Malitz, S., Esecover, H., Wilkens, B., and Hoch, P.H., 1960. Some observations on psilocybin, a new hallucinogen, in volunteer subjects. *Comprehensive Psychiatry*, 1, pp. 8–17.

Malone, T.C., Mennenga, S.E., Guss, J., Podrebarac, S.K., Owens, L.T., Bossis, A.P., Belser, A.B., Agin-Liebes, G., Bogenschutz, M.P., and Ross, S., 2018. Individual experiences in four cancer patients following psilocybin-assisted psychotherapy. *Frontiers in Pharmacology*, 9, p. 256.

Mangini, M., 1998. Treatment of alcoholism using psychedelic drugs: A review of the program of research. *Journal of Psychoactive Drugs*, 30(4), pp. 381–418.

Mann, T., 2011. Magnificent visions. *Vanity Fair*. < https://www.vanityfair.com/news/2011/12/amazon-201112 >. 18 July 2020.

Marsella, A. J., & Price-Williams, D. (1974). A note on epistemic organization and hallucinogens. *Bulletin of the Menninger Clinic*, 38(1), pp. 70–72.

Mason, N.L., Mischler, E., Uthaug, M.V., and Kuypers, K.P., 2019. Sub-acute effects of psilocybin on empathy, creative thinking, and subjective well-being. *Journal of Psychoactive Drugs*, 51(2), pp. 123–134.

Mason, N.L., Kuypers, K.P.C., Müller, F., Reckweg, J., Tse, D.H.Y., Toennes, S.W., Hutten, N.R.P.W., Jansen, J.F.A., Stiers, P., Feilding, A., and Ramaekers, J.G., 2020. Me, myself, bye: regional alterations in glutamate and the experience of ego dissolution with psilocybin. *Neuropsychopharmacology*, 45(12), pp. 2003–2011.

Masters, R. and Houston, J., 1966. *The Varieties of Psychedelic Experience*. Reprint, Rochester: Park Street Press, 2000.

McClelland, T., 2019. Against virtual selves. *Erkenntnis*, 84(1), pp. 21–40.

McGinn, C., 1989. Can we solve the mind-body problem? *Mind*, 98(391), pp. 349–366.

Medford, N., 2012. Emotion and the unreal self: Depersonalization disorder and de-affectualization. *Emotion Review*, 4(2), pp. 139–144.

Meikle, S.E., Liknaitzky, P., Rossell, S.L., Ross, M., Strauss, N., Thomas, N., Murray, G., Williams, M., and Castle, D.J., 2020. Psilocybin-assisted therapy for depression: How do we advance the field? *Australian & New Zealand Journal of Psychiatry*, 54(3), pp. 225–231.

Menon, V. and Uddin, L.Q., 2010. Saliency, switching, attention and control: A network model of insula function. *Brain Structure and Function*, *214*(5–6), pp. 655–667.

Mertens, L.J., Wall, M.B., Roseman, L., Demetriou, L., Nutt, D.J., and Carhart-Harris, R.L., 2020. Therapeutic mechanisms of psilocybin: Changes in amygdala and prefrontal functional connectivity during emotional processing after psilocybin for treatment-resistant depression. *Journal of Psychopharmacology*, *34*(2), pp. 167–180.

Metzinger, T., 2003. *Being No-one: The Self-Model Theory of Subjectivity*. Cambridge, MA: MIT Press.

Metzinger, T., 2009. *The Ego Tunnel: The Science of the Mind and the Myth of the Self*. Basic Books.

Metzinger, T., 2011. The no-self alternative. In Gallagher, S. (ed.) *The Oxford handbook of the self*, pp 279–296. Oxford University Press.

Metzinger, T., 2013a. Spirituality and intellectual honesty: an essay. < https://philarchive.org/archive/METSAI>. 3 July 2020.

Metzinger, T.K., 2013b. Why are dreams interesting for philosophers? The example of minimal phenomenal selfhood, plus an agenda for future research1. *Frontiers in Psychology*, *4*, p. 746.

Metzinger, T., 2014. How does the brain encode epistemic reliability? Perceptual presence, phenomenal transparency, and counterfactual richness. *Cognitive Neuroscience*, *5*(2), pp. 122–124.

Metzinger, T., 2020. Minimal phenomenal experience. *Philosophy and the Mind Sciences*, *1*(I), pp. 1–44.

Metzner, R., 1998. Hallucinogenic drugs and plants in psychotherapy and shamanism. *Journal of Psychoactive Drugs*, *30*(4), pp. 333–341.

Mian, M.N., Altman, B.R., and Earleywine, M., 2020. Ayahuasca's antidepressant effects covary with behavioral activation as well as mindfulness. *Journal of Psychoactive Drugs*, *52*(2), pp. 130–137.

Miller, M.J., Albarracin-Jordan, J., Moore, C., and Capriles, J.M., 2019. Chemical evidence for the use of multiple psychotropic plants in a 1,000-year-old ritual bundle from South America. *Proceedings of the National Academy of Sciences*, *116*(23), pp. 11207–11212.

Miller, W.R., 2004. The phenomenon of quantum change. *Journal of Clinical Psychology*, *60*(5), pp. 453–460.

Millière, R., 2017. Looking for the self: Phenomenology, neurophysiology and philosophical significance of drug-induced ego dissolution. *Frontiers in Human Neuroscience*, *11*, p. 245.

Millière, R., 2020. The varieties of selflessness. *Philosophy and the Mind Sciences*, *1*(I), p. 8. DOI: https://doi.org/10.33735/phimisci.2020.I.48

Millière, R., Carhart-Harris, R.L., Roseman, L., Trautwein, F.M., and Berkovich-Ohana, A., 2018. Psychedelics, meditation, and self-consciousness. *Frontiers in Psychology*, *9*, p. 1475.

Millière, R. and Metzinger, T., 2020. Radical disruptions of self-consciousness. *Philosophy and the Mind Sciences*, *1*(I), p. 1. DOI: https://doi.org/10.33735/phimisci.2020.I.50

Mitchell, S.W., 1896. Remarks on the effects of Anhelonium lewinii (the mescal button). *British Medical Journal*, *2*(1875), pp. 1625–1629.

Modak, T., Bhad, R., and Rao, R., 2019. A rare case of physical dependence with psychedelic LSD—A case report. *Journal of Substance Use*, *24*(4), pp. 347–349.

Moreno, F.A., Wiegand, C.B., Taitano, E.K., and Delgado, P.L., 2006. Safety, tolerability, and efficacy of psilocybin in 9 patients with obsessive-compulsive disorder. *Journal of Clinical Psychiatry*, *67*(11), pp. 1735–1740.

Móró, L., 2010. Hallucinatory altered states of consciousness. *Phenomenology and the Cognitive Sciences*, *9*(2), pp. 241–252.

Moutoussis, M., Fearon, P., El-Deredy, W., Dolan, R.J., and Friston, K.J., 2014. Bayesian inferences about the self (and others): A review. *Consciousness and Cognition*, *25*, pp. 67–76.

Mueller, F., Lenz, C., Dolder, P.C., Harder, S., Schmid, Y., Lang, U.E., Liechti, M.E., and Borgwardt, S., 2017. Acute effects of LSD on amygdala activity during processing of fearful stimuli in healthy subjects. *Translational psychiatry*, 7(4), p. e1084.

Müller, F., Liechti, M.E., Lang, U.E., Borgwardt, S., Wilson, M.R., Webb, A., Wylie, L.J., Vine, S.J., Weavil, J.C., Amann, M., and Lutz, K., 2018a. Advances and challenges in neuroimaging studies on the effects of serotonergic hallucinogens: Contributions of the resting brain. *Progress in Brain Research*, 242, pp. 159–177.

Müller, F., Dolder, P.C., Schmidt, A., Liechti, M.E., and Borgwardt, S., 2018b. Altered network hub connectivity after acute LSD administration. *NeuroImage: Clinical*, 18, pp. 694–701.

Murdoch, I., 1970. *The Sovereignty of Good*. London: Routledge & Kegan Paul.

Murphy, D., 2020. Philosophy of psychiatry. In Zalta, E.N. (ed.) *The Stanford Encyclopedia of Philosophy* (Fall 2020 edition). DOI: https://plato.stanford.edu/archives/fall2020/entries/psychiatry

Murphy-Beiner, A. and Soar, K., 2020. Ayahuasca's "afterglow": Improved mindfulness and cognitive flexibility in ayahuasca drinkers. *Psychopharmacology*, 237(4), pp. 1161–1169.

Muthukumaraswamy, S.D., Carhart-Harris, R.L., Moran, R.J., Brookes, M.J., Williams, T.M., Errtizoe, D., Sessa, B., Papadopoulos, A., Bolstridge, M., Singh, K.D., and Feilding, A., 2013. Broadband cortical desynchronization underlies the human psychedelic state. *Journal of Neuroscience*, 33(38), pp. 15171–15183.

Muttoni, S., Ardissino, M., and John, C., 2019. Classical psychedelics for the treatment of depression and anxiety: A systematic review. *Journal of Affective Disorders*, 258, pp. 11–24.

Nagel, T., 1974. What is it like to be a bat? *Philosophical Review*, 83(4), pp. 435–450.

Naragon-Gainey, K. and DeMarree, K.G., 2017. Structure and validity of measures of decentering and defusion. *Psychological Assessment*, 29(7), pp. 935–954.

Neff, K., 2003. Self-compassion: An alternative conceptualization of a healthy attitude toward oneself. *Self and Identity*, 2(2), pp. 85–101.

Nencini, P. and Grant, K.A., 2010. Psychobiology of drug-induced religious experience: From the brain "locus of religion" to cognitive unbinding. *Substance Use & Misuse*, 45(13), pp. 2130–2151.

Nicholas, C.R., Henriquez, K.M., Gassman, M.C., Cooper, K.M., Muller, D., Hetzel, S., Brown, R.T., Cozzi, N.V., Thomas, C., and Hutson, P.R., 2018. High dose psilocybin is associated with positive subjective effects in healthy volunteers. *Journal of Psychopharmacology*, 32(7), pp. 770–778.

Nichols, D.E., 1986. Differences between the mechanism of action of MDMA, MBDB, and the classic hallucinogens. Identification of a new therapeutic class: Entactogens. *Journal of Psychoactive Drugs*, 18(4), pp. 305–313.

Nichols, D.E., 2016. Psychedelics. *Pharmacological Reviews*, 68(2), pp. 264–355.

Nichols, D.E. and Grob, C.S., 2018. Is LSD toxic? *Forensic Science International*, 284, pp. 141–145.

Nichols, D.E., Johnson, M.W., and Nichols, C.D., 2017. Psychedelics as medicines: An emerging new paradigm. *Clinical Pharmacology & Therapeutics*, 101(2), pp. 209–219.

Nida-Rümelin, M. and O'Conaill, D., 2019. Qualia: The Knowledge Argument. In Zalta, E.N. (ed.) *The Stanford Encyclopedia of Philosophy* (Winter 2019 edition). DOI: https://plato.stanford.edu/archives/win2019/entries/qualia-knowledge/

Nielson, E.M., May, D.G., Forcehimes, A.A., and Bogenschutz, M.P., 2018. The psychedelic debriefing in alcohol dependence treatment: illustrating key change phenomena through qualitative content analysis of clinical sessions. *Frontiers in Pharmacology*, 9, p. 132.

Nolen-Hoeksema, S., 2000. The role of rumination in depressive disorders and mixed anxiety/depressive symptoms. *Journal of Abnormal Psychology*, 109(3), pp. 504–511.

Noorani, T., Garcia-Romeu, A., Swift, T.C., Griffiths, R.R., and Johnson, M.W., 2018. Psychedelic therapy for smoking cessation: Qualitative analysis of participant accounts. *Journal of Psychopharmacology, 32*(7), pp. 756–769.

Nour, M.M., Evans, L., Nutt, D., and Carhart-Harris, R.L., 2016. Ego-dissolution and psychedelics: Validation of the Ego-Dissolution Inventory (EDI). *Frontiers in Human Neuroscience, 10*, p. 269.

Nour, M.M., Evans, L., and Carhart-Harris, R.L., 2017. Psychedelics, personality and political perspectives. *Journal of Psychoactive Drugs, 49*(3), pp. 182–191.

Nozick, R., 1974/2013. *Anarchy, State, and Utopia*. New York: Basic Books.

Nutt, D., 2016. Psilocybin for anxiety and depression in cancer care? Lessons from the past and prospects for the future. *Journal of Psychopharmacology, 30*(12), pp. 1163–1164.

Nutt, D., 2019. Psychedelic drugs—a new era in psychiatry? *Dialogues in Clinical Neuroscience, 21*(2), pp. 139–147.

Nutt, D.J., King, L.A., and Phillips, L.D., 2010. Drug harms in the UK: A multicriteria decision analysis. *Lancet, 376*(9752), pp. 1558–1565.

Nutt, D.J., King, L.A., and Nichols, D.E., 2013. Effects of Schedule I drug laws on neuroscience research and treatment innovation. *Nature Reviews Neuroscience, 14*(8), pp. 577–585.

Nutting, S., Bruinsma, T., Anderson, M., and Jolly, T., 2020. Psychotic and still tripping—hallucinogen persisting perception disorder and first break psychosis in an adolescent. *International Journal of Mental Health and Addiction*. DOI: https://doi.org/10.1007/s11469-020-00338-5

O'Brien, G., 2011. Defending the semantic conception of computation in cognitive science. *Journal of Cognitive Science, 12*(4), pp. 381–399.

O'Brien, G. and Jureidini, J., 2002a. Dispensing with the dynamic unconscious. *Philosophy, Psychiatry, & Psychology, 9*(2), pp. 141–153.

O'Brien, G. and Jureidini, J., 2002b. The last rites of the dynamic unconscious. *Philosophy, Psychiatry, & Psychology, 9*(2), pp. 161–166.

O'Brien, G. and Opie, J., 2006. How do connectionist networks compute? *Cognitive Processing, 7*(1), pp. 30–41.

O'Brien, G. and Opie, J., 2015. A schizophrenic defense of a vehicle theory of consciousness. In Gennaro, R.J. (ed.) *Disturbed Consciousness: New Essays on Psychopathology and Theories of Consciousness*, pp. 265–292. Cambridge, MA: MIT Press.

O'Callaghan, C., Hubik, D.J., Dwyer, J., Williams, M., and Ross, M., 2020. Experience of music used with psychedelic therapy: A rapid review and implications. *Journal of Music Therapy*. DOI: https://doi.org/10.1093/jmt/thaa006

Olson, D.E., 2018. Psychoplastogens: A promising class of plasticity-promoting neurotherapeutics. *Journal of Experimental Neuroscience, 12*. DOI: https://doi.org/10.1177/1179069518800508

Ona, G., Kohek, M., Massaguer, T., Gomariz, A., Jiménez, D.F., Dos Santos, R.G., Hallak, J.E., Alcázar-Córcoles, M.Á., and Bouso, J.C., 2019. Ayahuasca and public health: Health status, psychosocial well-being, lifestyle, and coping strategies in a large sample of ritual ayahuasca users. *Journal of Psychoactive Drugs, 51*(2), pp. 135–145.

Osmond, H., 1957. A review of the clinical effects of psychotomimetic agents. *Annals of the New York Academy of Sciences, 66*(1), pp. 418–434.

Osório, F.D.L., Sanches, R.F., Macedo, L.R., dos Santos, R.G., Maia-de-Oliveira, J.P., Wichert-Ana, L., de Araujo, D.B., Riba, J., Crippa, J.A., and Hallak, J.E., 2015. Antidepressant effects of a single dose of ayahuasca in patients with recurrent depression: a preliminary report. *Revista Brasileira de Psiquiatria, 37*(1), pp. 13–20.

Osto, D., 2016. *Altered States: Buddhism and Psychedelic Spirituality in America*. Columbia University Press.

Pahnke, W.N., 1963. *Drugs and Mysticism: An Analysis of the Relationship Between Psychedelic Drugs and the Mystical Consciousness: A Thesis* (Doctoral dissertation, Harvard University) DOI: https://maps.org/images/pdf/books/pahnke/walter_pahnke_drugs_and_mysticism.pdf

Pahnke, W.N., 1966. Drugs and mysticism. *International Journal of Parapsychology*, 8(2), pp. 295–313.

Pahnke, W.N., 1967. LSD and religious experience. In DeBold, R.C. and Leaf, R. C. (eds) *LSD, Man and Society*. Wesleyan University Press.

Pahnke, W.N., 1969. The psychedelic mystical experience in the human encounter with death. *Harvard Theological Review*, 62(1), pp. 1–21.

Pahnke, W.N. and Richards, W.A., 1966. Implications of LSD and experimental mysticism. *Journal of Religion and Health*, 5(3), pp. 175–208.

Palhano-Fontes, F., Barreto, D., Onias, H., Andrade, K.C., Novaes, M.M., Pessoa, J.A., Mota-Rolim, S.A., Osório, F.L., Sanches, R., dos Santos, R.G., and Tófoli, L.F., 2019. Rapid anti-depressant effects of the psychedelic ayahuasca in treatment-resistant depression: A randomized placebo-controlled trial. *Psychological Medicine*, 49(4), pp. 655–663.

Papineau, D., 2016. Naturalism. In Zalta, E.N. (ed.) *The Stanford Encyclopedia of Philosophy* (Winter 2016 edition). DOI: https://plato.stanford.edu/archives/win2016/entries/naturalism

Parfit, D., 1984. *Reasons and Persons*. Oxford University Press.

Passie, T., Seifert, J., Schneider, U., and Emrich, H.M., 2002. The pharmacology of psilocybin. *Addiction Biology*, 7(4), pp. 357–364.

Paul, L.A., 2014. *Transformative Experience*. Oxford University Press.

Peters, S.K., Dunlop, K., and Downar, J., 2016. Cortico-striatal-thalamic loop circuits of the salience network: A central pathway in psychiatric disease and treatment. *Frontiers in Systems Neuroscience*, 10, p. 104.

Petrolini, V., 2017. *From Normality to Pathology: In Defense of Continuity*. (Doctoral dissertation, University of Cincinnati)

Phillips, M.L., Medford, N., Senior, C., Bullmore, E.T., Suckling, J., Brammer, M.J., Andrew, C., Sierra, M., Williams, S.C., and David, A.S., 2001. Depersonalization disorder: Thinking without feeling. *Psychiatry Research: Neuroimaging*, 108(3), pp. 145–160.

Piccinini, G., 2009. Computationalism in the Philosophy of Mind. *Philosophy Compass*, 4(3), pp. 515–532.

Piccinini, G. and Bahar, S., 2013. Neural computation and the computational theory of cognition. *Cognitive Science*, 37(3), pp. 453–488.

Piccinini, G. and Craver, C., 2011. Integrating psychology and neuroscience: Functional analyses as mechanism sketches. *Synthese*, 183(3), pp. 283–311.

Piff, P.K., Dietze, P., Feinberg, M., Stancato, D.M., and Keltner, D., 2015. Awe, the small self, and prosocial behavior. *Journal of Personality and Social Psychology*, 108(6), pp. 883–899.

Pisano, V.D., Putnam, N.P., Kramer, H.M., Franciotti, K.J., Halpern, J.H., and Holden, S.C., 2017. The association of psychedelic use and opioid use disorders among illicit users in the United States. *Journal of Psychopharmacology*, 31(5), pp. 606–613.

Pokorny, T., Preller, K.H., Kometer, M., Dziobek, I., and Vollenweider, F.X., 2017. Effect of psilocybin on empathy and moral decision-making. *International Journal of Neuropsychopharmacology*, 20(9), pp. 747–757.

Poland, J. and Tekin, S. (eds) 2017. *Extraordinary Science and Psychiatry: Responses to the Crisis in Mental Health Research*. Cambridge, MA: MIT Press.

Polito, V. and Stevenson, R.J., 2019. A systematic study of microdosing psychedelics. *PloS One*, 14(2), p. e0211023.

Pollan, M., 2015. The trip treatment. *The New Yorker*, February 9. DOI: https://www.newyorker.com/magazine/2015/02/09/trip-treatment

Pollan, M., 2018. *How to Change Your Mind: The New Science of Psychedelics*. New York: Penguin.

Preller, K.H. and Vollenweider, F.X., 2016. Phenomenology, structure, and dynamic of psychedelic states. *Current Topics in Behavioral Neurosciences, 36*, pp. 221–256.

Preller, K.H. and Vollenweider, F.X., 2019. Modulation of social cognition via hallucinogens and "entactogens". *Frontiers in Psychiatry, 10*, p. 881.

Prinz, J., 2003. Level-headed mysterianism and artificial experience. *Journal of Consciousness Studies, 10*(4–5), pp. 111–132.

Prinz, J.J., 2004. *Gut Reactions: A Perceptual Theory of Emotion*. Oxford University Press.

Putnam, Hilary, 1967. Psychological predicates. In Capitan, W.H. and Merrill, D.D. (eds) *Art, Mind, and Religion*, pp. 37–48. University of Pittsburgh Press.

Radden, J., 1994. Recent criticism of psychiatric nosology: A review. *Philosophy, Psychiatry, & Psychology, 1*(3), pp. 193–200.

Raichle, M.E., MacLeod, A.M., Snyder, A.Z., Powers, W.J., Gusnard, D.A., and Shulman, G.L., 2001. A default mode of brain function. *Proceedings of the National Academy of Sciences, 98*(2), pp. 676–682.

Rantamäki, T. and Yalcin, I., 2016. Antidepressant drug action—From rapid changes on network function to network rewiring. *Progress in Neuro-Psychopharmacology and Biological Psychiatry, 64*, pp. 285–292.

Ratcliffe, M., 2005. The feeling of being. *Journal of Consciousness Studies, 12*(8–9), pp. 43–60.

Ratcliffe, M., 2009. Existential feeling and psychopathology. *Philosophy, Psychiatry, & Psychology, 16*(2), pp. 179–194.

Reiche, S., Hermle, L., Gutwinski, S., Jungaberle, H., Gasser, P., and Majić, T., 2018. Serotonergic hallucinogens in the treatment of anxiety and depression in patients suffering from a life-threatening disease: A systematic review. *Progress in Neuro-psychopharmacology and Biological Psychiatry, 81*, pp. 1–10.

Rescorla, M., 2020. The computational theory of mind. In Zalta, E.N. (ed.) *The Stanford Encyclopedia of Philosophy* (Spring 2020 edition). DOI: https://plato.stanford.edu/archives/spr2020/entries/computational-mind

Revonsuo, A., 1999. Binding and the phenomenal unity of consciousness. *Consciousness and Cognition, 8*(2), pp. 173–185.

Revonsuo, A., 2006. *Inner Presence: Consciousness as a Biological Phenomenon*. Cambridge, MA: MIT Press.

Richards, W.A., 1978. Mystical and archetypal experiences of terminal patients in DPT-assisted psychotherapy. *Journal of Religion and Health, 17*(2), pp. 117–126.

Richards, W.A., 2008. The phenomenology and potential religious import of states of consciousness facilitated by psilocybin. *Archive for the Psychology of Religion, 30*(1), pp. 189–200.

Richards, W.A., 2015. *Sacred knowledge: Psychedelics and religious experiences*. Columbia University Press.

Richards, W.A., 2017. Psychedelic psychotherapy: Insights from 25 years of research. *Journal of Humanistic Psychology, 57*(4), pp. 323–337.

Roberts, T.B., 2006. *Psychedelic Horizons*. Reprint: Andrews UK Limited, 2015.

Rocha, J.M., Osório, F.L., Crippa, J.A.S., Bouso, J.C., Rossi, G.N., Hallak, J.E., and dos Santos, R.G., 2019. Serotonergic hallucinogens and recognition of facial emotion expressions: a systematic review of the literature. *Therapeutic Advances in Psychopharmacology, 9*, pp. 1–11.

Roche, G.T., 2010. Seeing snakes: On delusion, knowledge and the drug experience. In Jacquette, D. (ed.) *Cannabis Philosophy for Everyone*, pp. 35–49. Blackwell.

Romeo, B., Karila, L., Martelli, C., and Benyamina, A., 2020. Efficacy of psychedelic treatments on depressive symptoms: A meta-analysis. *Journal of Psychopharmacology*. DOI: https://doi.org/10.1177/0269881120919957

Roseman, L., Leech, R., Feilding, A., Nutt, D.J., and Carhart-Harris, R.L., 2014. The effects of psilocybin and MDMA on between-network resting state functional connectivity in healthy volunteers. *Frontiers in Human Neuroscience*, *8*, p. 204.

Roseman, L., Nutt, D.J., and Carhart-Harris, R.L., 2018a. Quality of acute psychedelic experience predicts therapeutic efficacy of psilocybin for treatment-resistant depression. *Frontiers in Pharmacology*, *8*, p. 974.

Roseman, L., Demetriou, L., Wall, M.B., Nutt, D.J., and Carhart-Harris, R.L., 2018b. Increased amygdala responses to emotional faces after psilocybin for treatment-resistant depression. *Neuropharmacology*, *142*, pp. 263–269.

Roseman, L., Haijen, E., Idialu-Ikato, K., Kaelen, M., Watts, R., and Carhart-Harris, R., 2019. Emotional breakthrough and psychedelics: Validation of the Emotional Breakthrough Inventory. *Journal of Psychopharmacology*, *33*(9), pp. 1076–1087.

Ross, S., Bossis, A., Guss, J., Agin-Liebes, G., Malone, T., Cohen, B., Mennenga, S.E., Belser, A., Kalliontzi, K., Babb, J., and Su, Z., 2016. Rapid and sustained symptom reduction following psilocybin treatment for anxiety and depression in patients with life-threatening cancer: A randomized controlled trial. *Journal of Psychopharmacology*, *30*(12), pp. 1165–1180.

Roth, B.L., Baner, K., Westkaemper, R., Siebert, D., Rice, K.C., Steinberg, S., Ernsberger, P., and Rothman, R.B., 2002. Salvinorin A: A potent naturally occurring nonnitrogenous κ opioid selective agonist. *Proceedings of the National Academy of Sciences*, *99*(18), pp. 11934–11939.

Rougemont-Bücking, A., Jungaberle, H., Scheidegger, M., Merlo, M.C., Grazioli, V.S., Daeppen, J.B., Gmel, G., and Studer, J., 2019. Comparing mental health across distinct groups of users of psychedelics, MDMA, psychostimulants, and cannabis. *Journal of Psychoactive Drugs*, *51*(3), pp. 236–246.

Ruck, C.A., R. G. Wasson, Bigwood, J., Ott, J., and Staples, D., 1979. Entheogens. *Journal of Psychedelic Drugs*, *11*(1-2), pp. 145–146.

Rucker, J.J., Iliff, J., and Nutt, D.J., 2017. Psychiatry and the psychedelic drugs. Past, present and future. *Neuropharmacology*, *142*, pp. 200–218.

Russ, S.L., Carhart-Harris, R.L., Maruyama, G., and Elliott, M.S., 2019a. States and traits related to the quality and consequences of psychedelic experiences. *Psychology of Consciousness: Theory, Research, and Practice*, *6*(1), pp. 1–21.

Russ, S.L., Carhart-Harris, R.L., Maruyama, G., and Elliott, M.S., 2019b. Replication and extension of a model predicting response to psilocybin. *Psychopharmacology*, *236*(11), pp. 3221–3230.

Russell, B., 1910. Knowledge by acquaintance and knowledge by description. *Proceedings of the Aristotelian Society*, *11*, pp. 108–128.

Russell, B., 1917. *Mysticism and Logic and Other Essays*. Reprint: Project Gutenberg, 2008. DOI: http://www.gutenberg.org/files/25447/25447-h/25447-h.htm

Russo, F. and Williamson, J., 2011. Epistemic causality and evidence-based medicine. *History and Philosophy of the Life Sciences*, *33*(4), pp. 563–581.

Ryle, G., 1945. Knowing how and knowing that: The presidential address. *Proceedings of the Aristotelian Society*, *46*, pp. 1–16.

Saarinen, J., 2014. The oceanic feeling: A case study in existential feeling. *Journal of Consciousness Studies*, *21*(5–6), pp. 196–217.

Sahakian, B.J. and Morein-Zamir, S., 2015. Pharmacological cognitive enhancement: Treatment of neuropsychiatric disorders and lifestyle use by healthy people. *Lancet Psychiatry*, *2*(4), pp. 357–362.

Saka, P., 2021. Pascal's wager about God. *The Internet Encyclopedia of Philosophy*, ISSN 2161-0002. https://iep.utm.edu/pasc-wag/. 12 February 2021.

Sampedro, F., de la Fuente Revenga, M., Valle, M., Roberto, N., Domínguez-Clavé, E., Elices, M., Luna, L.E., Crippa, J.A.S., Hallak, J.E., de Araujo, D.B., and Friedlander, P., 2017. Assessing the psychedelic "after-glow" in Ayahuasca users: Post-acute neurometabolic and functional connectivity changes are associated with enhanced mindfulness capacities. *International Journal of Neuropsychopharmacology, 20*(9), pp. 698–711.

Sanches, R.F., de Lima Osório, F., Dos Santos, R.G., Macedo, L.R., Maia-de-Oliveira, J.P., Wichert-Ana, L., de Araujo, D.B., Riba, J., Crippa, J.A.S., and Hallak, J.E., 2016. Antidepressant effects of a single dose of ayahuasca in patients with recurrent depression: A SPECT study. *Journal of Clinical Psychopharmacology, 36*(1), pp. 77–81.

Sander, D., Grafman, J., and Zalla, T., 2003. The human amygdala: An evolved system for relevance detection. *Reviews in the Neurosciences, 14*(4), pp. 303–316.

Sandison, R.A., 1954. Psychological aspects of the LSD treatment of the neuroses. *Journal of Mental Science, 100*(419), pp. 508–515.

Sandison, R.A., Spencer, A.M., and Whitelaw, J.D.A., 1954. The therapeutic value of lysergic acid diethylamide in mental illness. *British Journal of Psychiatry, 100*(419), pp. 491–507.

Savage, C., 1955. Variations in ego feeling induced by D-lysergic acid diethylamide (LSD-25). *Psychoanalytic Review, 42*(1), pp. 1–16.

Savage, C., Savage, E., Fadiman, J., and Harman, W., 1964. LSD: Therapeutic effects of the psychedelic experience. *Psychological Reports, 14*(1), pp. 111–120.

Schacter, D.L., Addis, D.R., and Buckner, R.L., 2007. Remembering the past to imagine the future: The prospective brain. *Nature Reviews Neuroscience, 8*(9), pp. 657–661.

Schachter, S. and Singer, J., 1962. Cognitive, social, and physiological determinants of emotional state. *Psychological Review, 69*(5), pp. 379–399.

Schenberg, E.E., 2018. Psychedelic-assisted psychotherapy: A paradigm shift in psychiatric research and development. *Frontiers in Pharmacology, 9*, p. 733.

Schliesser, E., 2019. Synthetic philosophy. *Biology & Philosophy, 34*(2), p. 19.

Schmid, Y. and Liechti, M.E., 2018. Long-lasting subjective effects of LSD in normal subjects. *Psychopharmacology, 235*(2), pp. 535–545.

Scott, G. and Carhart-Harris, R.L., 2019. Psychedelics as a treatment for disorders of consciousness. *Neuroscience of Consciousness.* DOI: https://doi.org/10.1093/nc/niz003

Sebastián, M.A., 2020. Perspectival self-consciousness and ego-dissolution: An analysis of (some) altered states of consciousness. *Philosophy and the Mind Sciences, 1*(I), pp. 1–27. DOI: https://doi.org/10.33735/phimisci.2020.I.44

Seeley, W.W., Menon, V., Schatzberg, A.F., Keller, J., Glover, G.H., Kenna, H., Reiss, A.L., and Greicius, M.D., 2007. Dissociable intrinsic connectivity networks for salience processing and executive control. *Journal of Neuroscience, 27*(9), pp. 2349–2356.

Seibt, J., 2020. Process philosophy. In Zalta, E.N. (ed.) *The Stanford Encyclopedia of Philosophy* (Summer 2020 edition). DOI: https://plato.stanford.edu/archives/sum2020/entries/process-philosophy

Sellars, W., 1963. Philosophy and the scientific image of man. In *Empiricism and the Philosophy of Mind*, pp. 1–40. Routledge & Kegan Paul.

Sessa, B., 2005. Can psychedelics have a role in psychiatry once again? *British Journal of Psychiatry, 186*(6), pp. 457–458.

Sessa, B., 2008. Is it time to revisit the role of psychedelic drugs in enhancing human creativity? *Journal of Psychopharmacology, 22*(8), pp. 821–827.

Sessa, B., 2012. *The Psychedelic Renaissance: Reassessing the Role of Psychedelic Drugs in 21st Century Psychiatry and Society.* London: Muswell Hill Press.

Sessa, B., 2014. Why psychiatry needs psychedelics and psychedelics need psychiatry. *Journal of Psychoactive Drugs, 46*(1), pp. 57–62.

Sessa, B., 2018. The 21st century psychedelic renaissance: Heroic steps forward on the back of an elephant. *Psychopharmacology, 235*(2), pp. 551–560.

Seth, A.K., 2013. Interoceptive inference, emotion, and the embodied self. *Trends in Cognitive Sciences, 17*(11), pp. 565–573.

Seth, A., 2016. The hard problem of consciousness is a distraction from the real one. Aeon. DOI: https://aeon.co/essays/the-hard-problem-of-consciousness-is-a-distraction-from-the-real-one

Sewell, R.A., Halpern, J.H., and Pope, H.G., 2006. Response of cluster headache to psilocybin and LSD. *Neurology, 66*(12), pp. 1920–1922.

Sha, Z., Wager, T.D., Mechelli, A., and He, Y., 2019. Common dysfunction of large-scale neurocognitive networks across psychiatric disorders. *Biological Psychiatry, 85*(5), pp. 379–388.

Shalit, N., Rehm, J., and Lev-Ran, S., 2019. Epidemiology of hallucinogen use in the US results from the National epidemiologic survey on alcohol and related conditions III. *Addictive Behaviors, 89*, pp. 35–43.

Shani, I., 2015. Cosmopsychism: A holistic approach to the metaphysics of experience. *Philosophical Papers, 44*(3), pp. 389–437.

Shanon, B., 2001. The divine within. *Journal of Consciousness Studies, 8*(2), pp. 91–95.

Shanon, B., 2002. *The Antipodes of the Mind: Charting the Phenomenology of the Ayahuasca Experience*. Oxford University Press.

Shanon, B., 2010. The epistemics of ayahuasca visions. *Phenomenology and the Cognitive Sciences, 9*(2), pp. 263–280.

Sierra, M. and David, A.S., 2011. Depersonalization: A selective impairment of self-awareness. *Consciousness and cognition, 20*(1), pp. 99–108.

Sierra-Siegert, M., & Jay, E.-L., 2020. Reducing oneself to a body, a thought, or an emotion: A measure of identification with mind contents. *Psychology of Consciousness: Theory, Research, and Practice, 7*(3), pp. 218–237. DOI: http://dx.doi.org/10.1037/cns0000233

Simpson, W., 2014. The mystical stance: The experience of self-loss and Daniel Dennett's "center of narrative gravity". *Zygon, 49*(2), pp. 458–475.

Sjöstedt-H, P., 2015. *Noumenautics: Metaphysics–Meta-ethics–Psychedelics*. London: Psychedelic Press.

Skryabin, V.Y., Vinnikova, M., Nenastieva, A., and Alekseyuk, V., 2018. Hallucinogen persisting perception disorder: A literature review and three case reports. *Journal of Addictive Diseases, 37*(3–4), pp. 268–278.

Smallwood, J. and Schooler, J.W., 2015. The science of mind wandering: Empirically navigating the stream of consciousness. *Annual Review of Psychology, 66*, pp. 487–518.

Smart, J.J.C., 1959. Sensations and brain processes. *Philosophical Review, 68*, pp. 141–156.

Smart, R.G. and Storm, T., 1964. The efficacy of LSD in the treatment of alcoholism. *Quarterly Journal of Studies on Alcohol, 25*(2), pp. 333–338.

Smigielski, L., Kometer, M., Scheidegger, M., Krähenmann, R., Huber, T., and Vollenweider, F.X., 2019a. Characterization and prediction of acute and sustained response to psychedelic psilocybin in a mindfulness group retreat. *Scientific Reports, 9*(1), pp. 1–13.

Smigielski, L., Scheidegger, M., Kometer, M., and Vollenweider, F.X., 2019b. Psilocybin-assisted mindfulness training modulates self-consciousness and brain default mode network connectivity with lasting effects. *NeuroImage, 196*, pp. 207–215.

Smigielski, L., Kometer, M., Scheidegger, M., Stress, C., Preller, K.H., Koenig, T., and Vollenweider, F.X., 2020. P300-mediated modulations in self–other processing under psychedelic psilocybin are related to connectedness and changed meaning: A window into the self–other overlap. *Human Brain Mapping*. DOI: https://doi.org/10.1002/hbm.25174

Smith, H., 1964. Do drugs have religious import? *Journal of Philosophy, 61*(18), pp. 517–530.

Smith, H., 2000. *Cleansing the Doors of Perception: The Religious Significance of Entheogenic Plants and Chemicals*. Reprint, Boulder: Sentient Publications, 2003.

Smith, W.R. and Sisti, D., 2020. Ethics and ego dissolution: The case of psilocybin. *Journal of Medical Ethics*. DOI: http://dx.doi.org/10.1136/medethics-2020-106070

Smythies, J.R., 1953. The mescaline phenomena. *British Journal for the Philosophy of Science*, 3(12), pp. 339–347.

Soler, J., Elices, M., Franquesa, A., Barker, S., Friedlander, P., Feilding, A., Pascual, J.C., and Riba, J., 2016. Exploring the therapeutic potential of Ayahuasca: Acute intake increases mindfulness-related capacities. *Psychopharmacology*, 233(5), pp. 823–829.

Soler, J., Elices, M., Dominguez-Clavé, E., Pascual, J.C., Feilding, A., Navarro-Gil, M., García-Campayo, J., and Riba, J., 2018. Four weekly ayahuasca sessions lead to increases in "acceptance" capacities: A comparison study with a standard 8-week mindfulness training program. *Frontiers in Pharmacology*, 9, p. 224.

Solomon, R.C., 2002. *Spirituality for the Skeptic: The Thoughtful Love of Life*. Oxford University Press.

Speth, J., Speth, C., Kaelen, M., Schloerscheidt, A.M., Feilding, A., Nutt, D.J., and Carhart-Harris, R.L., 2016. Decreased mental time travel to the past correlates with default-mode network disintegration under lysergic acid diethylamide. *Journal of Psychopharmacology*, 30(4), pp. 344–353.

Sridharan, D., Levitin, D.J., and Menon, V., 2008. A critical role for the right fronto-insular cortex in switching between central-executive and default-mode networks. *Proceedings of the National Academy of Sciences*, 105(34), pp. 12569–12574.

Stace, W.T., 1960. *Mysticism and Philosophy*. Reprint, Los Angeles: Jeremy P. Tarcher.

Stam, C.J., 2014. Modern network science of neurological disorders. *Nature Reviews Neuroscience*, 15(10), pp. 683–695.

Stein, D.J., 1991. Philosophy and the DSM-III. *Comprehensive Psychiatry*, 32(5), pp. 404–415.

Stolaroff, M.J., 1999. Are psychedelics useful in the practice of Buddhism? *Journal of Humanistic Psychology*, 39(1), pp. 60–80.

Stone, A.L., Storr, C.L., and Anthony, J.C., 2006. Evidence for a hallucinogen dependence syndrome developing soon after onset of hallucinogen use during adolescence. *International Journal of Methods in Psychiatric Research*, 15(3), pp. 116–130.

Stone, J.A., 2012. Spirituality for naturalists. *Zygon*, 47(3), pp. 481–500.

Strassman, R., 2001. *DMT: The Spirit Molecule: A Doctor's Revolutionary Research into the Biology of Near-Death and Mystical Experiences*. Rochester: Park Street Press.

Strassman, R.J., 1984. Adverse reactions to psychedelic drugs. A review of the literature. *Journal of Nervous and Mental Disease*, 172(10), pp. 577–95.

Studerus, E., Gamma, A., and Vollenweider, F.X., 2010. Psychometric evaluation of the altered states of consciousness rating scale (OAV). *PloS One*, 5(8), p. e12412.

Studerus, E., Gamma, A., Kometer, M., and Vollenweider, F.X., 2012. Prediction of psilocybin response in healthy volunteers. *PloS One*, 7(2), p. e30800. Studerus, E., Kometer, M., Hasler, F., and Vollenweider, F.X., 2011. Acute, subacute and long-term subjective effects of psilocybin in healthy humans: A pooled analysis of experimental studies. *Journal of Psychopharmacology*, 25(11), pp. 1434–1452.

Sturgeon, N., 2006. Moral naturalism. In Copp D. (ed.) *The Oxford Handbook of Ethical Theory*, pp. 91–121. Oxford University Press.

Sui, J. and Gu, X., 2017. Self as object: Emerging trends in self research. *Trends in Neurosciences*, 40(11), pp. 643–653.

Sui, J. and Humphreys, G.W., 2015. The integrative self: How self-reference integrates perception and memory. *Trends in Cognitive Sciences*, 19(12), pp. 719–728.

Swanson, L.R., 2016. The predictive processing paradigm has roots in Kant. *Frontiers in Systems Neuroscience*, 10, p. 79.

Swanson, L.R., 2018. Unifying theories of psychedelic drug effects. *Frontiers in Pharmacology*, 9, p. 172.

Swift, T.C., Belser, A.B., Agin-Liebes, G., Devenot, N., Terrana, S., Friedman, H.L., Guss, J., Bossis, A.P., and Ross, S., 2017. Cancer at the dinner table: Experiences of psilocybin-assisted psychotherapy for the treatment of cancer-related distress. *Journal of Humanistic Psychology*, 57(5), pp. 488–519.

Tagliazucchi, E., Carhart-Harris, R., Leech, R., Nutt, D., and Chialvo, D.R., 2014. Enhanced repertoire of brain dynamical states during the psychedelic experience. *Human Brain Mapping*, 35(11), pp. 5442–5456.

Tagliazucchi, E., Roseman, L., Kaelen, M., Orban, C., Muthukumaraswamy, S.D., Murphy, K., Laufs, H., Leech, R., McGonigle, J., Crossley, N., and Bullmore, E., 2016. Increased global functional connectivity correlates with LSD-induced ego dissolution. *Current Biology*, 26(8), pp. 1043–1050.

Tang, Y.Y., Hölzel, B.K., and Posner, M.I., 2015. The neuroscience of mindfulness meditation. *Nature Reviews Neuroscience*, 16(4), pp. 213–225.

Tennison, M.N., 2012. Moral transhumanism: The next step. *Journal of Medicine and Philosophy*, 37(4), pp. 405–416.

Terhune, D.B., Luke, D.P., Kaelen, M., Bolstridge, M., Feilding, A., Nutt, D., Carhart-Harris, R., and Ward, J., 2016. A placebo-controlled investigation of synaesthesia-like experiences under LSD. *Neuropsychologia*, 88, pp. 28–34.

Thagard, P., 2019. *Natural Philosophy: From Social Brains to Knowledge, Reality, Morality, and Beauty*. Oxford University Press.

Thakchoe, S., 2019. Buddhist philosophy of mind: Nāgārjuna's critique of mind-body dualism from his rebirth arguments. *Philosophy East and West*, 69(3), pp. 807–827.

Thiessen, M.S., Walsh, Z., Bird, B.M., and Lafrance, A., 2018. Psychedelic use and intimate partner violence: The role of emotion regulation. *Journal of Psychopharmacology*, 32(7), pp. 749–755.

Thomas, G., Lucas, P., Capler, N.R., Tupper, K.W., and Martin, G., 2013. Ayahuasca-assisted therapy for addiction: results from a preliminary observational study in Canada. *Current Drug Abuse Reviews*, 6(1), pp. 30–42.

Thompson, E., 2015. Dreamless sleep, the embodied mind, and consciousness—The relevance of a classical Indian debate to cognitive science. In Metzinger, T. and Windt, J.M. (eds) *Open MIND*: 37(T). Frankfurt am Main: MIND Group. DOI: https://doi.org/10.15502/9783958570351

Thomson, E. and Piccinini, G., 2018. Neural representations observed. *Minds and Machines*, 28(1), pp. 191–235.

Timmermann, C., Roseman, L., Williams, L., Erritzoe, D., Martial, C., Cassol, H., Laureys, S., Nutt, D., and Carhart-Harris, R., 2018. DMT models the near-death experience. *Frontiers in Psychology*, 9, p. 1424.

Timmermann, C., Kettner, H., Letheby, C., Roseman, L., Rosas, F. E., and Carhart-Harris, R. L., in preparation. Effects of psychedelics on metaphysical beliefs.

Tramacchi, D.T., 2006. *Vapours and visions: religious dimensions of DMT use*. Doctoral thesis. University of Queensland.

Tupper, K.W., 2002. Entheogens and existential intelligence: The use of plant teachers as cognitive tools. *Canadian Journal of Education/Revue canadienne de l'éducation*, 27, pp. 499–516.

Tupper, K.W., 2003. Entheogens and education: Exploring the potential of psychoactives as educational tools. *Journal of Drug Education and Awareness*, 1(2), pp. 145–161.

Uthaug, M.V., Van Oorsouw, K., Kuypers, K.P.C., Van Boxtel, M., Broers, N.J., Mason, N.L., Toennes, S.W., Riba, J., and Ramaekers, J.G., 2018. Sub-acute and long-term effects of ayahuasca on affect and cognitive thinking style and their association with ego dissolution. *Psychopharmacology*, 235(10), pp. 2979–2989.

Uthaug, M.V., Lancelotta, R., van Oorsouw, K., Kuypers, K.P.C., Mason, N., Rak, J., Šuláková, A., Jurok, R., Maryška, M., Kuchař, M., and Páleníček, T., 2019. A single inhalation of vapor from dried toad secretion containing 5-methoxy-N, N-dimethyltryptamine (5-MeO-DMT) in a naturalistic setting is related to sustained enhancement of satisfaction with life, mindfulness-related capacities, and a decrement of psychopathological symptoms. *Psychopharmacology*, *236*(9), pp. 2653–2666.

Uthaug, M.V., Lancelotta, R., Szabo, A., Davis, A.K., Riba, J., and Ramaekers, J.G., 2020. Prospective examination of synthetic 5-methoxy-N, N-dimethyltryptamine inhalation: effects on salivary IL-6, cortisol levels, affect, and non-judgment. *Psychopharmacology*, *237*(3), pp. 773–785.

van Mulukom, V., Patterson, R.E., and van Elk, M., 2020. Broadening your mind to include others: The relationship between serotonergic psychedelic experiences and maladaptive narcissism. *Psychopharmacology*. DOI: https://doi.org/10.1007/s00213-020-05568-y

Varga, S., 2012. Depersonalization and the sense of realness. *Philosophy, Psychiatry, & Psychology*, *19*(2), pp. 103–113.

Vaughan, F., 1983. Perception and knowledge: reflections on psychological and spiritual learning in the psychedelic experience. In Grinspoon, L. and Bakalar, J.B. (eds) *Psychedelic reflections*, pp. 108–114. Human Sciences Press.

Vivot, R.M., Pallavicini, C., Zamberlan, F., Vigo, D., and Tagliazucchi, E., 2020. Meditation increases the entropy of brain oscillatory activity. *Neuroscience*, *431*, pp. 40–51.

Vollenweider, F.X., Leenders, K.L., Scharfetter, C., Maguire, P., Stadelmann, O., and Angst, J., 1997. Positron emission tomography and fluorodeoxyglucose studies of metabolic hyperfrontality and psychopathology in the psilocybin model of psychosis. *Neuropsychopharmacology*, *16*(5), pp. 357–372.

Vollenweider, F.X., Vollenweider-Scherpenhuyzen, M.F., Bäbler, A., Vogel, H., and Hell, D., 1998. Psilocybin induces schizophrenia-like psychosis in humans via a serotonin-2 agonist action. *Neuroreport*, *9*(17), pp. 3897–3902.

Vollenweider, F.X. and Kometer, M., 2010. The neurobiology of psychedelic drugs: Implications for the treatment of mood disorders. *Nature Reviews Neuroscience*, *11*(9), pp. 642–651.

Waller, G., Shah, R., Ohanian, V., and Elliott, P., 2001. Core beliefs in bulimia nervosa and depression: The discriminant validity of Young's Schema Questionnaire. *Behavior Therapy*, *32*(1), pp. 139–153.

Walsh, Z., Hendricks, P.S., Smith, S., Kosson, D.S., Thiessen, M.S., Lucas, P., and Swogger, M.T., 2016. Hallucinogen use and intimate partner violence: Prospective evidence consistent with protective effects among men with histories of problematic substance use. *Journal of Psychopharmacology*, *30*(7), pp. 601–607.

Ward, A.M., Schultz, A.P., Huijbers, W., Van Dijk, K.R., Hedden, T., and Sperling, R.A., 2014. The parahippocampal gyrus links the default-mode cortical network with the medial temporal lobe memory system. *Human Brain Mapping*, *35*(3), pp. 1061–1073.

Wasson, R.G., 1957. Seeking the magic mushroom. *Life*, *42*(19), pp. 100–120.

Waters, R., 1975. Some epistemological questions concerning the non-medical use of drugs. *Revue de l'Université d'Ottawa*, *45*(4), pp. 518–540.

Watts, A., 1964. A psychedelic experience: Fact or fantasy. In Solomon, D. (ed.) *LSD: The Consciousness-Expanding Drug*. New York: G.P. Putnam's Sons. DOI: http://www. psychedelic-library.org/watts2.htm

Watts, A.W., 1960. The new alchemy. In *This is It, and Other Essays on Zen and Spiritual Experience*, pp. 127–153. New York: Pantheon.

Watts, A.W., 1962. *The Joyous Cosmology*. New York: Pantheon.

Watts, R., Day, C., Krzanowski, J., Nutt, D., and Carhart-Harris, R., 2017. Patients' accounts of increased "connectedness" and "acceptance" after psilocybin for treatment-resistant depression. *Journal of Humanistic Psychology*, *57*(5), pp. 520–564.

Watts, R. and Luoma, J., 2020. The use of the psychological flexibility model to support psychedelic assisted therapy. *Journal of Contextual Behavioral Science*, *15*, pp. 92–102.

West, R., Raw, M., McNeill, A., Stead, L., Aveyard, P., Bitton, J., Stapleton, J., McRobbie, H., Pokhrel, S., Lester-George, A., and Borland, R., 2015. Health-care interventions to promote and assist tobacco cessation: A review of efficacy, effectiveness and affordability for use in national guideline development. *Addiction, 110*(9), pp. 1388–1403.

Wheeler, S. W. and Dyer, N. L., 2020. A systematic review of psychedelic-assisted psychotherapy for mental health: An evaluation of the current wave of research and suggestions for the future. *Psychology of Consciousness: Theory, Research, and Practice.* DOI: http://dx.doi.org/10.1037/cns0000237

Whitfield-Gabrieli, S. and Ford, J.M., 2012. Default mode network activity and connectivity in psychopathology. *Annual Review of Clinical Psychology, 8*, pp. 49–76.

Wielgosz, J., Goldberg, S.B., Kral, T.R., Dunne, J.D., and Davidson, R.J., 2019. Mindfulness meditation and psychopathology. *Annual Review of Clinical Psychology, 15*, pp. 285–316.

Wiese, W., 2019. Explaining the enduring intuition of substantiality: The phenomenal self as an abstract 'Salience Object'. *Journal of Consciousness Studies, 26*(3–4), pp. 64–87.

Windt, J.M., 2011. Altered consciousness in philosophy. In Cardeña, E. and Winkelman, M. (eds) *Altering Consciousness: Multidisciplinary Perspectives*, pp. 229–254. Santa-Barbara, CA: Praeger.

Windt, J.M., Nielsen, T., and Thompson, E., 2016. Does consciousness disappear in dreamless sleep? *Trends in Cognitive Sciences, 20*(12), pp. 871–882.

Winkelman, M.J., 2017. The mechanisms of psychedelic visionary experiences: Hypotheses from evolutionary psychology. *Frontiers in Neuroscience, 11*, p. 539.

Winter, U., LeVan, P., Borghardt, T.L., Akin, B., Wittmann, M., Leyens, Y., and Schmidt, S., 2020. Content-free awareness: EEG-fcMRI correlates of consciousness as such in an expert meditator. *Frontiers in Psychology, 10*, p. 3064.

Wolff, M., Evens, R., Mertens, L.J., Koslowski, M., Betzler, F., Gründer, G., and Jungaberle, H., 2020. Learning to let go: A cognitive-behavioral model of how psychedelic therapy promotes acceptance. *Frontiers in Psychiatry, 11*, p. 5.

Wright, R., 2017. *Why Buddhism is True: The Science and Philosophy of Meditation and Enlightenment.* New York: Simon and Schuster.

Yaden, D.B., Le Nguyen, K.D., Kern, M.L., Belser, A.B., Eichstaedt, J.C., Iwry, J., Smith, M.E., Wintering, N.A., Hood Jr, R.W., and Newberg, A.B., 2017. Of roots and fruits: A comparison of psychedelic and nonpsychedelic mystical experiences. *Journal of Humanistic Psychology, 57*(4), pp. 338–353.

Yang, C., Shirayama, Y., Zhang, J.C., Ren, Q., Yao, W., Ma, M., Dong, C., and Hashimoto, K., 2015. R-ketamine: A rapid-onset and sustained antidepressant without psychotomimetic side effects. *Translational Psychiatry, 5*(9), p.e632.

Yon, D., de Lange, F.P., and Press, C., 2019. The predictive brain as a stubborn scientist. *Trends in Cognitive Sciences, 23*(1), pp. 6–8.

Zachar, P. and Kendler, K.S., 2017. The philosophy of nosology. *Annual Review of Clinical Psychology, 13*, pp. 49–71.

Zahavi, D., 2011. The experiential self: Objections and clarifications. In Siderits, M., Thompson, E., and Zahavi, D. (eds) *Self, no self?: Perspectives from analytical, phenomenological, and Indian traditions*, pp. 56–78. Oxford University Press.

Zahavi, D., 2014. *Self and other: Exploring subjectivity, empathy, and shame.* Oxford University Press.

Zahavi, D. and Kriegel, U., 2015. For-me-ness: What it is and what it is not. In Dahlstrom, D.O., Elpidorou, A., and Hopp, W. (eds) *Philosophy of Mind and Phenomenology: Conceptual and Empirical Approaches*, pp. 48–66. New York: Routledge.

Zeki, S., 1991. Cerebral akinetopsia (visual motion blindness) a review. *Brain, 114*(2), pp. 811–824.

Zhao, W., Luo, L., Li, Q., and Kendrick, K.M., 2013. What can psychiatric disorders tell us about neural processing of the self? *Frontiers in Human Neuroscience, 7*, p. 485.

Index